Macrophages and Cancer

T0200553

Editors

Gloria H. Heppner, Ph.D.
Senior Vice President and Chairman
Department of Immunology
Michigan Cancer Foundation
Detroit, Michigan

Amy M. Fulton, Ph.D.
Associate Member
Department of Immunology
Michigan Cancer Foundation
Detroit, Michigan

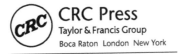

CRC Press
Taylor & Francis Group
Boca Raton London New York

CRC Press is an imprint of the
Taylor & Francis Group, an **informa** business

CRC Press
Taylor & Francis Group
6000 Broken Sound Parkway NW, Suite 300
Boca Raton, FL 33487-2742

Reissued 2019 by CRC Press

© 1988 by Taylor & Francis Group, LLC
CRC Press is an imprint of Taylor & Francis Group, an Informa business

No claim to original U.S. Government works

A Library of Congress record exists under LC control number:

Publisher's Note
The publisher has gone to great lengths to ensure the quality of this reprint but points out that some imperfections in the original copies may be apparent.

Disclaimer
The publisher has made every effort to trace copyright holders and welcomes correspondence from those they have been unable to contact.

ISBN 13: 978-0-367-22639-8 (hbk)
ISBN 13: 978-0-367-22641-1 (pbk)
ISBN 13: 978-0-429-27614-9 (ebk)

Visit the Taylor & Francis Web site at http://www.taylorandfrancis.com and the
CRC Press Web site at http://www.crcpress.com

PREFACE

The role of macrophages in cancer has received much attention in recent years without a consensus being reached regarding the precise mechanisms and influences operating on the interactions between macrophages and tumor cells. Nevertheless, macrophage biologists have made notable advances in understanding the complexity of macrophage phenotypes and functions. This complexity has multiple origins. One is the phenotypic heterogeneity of the group of cells collectively referred to as macrophages. As Morahan et al. discusses in Chapter 1 whether the underlying basis of this heterogeneity reflects the differentiation lineage of a single cell type or whether macrophages are multiple, unrelated populations is not yet known. Irregardless, it is necessary to appreciate that such heterogeneity exists and that "macrophages" are mixed populations of cells with quite different functions and potentials.

A second basis for the complexities of macrophage-tumor cell interactions is the multiple mechanisms involved in macrophage activation and effector function. Two groups of investigators, Adams and Hamilton and Stewart et al., both here review in Chapters 2 and 3 the molecular mechanisms of macrophage activity but, interestingly, from two very different and novel perspectives: one focuses on the events occurring in the macrophage, the other on macrophage induced responses in the tumor cell.

An important class of regulatory mediators of macrophage function, and one which can be affected by tumor cells, are the prostaglandins. Zwilling and Justement discuss in Chapter 4 the positive and negative regulatory effects of these molecules and their coupling to adenyl cyclase activation in the macrophage. Of course, the relationship between macrophages and tumor cells is subject to numerous regulatory influences. The genetic basis for control of macrophage function is being unraveled by a combination of classical genetic experiments and molecular approaches, as described by Stevenson and Skamene in Chapter 5.

Although it is apparent that our general understanding of macrophage biology is increasing, our ability to realize the therapeutic potential of this class of inflammatory cells in the treatment of cancer depends upon a parallel understanding of the biology of cancer cells. The heterogeneity of macrophages is matched, if not exceeded, by that of tumor cell populations. Indeed, as discussed by Fulton in Chapter 6, these two types of heterogeneity can impact upon each other in influencing the types of macrophages which infiltrate different tumors. Other players in the host tumor cell scenario are lymphocytes, which independently affect tumor cells, macrophages, and the interactions between them. Urban et al. describe in Chapter 7 an example of this latter principle in which T cells mediate the appearance of macrophage-resistant tumor cell variants. The theme of the interrelationship of tumor cell heterogeneity and macrophage heterogeneity is also taken up by North et al. who describe in Chapter 8 the biologic consequences of tumor cell heterogeneity in regard to susceptibility to macrophage effector functions.

Despite the formidable problems posed by multiple regulatory mechanisms and by macrophage and tumor heterogeneity, there have been some remarkable advances in the therapeutic use of macrophages. Fogler and Fidler describe in Chapter 9 the preclinical development of effective macrophage-based therapies, and Kirsh et al. discuss in Chapter 10 some of the strategies necessary to bring these new treatments to clinical reality.

The final chapter (Heppner and Dorcey) of this book is concerned with a role different from the primarily defensive activities of macrophages in tumor development. There is increasing evidence that macrophages might be a driving influence in the development and heterogeneity of tumor cell populations. The mechanisms by which this occurs, although incompletely understood, may be related, paradoxically, to those which mediate the defense reactions. Macrophages are also the sources of angiogenic factors, growth factors and invasion related proteases that may contribute positively to tumor growth and metastasis.

The relationship between tumor cells and macrophages is not a simple bidirectional interaction, but rather a complex network of multifactorial processes. The topics in this book have been selected to highlight recent advances in our knowledge of these processes and to illustrate how this knowledge may ultimately be used to help control neoplastic growth.

Gloria H. Heppner
Amy M. Fulton

THE EDITORS

Gloria H. Heppner, Ph.D., is the Senior Vice President of the Michigan Cancer Foundation in Detroit. She is also an Adjunct Professor of Pathology, Immunology, and Biological Sciences at Wayne State University.

Dr. Heppner received her B.A., M.A., and Ph.D. degrees from the University of California, Berkeley in 1962, 1964, and 1967, respectively. Her graduate training was in the Cancer Research Genetics Laboratory under the direction of Dr. David Weiss. She was a post-doctoral fellow from 1967 to 1969 at the University of Washington, Seattle in the laboratories of Drs. Karl-Eric and Ingegerd Hellstrom.

Before joining the Michigan Cancer Foundation in 1979, Dr. Heppner was on the faculty of Brown University, Providence, Rhode Island and was an Associate Director of the Brown-Roger Williams General Hospital Cancer Center. She is a member of several scientific societies, including the American Association of Immunologists and the American Association for Cancer Research. She has been a member of several study sections of the National Institutes of Health and a Chairman of the Bladder Cancer Working Group of the Organ Sites Program of the National Cancer Institute.

Dr. Heppner's research interests have centered on two areas: the immune and inflammatory responses to cancers and the development and consequences of cellular heterogeneity in murine mammary tumors.

Amy M. Fulton, Ph.D. is Associate Member and Chief of the Laboratory of Immunobiology in the Department of Immunology at the Michigan Cancer Foundation in Detroit, Michigan. She is an Adjunct Assistant Professor in the Department of Pathology at the Wayne State University Medical School.

She received her B.A. at the University of Kansas in Lawrence in 1972 where she was elected to Phi Beta Kappa. She received her Ph.D. in Medical Microbiology from the University of Wisconsin, Madison in 1977. Dr. Fulton was a National Institutes of Health post-doctoral fellow at the University of British Columbia, Vancouver, Canada for 2 years. She is a member of the American Association for Cancer Research and the American Association of Immunologists.

Since 1980, Dr. Fulton's research efforts have involved the study of the immunologic response to breast cancer and the role that inflammatory mediators (prostaglandins and reactive-oxygen intermediates) play in tumor growth and metastasis.

CONTRIBUTORS

Dolph O. Adams, M.D., Ph.D.
Professor and Director
Department of Pathology and
 Immunology
Duke University Medical Center
Durham, North Carolina

Peter J. Bugelski, Ph. D.
Smith Kline and French Laboratories
Philadelphia, Pennsylvania

Walla L. Dempsey, Ph.D.
Assistant Professor
Department of Microbiology and
 Immunology
Medical College of Pennsylvania
Philadelphia, Pennsylvania

Leslie Dorcey, B.S.
Department of Immunology
Michigan Cancer Foundation
Detroit, Michigan

Isaiah J. Fidler, D.V.M., Ph.D.
Chairman and Professor
Department of Cell Biology
M. D. Anderson Hospital
 and Tumor Institute
Houston, Texas

William E. Fogler, Ph.D.
Senior Research Scientist
Department of Immunobiology
 Research and Development
Centocor Incorporated
Malvern, Pennsylvania

Amy M. Fulton, Ph.D.
Associate Member
Department of Immunology
Michigan Cancer Foundation
Detroit, Michigan

Thomas A. Hamilton, Ph.D.
Section on Atherosclerosis
Cleveland Clinic Foundation
Cleveland, Ohio

Gloria Heppner, Ph.D.
Senior Vice President
Department of Immunology
Michigan Cancer Foundation
Detroit, Michigan

John B. Hibbs, Jr., M.D.
Professor
Department of Medicine
University of Utah School of Medicine
Salt Lake City, Utah

Tatsuro Irimura, Ph.D.
Assistant Professor
Department of Tumor Biology
M. D. Anderson Hospital
 and Tumor Institute
Houston, Texas

William J. Johnson, Ph. D.
Smith Kline and French Laboratories
Philadelphia, Pennsylvania

Louis B. Justement, Ph.D.
Divisional Immunology
National Jewish Center for
 Immunology and Respiratory Medicine
Denver, Colorado

Richard Kirsh, Ph.D.
Department of Immunology
Smith Kline and French Laboratories
Philadelphia, Pennsylvania

Meryle J. Melnicoff, M.S.
Senior Scientist
Department of Immunology and Anti-
 Infectives
Smith Kline and French Laboratories
Swedeland, Pennsylvania

Page S. Morahan, Ph.D.
Professor and Chairman
Department of Microbiology and
 Immunology
Medical College of Pennsylvania
Philadelphia, Pennsylvania

Garth Nicolson, Ph.D.
Professor and Chairman
Department of Tumor Biology
University of Texas
M. D. Anderson Hospital and Tumor
 Institute
Houston, Texas

Susan M. North, Ph.D.
Assistant Professor
Department of Tumor Biology
M. D. Anderson Hospital and Tumor
 Institute
Houston, Texas

George Poste, D.V.M., Ph.D.
Department of Research and Development
Smith Kline and French Laboratories
Philadelphia, Pennsylvania

Jay L. Rothstein
Department of Pathology
Immunology Group
University of Chicago
Chicago, Illinois

Hans Schreiber, M.D., Ph.D.
Professor
Department of Pathology
University of Chigago
Chicago, Illinois

Emil Skamene, Ph.D.
Professor
Faculty of Medicine
McGill University
Montreal, Quebec, Canada

Anita P. Stevenson, M.S.
Experimental Pathology Group
Life Sciences Division
Los Alamos National Laboratory
Los Alamos, New Mexico

Mary M. Stevenson, Ph.D.
Assistant Professor
Department of Medicine
McGill University
Montreal, Quebec, Canada

Carleton C. Stewart, Ph.D.
Experimental Pathology Group
Life Sciences Division
Los Alamos National Laboratory
Los Alamos, New Mexico

James Loron Urban, Ph.D.
Postdoctoral Fellow
Department of Biology
Leukemia Society of America
California Institute of Technology
Pasadena, California

Alvin Volkman, Ph.D.
Professor
Department of Pathology
East Carolina University School of Medicine
Greenville, North Carolina

Bruce S. Zwilling, Ph.D.
Professor
Department of Microbiology
Ohio State University
Columbus, Ohio

TABLE OF CONTENTS

Chapter 1

MACROPHAGE HETEROGENEITY

Page S. Morahan, Alvin Volkman, Meryle Melnicoff, and Walla L. Dempsey

TABLE OF CONTENTS

I. INTRODUCTION

Mononuclear phagocytes (MPs) have been demonstrated for over a decade to be potent effectors of natural and specific immune responses against neoplasia.[1-7] Therefore, there has been considerable interest in the use of MPs in cancer diagnosis and immunotherapy.[8-11] This clinical potential has not yet been realized, partially because of the heterogeneity that exists within the population of cells broadly classified as MPs. But not all MPs are effective against neoplasia; it appears necessary to have a particular kind of MP in the right place at the right time in tumor development. In this chapter, we will review the evidence documenting MP heterogeneity, current hypotheses for the origins of the heterogeneity, promising investigational approaches, and comment on the implications MP heterogeneity has in cancer diagnosis and immunotherapy.

The accepted features that have been recommended since 1970 to describe MPs[12,13] are ultimate origin from a single hemopoietic stem cell, Fc receptor-mediated phagocytosis, and a single nucleus — hence the name, mononuclear phagocyte. These criteria are somewhat broad, and exceptions can be found. It has been clearly established that MPs exist throughout the body, and are represented by precursor pools in hemopoietic tissues, blood monocytes, and fixed and free tissue macrophages (MOs) in the bone marrow, thymus, lymph nodes, spleen, liver (Kupffer cells), lung, intestine, and serosal cavities (e.g., peritoneal, pleural).[14,15] It is estimated that the total MP compartment in the mouse consists of about 10^8 cells.[16] The wide dispersion of MPs makes these cells uniquely suited to provide a "first line of defense" against foreign elements before leukocytic emigration can take place, and also provides mobile inflammatory monocytes. MPs also provide a homeostatic function by virtue of their synthetic and secretory activities. Additional cells share some MP characteristics, but their lineage has not been definitively established. These cells include the nonphagocytic Langerhans cells in the epidermis, the dendritic cells in lymphoreticular organs, the phagocytic microglial cells in the central nervous system, and the osteoclasts in bone.[12,17-19,220]

When discussing heterogeneity of MP populations, it is important to distinguish between the diversity that is (1) present in the steady state under normal homeostatic control and (2) induced by tumor growth, inflammatory processes, and immunomodulatory treatments. In the steady state there is the question of what part of the expressed heterogeneity is genetically and ontogenetically endowed, and what part is environmentally induced. It is easy to appreciate the vast differences among the environments to which tissue MO compartments are exposed. As examples, peritoneal MOs are lodged in an anaerobic environment, whereas pulmonary alveolar MO reside in an aerobic environment which is in continuity with the external mileau. Kupffer cells, although regarded as tissue MOs, are normally intravascular, but they may be capable of being mobilized into tissues during early stages of microbial invasion.[20] Kupffer MOs have a lower oxidative metabolism than other MOs,[21,22] and it is still not clear whether this metabolic state is ontogenetically determined or locally regulated.[23]

An additional aspect of heterogeneity is that caused by mixing cells of different ages. The loss of MPs from the blood[55,57,59] and tissues[122-124] appears to take place in a stochastic manner, that is, randomly or irrespective of ages of the cells being lost. This common mechanism of cell loss will naturally give rise to residual cell populations of mixed ages. It is reasonable to assume that the functional capacities of cells of varying age may be distinctly different. As discussed later, local proliferation may also be an important mechanism of tissue MO renewal with or without monocyte influx.[56,125] This obviously provides another mechanism for the generation of MP populations consisting of cells of different ages.

In brief, heterogeneity is a collective term for a variety of complex biological phenomena, some of which are readily understandable and some of which are obscure. Multidirectional experimental approaches will be necessary to uncover the mechanisms underlying or regulating the different expressions of functional diversity. The literature concerning MP heterogeneity is filled with so much controversy that we can identify only two issues on which consensus exists. (1) MPs are indeed heterogeneous, both among and within various anatomic compartments. This point is addressed in Section III and Tables 1 and 2. (2) There exists a pluripotent stem cell (colony forming units, CFU-s) from which the heterogeneous MPs are derived.[126,127] All other events between the beginning of MP development and the appearance of the final heterogeneous population(s) are topics of debate.

II. TERMS USED IN DISCUSSING MP HETEROGENEITY

We feel it is prudent to propose working definitions of two terms which are widely used in discussing MP heterogeneity — differentiation and activation.

Differentiation is the process which occurs as part of normal development and homeostasis, and reflects narrowing or limitation of expression of a cell's genetic potential.[24,25] Differentiation is not reversible under normal conditions, may or may not involve cell division, and is mediated by microenvironments. Defining MP differentiation would be facilitated if MPs contained identifiable, nonreversible events comparable to the genomic rearrangement which occurs during lymphocyte differentiation,[26,27] but no such events have been described in MP differentiation. Gene rearrangement of this type may be limited to lymphocytes, whereas MP differentiation may involve nonreversible changes at the level of expression of a coordinated set of genes,[13,28,29] as observed in other cell types.[30] Understanding the events which accompany MP differentiation, at the levels of both the DNA genome and mRNA genomic expression, is a crucial step in defining the origins of MP heterogeneity.

We will define MP activation broadly, as any process that causes reversible changes in MP phenotype and functions, mediated by altered expression of one gene or a coordinated set of genes.[28,31,32] There is evidence that activation in vitro is reversible and may regress with time or with the removal or neutralization of the activating signal.[33-35,49] Different types of activation exist, and the activation process appears to involve more than one cascade of events.[31,36] Many investigators reserve the term activation for the enhanced expression of antitumor and antimicrobial activity,[37-39] and use the term stimulation for other forms of altered expression of MP function (e.g., secretory, antigen presenting). The term priming is used by some workers to describe a step enabling MP activation.[23,40]

Distinguishing MP activation from differentiation is complicated by the fact that activating signals such as interferons, may also regulate differentiation (granulocyte-macrophage colony-forming unit, CFU-GM, etc.).[41-46] Differentiation and activation may occur virtually simultaneously, as in the recruitment of blood monocytes to tissues during an inflammatory response to an activating agent. Both processes may be enhanced or depressed within the microenvironment under the influence of hormones and cytokines.[35,46,188] A highly regulated interacting network of signals that may synergise or antagonize has been suggested.[47-52,228] There is some evidence that steady-state tissue MOs may be under active suppression to prevent full differentiation.[23]

A variety of additional terms, maturation, terminal differentiation, and dedifferentiation, have been applied inconsistently to describe altered states of MP function. We recommend that these terms should be restricted to their accepted use in current developmental biology. For example, maturation is used very specifically by developmental biologists to describe the oocyte's attainment of full potential for fertilization,[30] or by cell kineticists to describe the interval between mitosis in actively dividing populations.[53] The term maturation, which has been used to suggest implicit senescence in the change of the monocyte to resident MO, is imprecise. In certain cell renewal systems, the maturation compartment is intermitotic and is part of an amplification mechanism. This subject is well discussed by Cleaver.[128] The term, terminal differentiation, has sometimes been used to imply that the resident MO

Table 1
REFERENCES DEMONSTRATING HETEROGENEITY OF MPS IN SMALL ANIMALS

Macrophage Populations

Methods	Resident MO				Activated MO					Cultured MO		
	Peritoneal	Lung	Liver	Other	Peritoneal	Lung	Liver	Other	Monocytes	BMDMO[a]	Cell lines[b]	Stem cells
Physical methods (size, morphology, ultrastructure)	60, 61, 62, 63, 64, 65, 66	67, 68, 69, 70, 164		72	61, 64, 66, 74, 75, 16, 76, 77, 78, 79	80		81, 82	71, 72, 73, 25	61, 66	63	83
Surface markers (MoAb, enzymes, Ia antigens, receptors)	63, 65, 66, 74, 60, 230	69, 84, 67, 85, 86	84	84, 87, 88, 82, 72, 189	74, 76, 78, 84, 89, 36			81, 89, 90	71, 72, 84, 87, 36	66, 91	93	92
Secreted products (IL-1, CSF, PGE, proteases)	66, 60				94, 95	80					93, 96	
Function (antitumor, antimicrobial, chemotaxis, phagocytosis, antigen presentation)	60, 62, 63, 64, 66, 21, 97, 61	68, 70, 69, 164	21,	97, 98	64, 66, 74, 162, 76, 78, 79, 95, 97, 94	80		81	97, 98	66, 98, 61, 266	93, 63, 225	
Growth characteristics (CSF responsiveness, lymphokine responsiveness)	61, 64	67			61, 64, 75				25	61		83, 41
Intracellular changes (RNA, DNA, protein)	99	69			77, 99							

[a] BMDMO represents bone marrow-derived macrophages obtained by culturing bone marrow stem cells with CSF-1.

[b] Includes cell lines, clones, and macrophage hybridomas.

Table 2
REFERENCES DEMONSTRATING HETEROGENEITY OF MPS IN HUMANS

Macrophage Populations

| Methods | Resident MO | | | | | Cultured MO | | Stem cells |
	Peritoneal	Lung	Liver	Other	Monocytes	BMDMO[a]	Cell lines[b]	
Physical methods (size, morphology, ultrastructure)	100, 101	221	101		107, 108, 109, 110, 121, 221, 241			119, 120
Surface markers (MoAb, enzymes, Ia antigens, receptors)	100, 101, 102, 103, 104	103, 104, 105, 106	101, 106	103, 104, 106, 115, 20, 119	103, 108, 110, 111, 109, 112, 113, 114, 115, 243		104	
Secreted products (IL-1, CSF, PGE, proteases)		221			110, 112, 113, 221			
Function (antitumor, antimicrobial, chemotaxis, phagocytosis, antigen presentation)		105, 116		118	109, 110, 112, 113, 116, 117, 118, 121			
Intracellular changes (RNA, DNA protein)	101		101					

Note: No data were available for activated macrophage populations growth characteristics.

[a] BMDMO represents bone marrow-derived macrophages obtained by culturing bone marrow stem cells with CSF-1.

[b] Includes cell lines, clones, and macrophage hydridomas.

is an "end-stage" MO. Resident MOs, however, can clearly be activated and can proliferate under certain conditions.[56-58]

III. EXPERIMENTAL APPROACHES USED TO DOCUMENT MP HETEROGENEITY

Tables 1 and 2 document some of the literature on MP heterogeneity within, as well as among, anatomic compartments. Most studies have used small animals (rats, mice, guinea pigs, and rabbits) (Table 1). Much less is known about MP in humans because the majority of work has been limited to monocytes (Table 2). While heterogeneity within MPs is now well appreciated, it has been much more difficult to determine the causative mechanisms.

MP heterogeneity has been demonstrated often by physical separation of cells by size or density (Tables 1 and 2). These studies have shown that MPs within a single anatomic compartment often vary in size, which, according to many reports, is correlated with differences in functions and expression of surface phenotypes. These correlations, unfortunately, are mostly associative and not definitive. Thus, this experimental approach cannot adequately address the source of MP heterogeneity. It is still not clear what proportion of heterogeneity is attributable to differences in the ages within the MP population, to mixtures of tissue MPs, and MPs in transit through the particular tissue compartment, or to whether the subpopulations express phenotypic fidelity, or whether any of the subpopulations can be induced to resemble one another. Moreover, most of these studies documented heterogeneity within a limited number of easily accessible MP compartments. It is not known whether equivalent heterogeneity exists within all sites. For example, liver Kupffer MPs appear to be less heterogeneous than splenic MOs.[21,92,129]

Antibodies (polyclonal and monoclonal) to cell surface markers have also been used to identify MP subpopulations. Evidence from immunocytochemistry and immunofluorescence studies has, in general, added support for the concept of MP heterogeneity, but has not been of great help in resolving the origins of heterogeneity. Whether markers are common to all MOs, as they appear to be in the case of the F4/80 antigen,[17,130] or detectable only on certain anatomically or functionally distinct MPs, one can argue that some surface markers may signify conservation of an antigen from a common ancestor. Another possibility is that certain surface antigens become expressed under local influences well after the emergence of cells from formative compartments. An additional problem with this experimental approach is that the use of the antigen characterization techniques usually has not allowed further functional analysis. Recently, identification and separation of MP subpopulations by flow cytometry has begun to be employed. This technology should permit assays of functions and responses to stimuli to be performed.

In vitro derived or cultured MPs, such as MO-like cell lines, MO hybridomas, and bone marrow derived MOs (from CSF-1 stimulated bone marrow stem cells) also demonstrate heterogeneity, but these experimental approaches, like the others, have provided few clues as to the origin of heterogeneity. The populations have been used to establish phenotypic and genotypic responses of MPs to cellular signals. Apparently stable subpopulations have been identified within some of these MP sources, thus documenting heterogeneity among transformed MPs. Because these populations divide readily, cloned subpopulations can be established and used to determine the range of responses of a single MP phenotype to a variety of activational or differentiation signals. Comparison of cloned phenotypes may establish inherent differences in MP responsiveness. Caution must be exercised in interpreting these types of studies because cultured MPs are not identical to steady-state MPs in vivo. Nevertheless, although extrapolation back to the in vivo situation is limited, analysis of cloned MPs should continue to be a fruitful experimental approach.

In vivo models, in which certain MP populations are depleted or permanently labeled, have not been used extensively in identifying MP heterogeneity. Models which have been used include total or partial body irradiation, radiation chimeras, parabiosis systems, and induced MP depletion, as well as animals with genetic deficiencies in hemopoiesis or MPs. These systems are yielding important information regarding the origin of MP heterogeneity within a given compartment.

It is evident, then, that a multifactorial approach will be the most fruitful in providing answers to the many questions regarding MP heterogeneity. Systematic documentation of MP populations within each anatomical compartment needs to be completed under steady state and tumor inflammatory states. There is a need to distinguish between status, traffic, and renewal of MP populations. These investigations should include contemporary methodologies such as analysis at the DNA, mRNA, and protein levels, in addition to functional and surface marker assays. Studies using cloned MO or MO-like cell lines should also be useful. Analysis at the single-cell level, using appropriate probes, should aid in determining which MP characteristics are common to all MPs, regardless of anatomic origin. Finally, whole animal models which exhibit depletion or permanent labeling of selected MP populations will be useful in addressing the question of the role of microenvironments, and of the mobile monocytes, as compared with tissue MPs, in generation of the total MP heterogeneity.

IV. UNANSWERED QUESTIONS CONCERNING THE ORIGIN OF MP HETEROGENEITY

The, as yet, incompletely answered questions concerning the origins of MP heterogeneity include:

1. In homeostasis (i.e., in the absence of inflammation or tumor burden) is there a single or are there multiple MP lineages derived from the pluripotent stem cell?
2. If there are multiple MP lineages, are these lineages ontogenetically determined to home to a particular anatomic compartment, and is such localization a random event with the subsequent differentiated phenotype determined solely by the local environment, or is a combination of these events involved, with cell receptors and stages of differentiation being critical determinants to anatomic localization?
3. Once situated within an anatomic compartment, do MPs exhibit phenotypic fidelity? In other words, does a resident peritoneal MO have the capacity to become an alveolar MO if transplanted to the lung?
4. After MP commitment (whether single or multiple lineages), is the observed heterogeneity within the lineage due to: a continuum of differentiation stages, differentiation into distinct subpopulations; random loss of different stage or subset members; a mixture of different aged, recirculating, and sessile tissue MPs; or transient activation? It is of course plausible that all may be operative.

The questions above are directed at the ideal homeostatic state. It is important to keep in mind that normal homeostatic regulation of MP origin, renewal, and traffic is a process quite distinct from regulation in a physiologic state altered by a tumor burden. Even normal homeostasis, however, can be interrupted by intermittent events which result in differentiation, activation, and mixing or replacement of various MP populations.

V. EXPERIMENTAL EVIDENCE CONCERNING THE ORIGIN OF MP HETEROGENEITY

A. Historical Comments

Most of the information concerning the ontogeny of MPs relates to mammals, particularly rodents and humans, although interesting studies have been conducted in a variety of vertebrates and invertebrates. Perhaps the earliest studies on MP differentiation were made by Metchnikoff, who convincingly described a series of transitional forms in inflammatory exudates, beginning with the small lymphocyte, developing into a monocyte, and ultimately into an MO.[131] The belief that the lymphocyte "hypertrophied" and "transformed" into a MO was reinforced and widely espoused for well over 50 years, until the mid-1960s. This concept was derived largely on the basis of inference from sampling experimentally induced foci of inflammation at intervals, and finding variations in cellular morphology. There were a few notable exceptions. Lewis, who contended that continuous observation of living cells was a more objective approach to the problem than using fixed cells and tissues, demonstrated by means of time lapse cinephotomicrography that chick monocytes developed into MOs.[132] Ebert and Florey took turns observing in a rabbit ear chamber, the emigration of carbon-labeled blood monocytes into traumatized tissues.[133] Unfortunately, the soundness of these pioneering studies was not widely appreciated.

The use of radioactive isotopes in biomedial research following World War II provided another highly objective method for studying cell lineage, cell kinetics, and pathways of cellular migration. It was soon established that tritiated thymidine is a specific precursor for DNA, and is rapidly incorporated into the DNA molecule during the synthesis phase of the cell cycle. This procedure provides a stable marker for the parent cell and three or more generations of progeny.[134] Through the use of this indelible marker, the monocytic origin of inflammatory (immigrant) MOs was definitively established.[135,136] Blood monocytes, in turn, were traced to a rapidly proliferating precursor pool in the bone marrow and, to a lesser extent, in the spleen. Monocytoid cells capable of proliferation were later isolated from the bone marrow and named monoblasts and promonocytes.[137] Their precise position in the scheme of monocyte ontogeny has not been firmly established.

This brief historical account has been included partly to provide background and, in addition, to underscore two interesting points. One is that scientists are tempted to formulate global explanations based on limited observations even when the available technology is unable to provide complete answers to the question being posed. That is, scientists, like other mortals, attempt to explain natural phenomena in terms of their current knowledge despite the awareness that this knowledge is incomplete. Secondly, traditional views among scientists are difficult to overcome, even when confronted with contradictory findings.[202,203]

B. Phylogenetic Considerations

Irrespective of the relative paucity of phylogenetic studies of MOs, it is clear that MPs appeared many phyla before any organized hemopoietic systems. It is worth considering whether there has been any persistence of these primitive MPs to the mammalian level. If so, which MP populations and which precursors represent the early forms? Current evidence in mammals suggests that MPs in the higher phyla have an ancestry in common with the granular leukocytes or myeloid series.[138,141] For example, data from culture of bone marrow cells indicate the simultaneous appearance of granulocytes and MPs from the same precursor cell. Myeloid cells, however, clearly originated later in phylogenesis than did MPs. These facts could mean that the primitive MP lineage has been deleted and that the myeloid series evolved in its place. An alternative idea is that primitive precursors of mobile phagocytes evolved into a more highly complex system. In the latter case, a tempting speculation is that the primitive MPs have been conserved as the MOs of tissues and tissue spaces, and that the myeloid-monocyte pathway represents the later development. This latter concept ontogenetically recapitulates, in part, the phylogeny, but becomes more highly specialized in step with evolution of the immune system. This leads to the provocative hypothesis that both the early type of tissue MP, and the "modern" type MP exist in mammals, as distinct MP lineages. It would be of obvious interest to expand the use of probes for MP cell surface markers to phylogenetic studies.

C. Role of Ontogeny in MP Heterogeneity

The subject of MP ontogeny merits discussion in connection with its possible contribution to MP heterogeneity. Information on the ontogeny of the hemopoietic system in general has been reported in the classic studies of Moore and Owen,[139,140] who proposed a scheme of hemopoiesis beginning with the differentiation of hemopoietic stem cells in the extra-embryonic yolk sac by day 8, and successive colonization of the liver on day 10, and then the spleen and bone marrow.

Exactly when MPs appear in the course of embryogenesis and hemopoiesis remains uncertain. Gordon and co-workers cite experiments employing the monoclonal antibody to antigen F4/80, said to be a specific marker for all MPs.[17] F4/80 positive stellate stromal-like MP cells are present in the fetal liver stage of hemopoiesis, before apparent erythrocyte production. Subsequently, monocyte-like F4/80 positive cells are reported to be detectable after erythrocytes are present. Without knowing more about the origin and nature of the F4/80 marker, one cannot be certain of its significance for developmental heterogeneity.

The ontogeny of microglia cells in the brain, and their relationship to MPs, is a particularly intriguing and controversial area. These putative MPs are sequestered within the blood-brain barrier; the endothelium of which is normally poorly permeable to macromolecules and cells. Microglia have been reported to react positively with antibody to MP-specific antigens such as F4/80.[17,18,189] This fact provides insight into the embryonal ancestry of microglia, but yields no information about their mechanism of population renewal. That is, are microglia cells maintained by local proliferation or from monocytes? It seems reasonable to ask for objective evidence that blood monocytes breach the blood-brain barrier under physiologic conditions before making any inference about a monocyte to microglia relationship. A detailed review of experimental approaches to the study of microglia makes it clear that failure to exclude injury and inflammation (which invariably disrupt the blood-brain barrier), is a common problem in experimental design.[142] Gillian[244] has recently presented evidence for the origin of microglia from monocyte-like cells in the tissue early in embryonic development, and evidence against the origin of microglia from blood monocytes has recently been presented.[143]

In studies on MP ontogeny in the rat, Takahashi and his colleagues have described fetal MOs which they identified in the subepidermal mesenchyme and in the liver before the induction of bone marrow hemopoiesis.[144-146] Such fetal MOs, some of which were identified as early as the 12th day of gestation, were actively phagocytic with high levels of incorporation of tritiated thymidine, but were generally negative for peroxidase and α-naphthylbutyrate esterase activity. MPs arising from possibly distinct sources have also been reported in human, chicken, rat, rabbit, hamster, and mouse fetuses.[119,147,148,173,246] Some of these fetal MPs possess complement receptors, are capable of immune phagocytosis, and become increasingly ameboid; but they do not develop nonspecific esterase or endogenous peroxidase activities in extended culture.

The problems of Kupffer cell ontogeny and population renewal are complicated by the issue of peroxidative activity in the nuclear envelope and rough endoplasmic reticulum.[149,150] Some contend that this activity is modulatable and is not a critical means of distinguishing between MPs originating from blood monocytes rather than from a pre-existing self-sustaining cell population.[151] Additional observations on Kupffer cell ontogeny were made by Deimann and Fahimi who suggested that Kupffer cells may become established before hepatic hemopoiesis and blood monocytes are detectable.[152] Overall, the findings from the various fetal studies suggest ontogenetic events that reflect distinctly different pathways of development for tissue MOs and blood monocytes.

Evidence at the hemopoietic level for the development of more than one line of MPs is relatively scarce. A number of investigators have reported apparent clonal differences among MO colony-forming cells from bone marrow with respect to certain characteristics such as cell density, 5'nucleotidase ectoenzyme activity, and Ia antigen expression.[83,91,153,187] In some other studies, however, expression of some of these markers appears to be modulable.[89] Thus, the evidence is inconclusive.

On the basis of receptors for colony-stimulating factor-1 (CSF-1), progenitors of MOs appear to behave as a uniform population.[141] Even within such a putative common lineage, differentiational factors could determine the expression of function, the destination, and the fate of MPs. For example, progenitor cells, even stem cells, may be widely distributed, maintain themselves, and differentiate under local influences into the type of MP characteristic to that compartment. Indeed, Goodman unequivocally demonstrated the presence of hemopoietic stem cells in the peritoneal cavity of the mouse,[154,155] and Stewart and co-workers have demonstrated the presence of MO progenitor cells in that site.[153] In brief, there is, at least at the same loci, the capacity to generate MOs and to maintain local populations.

Others have presented data which suggest that a proliferative compartment for the formation of peritoneal MOs is present in the milky spots of the omentum and mesentery.[156-160] These examples suggest that there is a complexity in the formation of MPs which could have some influence on developmental divergences. Evidence that resident peritoneal and pulmonary alveolar MOs are unaffected by profound sustained monocytopenia is consonant with this idea.[56,161] Overall, it appears reasonable to suggest that the possibilities of an ontogenetic contribution to MP heterogeneity should not be dismissed, and to consider whether the importance of the blood monocyte in the formation of tissue MPs may have been overestimated.

D. Role of the Blood Monocyte in MP Heterogeneity

How do the above observations, from phylogenetic and ontogenetic lines of investigation, reconcile with the idea that all MPs are derived from blood monocytes or perhaps by local proliferation of an immigrant monocyte limited to one or two generations? This popular and comfortable theory is based largely on observations in adult animals, and merits some re-examination.

The blood monocyte, according to currently prevailing theory, serves all functions dependent upon a mobile pool of incompletely differentiated MPs. These include renewal of tissue MO populations, and in addition, the response to signals generated in the inflammatory response. Further differentiation, according to this hypothesis, is regulated by the intracompartmental environment. By inference, this means that circulating monocytes emerge from the bone marrow with no commitment with respect to destination or to characteristic function. Much of the fate of the circulating blood monocyte is determined stochastically until the monocyte becomes associated with a particular MO population. An immigrant monocyte would then become subject to whatever steady-state mechanisms regulate that particular MO population. At present, there is virtually no information concerning the nature or even the existence of the signals required for such an ongoing influx of monocytes into normal tissues under steady-state conditions.

There is much that is appealing about this simple unitarian concept of monocytes providing all MOs. It reconciles well with the many similarities displayed by MS throughout the vertebrate body. For it must be said that despite the great interest in heterogeneity (morphological as well as functional), the many similarities that are distinguished only by quantitative differences would seem to make the argument for a unitary MP system virtually unassailable. Such similarities include the expression of surface antigens such as MAC-1, MAC-3, and F4/80; constitutive secretion of lysozyme; the expression of Fc receptors and complement receptors; and the secretion of bioactive peptides that differ only quantitatively among certain MP populations which can be stimulated to higher outputs.

The principal problem with this concept is the notion that the immediate pool for population maintenance of all resident type MOs is represented by the blood monocyte. One might ask the question whether blood monocytes themselves are an autonomous and homogeneous population. There is considerable evidence that the blood monocytes are heterogeneous (Tables 1 and 2); thus, emigration may well be a selective process. The circulating monocyte pool is normally mixed with respect to age because of cytokinetic mechanisms, but whether heterogeneity in age distribution can account for all the observations of monocyte heterogeneity is uncertain. In detailed studies of guinea pig monocytes, Normann and Noga have shown that the peripheral blood monocytes exist in four subsets which differ in size, cytochemistry, function, cytokinetics, rate of production, and time in circulation.[71-73,117,163] Inflammation was found to affect most profoundly large monocytes which were highly responsive to chemoattractant stimuli, actively phagocytic, and microbicidal, but did not possess native tumoricidal activity and were less readily activated for tumoricidal activity than were small monocytes. The majority of MOs in early inflammatory exudates proved to be derived from the large monocytes. These investigators also found evidence for a reserve pool of the large monocytes which probably exists as a marginated pool of cells.

The distribution of human neutrophil granulocytes into circulating and marginating pools was demonstrated by Athers and his colleagues in a series of kinetic studies.[165,166] Thus, conventional blood samples tap the circulating granulocyte pool which is represented in the axial flow of blood, whereas the marginal granulocyte pool is poorly sampled by traditional methods. Cells in the marginal pool are slowly moving along the endothelium, and pool in regions of static flow. The ratio of the circulating to marginal granulocyte pool is said to be about 1:1 in the steady state. Data supporting the existence of a marginal monocyte pool in humans were later published by Meuret,[167] who estimated that the circulating blood monocyte pool is approximately three to four times the size of the marginal blood monocyte pool. Closely corresponding data for marginal and circulating monocyte pools in the rat were presented by Volkman.[125] More recently, Van Furth and Sluiter reported data estimating that the circulating and marginal monocyte pools in the mouse were in a 1:1 ratio.[168] One implication of these data is that calculations of monocyte kinetics and putative influx have to take into account the marginal blood monocyte pool. Studies of monocyte depletion must likewise consider the pitfall of a marginal monocyte pool when estimating the effect of depletion protocols based on the number of circulating blood monocytes. This problem can be dealt with effectively by estimating the availability of residual blood monocytes for emigration in response to eliciting agents.[56]

What in fact is the evidence that favors the monocytic derivation of all tissue MOs? One point is that it makes good common sense that the relatively sessile pools of tissue MOs depend upon the blood-borne monocyte for the delivery of new members. Some of the other supporting evidence is that, in labeling mice or rats with tritiated thymidine and then studying changes in the labeling indexes in monocytes and peritoneal or alveolar MOs, a correspondence of peak labeling may be seen, although there is relatively little labeling among the resident MOs.[59] Unfortunately, this is not sufficient evidence because one could probably find many other samples of clearly unrelated cell populations that have a concordance of labeling kinetics. Additional support for the monocyte to MO concept has come from the numerous studies in radiation chimeras in which restoration with genetically marked bone marrow was used, so that derivative cells in the recipients could be identified with respect to their source, whether donor or recipient.[169,242] Chimeras are very drastic experiments, involving massive destruction of many populations of cells in the irradiated adult recipients. It is, therefore, not surprising that in most of these experiments, the majority of cells related in any way to the hemopoietic elements bear the genotype of the donor. The relevance of such chimera experiments for normal physiologic population renewal and normal ontogeny remains uncertain. There are no objective experiments to show that monocytes emigrate under physiologic conditions to provide complete replacement of effete tissue MOs. At best, one can say that the chimera experiments strongly suggest an ultimate common origin for MPs.

Experiments with parabiotic rats have also addressed the issue of monocyte renewal of tissue MO populations. No support was found for renewal of peritoneal MOs or Kupffer cells by blood monocytes, but the derivation of inflammatory MOs from blood monocytes was confirmed.[170] The findings were contended by Parawaresch and Walker in cross circulation studies; however, the use of tritiated thymidine with very high specific activity makes the results of these experiments difficult to interpret.[171]

The alternative view, based upon observations in monocyte-depleted mice, suggests that tissue MO compartments are independent of the blood monocyte, at least under steady-state conditions in adult mammals.[56-58,123,172,235-237] There is evidence that tissue MO compartments have the capacity for self-renewal. For example, the presence of pluripotential hemopoietic stem cells and of MO progenitor cells have been demonstrated in the unstimulated peritoneal cavity of the mouse.[153-155] Other studies have shown consistent, instantaneous, and sustained incorporation of tritiated thymidine by resident peritoneal and pulmonary alveolar MOs in normal and monocyte-depleted mice.[123,172] Cytokinetic data for the expansion of the Kupffer cell population in the rat have been published.[174] A portion of the splenic MO population in the mouse also appears to be formed by local proliferation.[129] Two interesting concepts emerge from these data. One is that the blood monocyte is a cell committed to respond to inflammatory stimuli and not to population maintenance. The second is that tissue MO populations are self-maintaining. These data suggest that the contribution of local proliferation to the maintenance of tissue MO populations has been underestimated and could provide a means of continuity of functional phenotypic expression characteristic of the compartment.

In summary, limitations in the presently available technology prevent us from answering definitively the question of the role of the monocyte in the development and maintenance of resident type tissue MOs. At this point, the data are inconclusive to prove or disprove the issue of whether the heterogeneity among tissue MOs is derived solely from monocytes, solely from a nonmonocyte source, or whether there is a dual source.[129,175,176] This complex issue needs to be readdressed with newer technologies.

E. Studies on the Role of the Monocyte in Inflammation

The best substantiated in vivo activity of the blood monocyte is its emigration from the blood stream in response to injurious stimuli and chemoattractant agents. Several terms have been applied to MOs that accumulate in a focus of inflammation as a result of emigration from the blood. Many investigators prefer the term monocyte-MO to connote, quite correctly, that these cells are monocytes which have developed into active effector cells in the tissues.

In many types of inflammation, large numbers of monocytes emigrate from the blood to the affected tissue. The MOs within such a compartment rapidly become heterogeneous, and the compartment becomes distinctly different from the unaffected MP compartments. In uncomplicated inflammation, the enlarged MO mass diminishes over a series of days and the compartment approaches normal. One of the most dramatic examples of massive accumulation of MOs, followed by their remarkably rapid disappearance (commonly in less than a week), was found in untreated pneumococcal pneumonia.[177,178] Persistence of MOs in sites of previous inflammation may occur, however, under certain conditions. The presence of insoluble intracellular particulate material may predispose to persistence. In granulomatous inflammation and chronic inflammation of certain types, monocyte influx into a compartment may be sustained for long periods with abundant monocyte-MOs present in the tissues or tissue spaces.[133,224] Thus, a variety of different types of MP inflammatory responses may be generated against tumors. For the most part, these have not been systematically categorized.

An important and practical aspect of the subject of MP heterogeneity is really its relevance to the therapeutic utilization of MPs in the control of malignancy. It is likely that blood monocytes are of great importance in this context. The emigration of monocytes from the blood into tissues where they develop further into highly active inflammatory MOs has been well documented.[59,135,136] These facts bring up the theoretical considerations that when mobilizing the monocyte for therapeutic purposes, chemotherapy which may suppress bone marrow would be an unsound adjunct. However redundant this comment may seem, there is the possibility that some currently popular regimens may represent such a two-edged sword. It is also important for workers in this field to consider that the blood monocytes are functionally heterogeneous when planning experiments or interpreting data.

VI. IMPLICATIONS OF MP HETEROGENEITY FOR CANCER

A. Theoretical Implications

The preceding sections have clearly documented the heterogeneity that exists in MPs, and shown that there is insufficient information to determine the origins of this heterogeneity. When one adds the complexity of tumor heterogeneity, the problem of defining the interaction of MPs with tumors is formidable indeed. It is plain that many complexities remain to be unraveled before clinical applications can be employed predictably and optimally.

On the teleological level, one might consider why there is so much heterogeneity among MPs. Perhaps this system evolved to provide protective redundancy for host resistance. Different MPs may differ quantitatively in their capacity for surveillance[179] of tumor initiation, micrometastases, carcinoma *in situ,* early invasive cancers, and in inhibition of well established tumors.[215] Having multiple types of MPs may also provide a more rapid response than otherwise available, with certain MPs being effective earlier than other MPs. Finally, the last 5 years have established that there is a complex network of positive and negative immunoregulatory circuits, that apparently is required to maintain normal physiologic homeostasis. The heterogeneity of MPs undoubtedly has significance, as yet incompletely defined, in these immunoregulatory circuits.

B. Practical Considerations for Tumor Diagnosis, Immunity, Infection, and Immunotherapy

1. Are the MPs within Tumors Primarily Derived from Inflammatory Monocytes or from Proliferation and Differentiation/Activation of Resident MOs?

The inflammatory influx of monocytes appears predominant in many tumors; but the present consensus appears to be that tumor-associated MOs may arise from both sources.[6,9,54,180-183] The precise roles of tumor-associated inflammatory monocyte-MOs and proliferating tissue MOs remain to be delineated. More investigation in animal models with selective depletion of certain types of MPs, such as depression of monocytes with ^{89}Sr,[123] or with selective labeling of certain types of MP,[184,185] are necessary to establish the precise relationships between emigrant and *in situ* MOs in tumor biology. A recent report indicated that local activation of alveolar MOs by *Corynebacterium parvum* did not provide resistance against intravenous (i.v.) injection of tumor cells, while systemic activation provided significant resistance, possibly due to activated monocytes.[186] The data suggest that activated pulmonary MOs alone are not effective, perhaps because of anatomic compartmentalization, in conferring resistance to pulmonary tumor nodule formation. Thus, the question remains as to whether emigrant monocytes or MOs, or local MOs will exert the greatest antitumor effects.[4,206,222] The resolution of this issue has obvious important implications for tumor immunotherapy. Should it be directed primarily at local MOs by using procedures such as activation of local MOs by liposome-encapsulated MO-activating agents? Conversely, should immunotherapy be directed primarily at monocytes?

Considerable differences have been reported in the pattern of tumor-associated MOs among tumor variants.[190,215] The particular heterogeneous pattern of tumor-associated MOs appears to be similar for a given tumor variant, suggesting the particular MO response is regulated by the tumor or host immunologic/nonimmunologic response to the tumor.[54] The total number of MPs appears to be less important than the particular proportions of subsets of cells. This is another reason why individual cell analysis of tumor-associated MPs is needed in addition to total population analysis. The particular profile of tumor-associated MOs obviously depends upon a complex interaction of such factors as: chemotactic attractants and antagonists produced by the tumor or host antitumor response, MP growth and growth inhibitory factors present within the tumor, and nonselective and selective mechanisms of trapping MPs within the tumor.

2. Do the Tumor-Associated MO Populations Change During Tumor Development?

The limited data in this area suggest there are definite differences in the heterogeneous MOs profile present at various times during tumor growth.[9] The relationships of these changes to tumor progression will not be clear until we have more knowledge of the source, survival, and turnover time of tumor associated MOs. A related issue is whether tumor cells vary in sensitivity to MO-mediated cytolysis during tumor progression. There is a recent report of host-selected tumor progressor variants that lost their tumor-specific antigen as well as sensitivity to cytotoxic MOs.[191] Such a relationship between tumor progression and decreased sensitivity to MO cytolysis is observed in some but not all tumor systems.[54,185,192-194]

3. Which Types of MPs will "Home" the Most Selectively to Tumors?

These MPs are the best candidates for tumor diagnosis through the use of labeled MPs, or for tumor immunotherapy using cytotoxic MPs or MPs that contain encapsulated toxins.[4,195]

4. Do Certain MPs Enhance Tumor Progression?

The importance of MP heterogeneity in tumor biology is shown by the observations that while MPs can inhibit tumors, they can also enhance tumor growth and indeed, in a few cases, appear to be actually "required" for tumor growth.[196-200] Exactly which MPs are responsible for these opposing activities is not clear. A related issue is whether MPs can enhance carcinogenic processes. Certain activated MPs are potent sources of oxygen metabolites which have been shown to act as mutagens, tumor promoters, and carcinogens.[54] Moreover, MOs might harbor toxic carcinogenic substances, such as asbestos. One current hypothesis is that tumor associated MOs, through oxygen metabolites, increase the instability of certain tumor cells, resulting in higher rates of metastasis or drug resistance.[54,200,201] If these MPs can be separated and characterized, immunotherapy could be aimed to selectively inhibit or delete these MP populations.

5. In MP Populations that Exhibit Apparently Antagonistic Functions, do the Same MPs Exhibit these Functions Simultaneously or is the Apparent Antagonism due to Mixed MP Populations?

Certain MP populations have been described that are tumoricidal in vitro, yet immunosuppressive.[204-207] Human monocytes have been reported to exhibit concurrently both augmentative and suppressive activities for natural killer (NK) cells.[208] Human monocytes activated by gamma interferon in vitro have been described to be tumoricidal and leishmanicidal, but they enhance the intracellular growth of mycobacteria.[209] Most of these functions have been described in vitro. The relevance of such different functioning MPs in vivo is still not clear.

Relatively little evidence is available to indicate whether separable, phenotypically stable MP subpopulations are responsible for the diverse functions. We have demonstrated that when *Corynebacterium parvum* elicited peritoneal rat MO populations are separated into subpopulations based upon size, the subpopulation with the smallest sized cells enhanced tumor growth in vivo compared with the unseparated *C. parvum* MOs, whereas the subpopulation containing the largest sized MOs suppressed tumor growth.[74] Holden et al. demonstrated two MP populations within primary murine sarcoma virus-induced tumors; both exhibited tumor growth inhibitory activity.[210] Mahoney et al. demonstrated that tumor-associated MOs showed considerable heterogeneity in size, density, and function.[190] How these various MP subpopulations are related and inter-regulated remains a question.

6. How do Tumors Change MP Trafficking and MP Functions for Nonantitumor Functions?
Tumor-induced alterations in MP populations obviously may affect host resistance, possibly increasing susceptibility to infection in cancer patients.[9] In this regard, it is interesting that considerable monocytopenia can occur in mice or in clinical situations without necessarily impairing host resistance,[211,283] suggesting an important role for tissue MOs in such resistance. How the tumor burden ultimately affects tissue MOs remains to be defined; both enhancement and inhibition of MP functions have been observed.[9] Tumors, as demonstrated for many viral infections,[212] may also affect MP physiologic functions so that levels of biologically potent secretory products (complement components, tumor necrosis factor, interleukin-1 (IL-1), and neutral proteases) are altered. Such changes can have profound effects on the normal physiology of cancer patients.

VI. CONCLUSIONS AND FUTURE APPROACHES

It is obvious that new investigational approaches will be necessary to elucidate the origin of heterogeneity in MPs, and to make use of this information for better use of MPs in the diagnosis and treatment of cancer. The experimental approaches focused on parallels with lymphocyte, granulocyte, and erythrocyte differentiation are probably too simplistic because of the unique pleiotropic nature and plasticity of MPs. Appreciation of the importance of microenvironments (of the bone marrow, lymphoreticular organs, tumors) for MP differentiation and activation is becoming increasingly recognized.

We need to establish exactly which MPs are involved in a given activity against tumors. Unfortunately, most studies have analyzed entire MP populations rather than individual cells. We need to be able to label MPs with permanent, innocuous markers, separate the cells into defined groups, and assess localization and function of individual MP cells. The newer technologies of radiolabeling cells,[213,229] stable transfection with genetic or other markers,[214,245] differential staining,[184] and the use of cloned MP lines[219,225] should help us discover which MPs are really present at certain sites and are performing which functions. A requirement for such individual cell analysis is a more complete delineation of MP developmental patterns. Caution should be exercised in making neat developmental schemes with the presently available cell surface or oncogene markers; we still lack a comprehensive array of differentiation markers.[217,218,223,227]

What other experimental methods may enhance our insights? Some that appear promising include: exogenous or genetic models of selective depletion of certain MP populations;[122,176,232-240] comparative studies of MPs in normal physiology and in various tumor and inflammatory situations; use in vivo of purified biologic mediators such as IL-1, gamma interferon, CSF-1, and combinations to provide multiple signals that may be necessary for MO activation and differentiation; and identification of additional developmental markers at the molecular level, such as specific mRNA probes.

In conclusion, it is clear that the expressions of MP heterogeneity are more complex than formerly appreciated. We seem to be almost as remote from understanding the underlying mechanisms and significance of the heterogeneity as we were in 1980.[231] Our lack of understanding complicates the use of MPs for tumor diagnosis or tumor immunotherapy.[215,216] At present, there does not appear to be one technology that can meet the criteria required for elucidation of the origins of MP heterogeneity without imposing adventitious alterations in the cells under study. One further requirement is that the technology must be applicable to the "black box", to the ultimate proving ground, that is, the intact animal.

ACKNOWLEDGMENTS

This work was partially supported by research grants CA 35961 and AI 17162, and by contracts N00014-82-K-0669 from the Office of Naval Research and DAMD 17-86-C-6117 from the Army Medical Development Command.

REFERENCES

1. **Russell, S. W., Gillespie, C. Y., and Pace, J. L.,** Evidence for mononuclear phagocytes in solid neoplasms and appraisal of their nonspecific cytotoxic capabilities, *Contemp. Top. Immunobiol.,* 10, 143, 1980.
2. **Mantovani, A., Ming, W. J., Balotta, C., Abdeljalil, B., and Bottazzi, B.,** Origin and regulation of tumor-associated macrophages: the role of tumor derived chemotactic factor, *Biochim. Biophys. Acta,* 865, 59, 1986.
3. **Freedman, V. H., Valvell, T. A., Silagi, S., and Silverstein, S. C.,** Macrophages elicited with heat killed bacillus Calmette Guerin protect C57B1/6J mice against a syngeneic melanoma, *J. Exp. Med.,* 152, 657, 1980.
4. **Fidler, I. J.,** Inhibition of pulmonary metastasis by intravenous injection of specifically activated macrophages, *Cancer Res.,* 34, 1074, 1974.
5. **Marcelleti, J. and Furmanski, P.,** Spontaneous regression of Friend virus induced erythroleukemia. III. Role of macrophages in regression, *J. Immunol.,* 120, 1, 1978.
6. **Haskill, J. S., Proctor, J. W., and Yamamura, Y.,** Host responses within solid tumors. I. Monocytic effector cells within rat sarcomas, *J. Natl. Cancer Inst.,* 54, 387, 1975.
7. **Zarling, J. M. and Tevethia, S. S.,** Transplantation immunity to simian virus 40 transformed cells in tumor bearing mice. II. Evidence for macrophage participation at the effector level of tumor cell, *J. Natl. Cancer Inst.,* 50, 149, 1973.
8. **Fidler, I. J.,** Macrophages and metastasis — a biological approach to cancer therapy, *Cancer Res.,* 45, 4714, 1985.
9. **Norman, S. J.,** Macrophage infiltration and tumor progression, *Cancer Metastasis Rev.,* 4, 277, 1985.
10. **Evans, R. and Eidlen, D. M.,** Macrophage accumulation in transplanted tumors is not dependent on host immune responsiveness or presence of tumor-associated rejection antigens, *J. Reticuloendothel. Soc.,* 30, 425, 1981.
11. **Wang, B. S., Lumanglas, A. L., and Durr, F. E.,** Immunotherapy of a murine lymphoma by adoptive transfer of syngeneic macrophages activated with bisantrene, *Cancer Res.,* 46, 503, 1986.
12. **Van Furth, T., Cohn, Z. A., Hirsch, J. G., Humphrey, J. H., Spector, W. G., and Langevoort, H. L.,** The mononuclear phagocyte system: a new classification of macrophages, monocytes and their precursor cells, *Bull. WHO,* 46, 845, 1972.
13. **Morahan, P. S.,** Macrophage nomenclature: where are we going?, *J. Reticuloendothel. Soc.,* 27, 223, 1980.
14. **Hirsch, S. and Gordon, S.,** Surface antigens as markers of mouse macrophage differentiation, *Annu. Rev. Immunol.,* 999, 51, 1983.
15. **Hume, D. A. and Gordon, S.,** Mononuclear phagocyte system of the mouse defined by immunohistochemical localization of antigen F4/80, *J. Exp. Med.,* 157, 1704, 1983.
16. **Lee, S. H.,** Quantitative analysis of total macrophage content in adult mouse tissues. Immunochemical studies with monoclonal antibody FY/80, *J. Exp. Med.,* April-June, 161, 1985.
17. **Gordon, S., Crocker, P. R., Morris, L., Lee, S. H., Perry, V. H., and Hume, D. A.,** Localization and function of tissue macrophages, *Ciba Found. Symp.,* 118, 54, 1986.
18. **Gordon, S.,** Biology of the macrophage, *J. Cell Sci.,* 4, 267, 1986.
19. **North, R. A.,** The mitotic potential of fixed phagocytes in the liver as revealed during the development of cellular immunity, *J. Exp. Med.,* 130, 315, 1969.
20. **Hogg, N., Selvendran, Y., Dougherty, G., and Allen, C.,** Macrophage antigens and the effect of a macrophage activating factor, interferon-γ, *Ciba Found. Symp.,* 118, 66, 1986.
21. **Lepay, D. A., Nathan, C. F., Steinman, R. M., Murray, H. W., and Cohn, Z. A.,** Murine Kupffer cells. Mononuclear phagocytes deficient in the generation of reactive oxygen intermediates, *J. Exp. Med.,* 161, 1079, 1985.

22. **Arthur, M. J. P., Kowalski-Saunders, P., and Wright, R.,** *Corynebacterium parvum*-elicited hepatic macrophages demonstrate enhanced respiratory burst activity compared with resident Kupffer cells in the rat, *Gastroenterology*, 91, 174, 1986.
23. **Adams, D. O. and Hamilton, T. A.,** The cell biology of macrophage activation, *Annu. Rev. Immunol.*, 2, 283, 1984.
24. **O'Malley, B. W., Towle, H. C., and Schwartz, R. J.,** Regulation of gene expression in eukaryotes, *Annu. Rev. Genet.*, 11, 239, 1977.
25. **O'Malley, B. W., Tasai, S. Y., Tasai, M. J., and Towele, H.,** Regulation of gene expression in eukaryotes, in *Cell Differentiation and Neoplasia*, Sanders, G. F., Ed., Raven Press, New York, 1978, 473.
26. **Bauer, S. R., Homes, K. L., Moorse, H. C., III, and Potter, M.,** Clonal relationship of the lymphoblastic cell line P388 to the macrophage cell line P388D1 as evidenced by immunoglobulin gene rearrangement and expression of cell surface antigens, *J. Immunol.*, 136, 4695, 1986.
27. **Leder, P.,** Genetics of antibody diversity, *Sci. Am.*, 246, 102, 1982.
28. **Strunk, R. C., Cole, F. S., Perlmutter, D. H., and Colten, J. R.,** Y-interferon increases expression of class III complement genes C2 and factor B in human monocytes and in murine fibroblasts transfected with human C2 and factor B genes, *J. Biol. Chem.*, 260, 15280, 1985.
29. **Cole, F. S., Auerbach, H. W., Goldberger, G., and Colten, H. R.,** Tissue-specific pretranslation regulation of complement production in human mononuclear phagocytes, *J. Immunol.*, 134, 2610, 1985.
30. **DiBeradina, M. A., Hoffner, N. J., and Etkin, L. D.,** Activation of dormant genes in specialized cells, *Science*, 224, 946, 1984.
31. **Stevenson, H. C., Miller, P., Oldham, R., Kanapa, D. J., and Sen, A.,** Characterization of 3H-uridine incorporation and messenger RNA synthesis in human monocytes activated to secrete alpha interferon or monocyte derived fibroblast growth factor, *J. Leukocyte Biol.*, 37, 585, 1985.
32. **Paulnock-King, D., Sizer, K. C., Freund, Y. R., Jones, P. P., and Barnes, J. R.,** Coordinate induction of Ia alpha, beta and Ii mRNA in a macrophage cell line, *J. Immunol.*, 135, 632, 1985.
33. **Ruco, L. P. and Meltzer, M. S.,** Macrophage activation for tumor cytotoxicity: induction of tumoricidal macrophages by supernatants of PPD-stimulated Bacillus Calmette-Guerin-immune spleen cells, *J. Immunol.*, 119, 889, 1977.
34. **Ruco, L. P. and Meltzer, M. S.,** Macrophage activation for tumor cytotoxicity: development of macrophage cytotoxicity requires completion of a sequence of short-lived intermediary reactions, *J. Immunol.*, 121, 2035, 1978.
35. **Hibbs, J. B., Chapman, H. A., and Weinberg, J. B.,** The macrophage as an antineoplastic surveillance cell: biological perspectives, *J. Reticuloendothel Soc.*, 24, 549, 1978.
36. **Strassmann, G., Springer, T. A., Haskill, S. J., Mirgalia, C. C., Lanier, L. L., and Adams, D. O.,** Antigens associated with the activation of murine mononuclear phagocytes in vivo: differential expression of lymphocyte function-associated antigen in the several stages of development, *Cell. Immunol.*, 94, 265, 1985.
37. **Cohn, Z. A.,** The activation of mononuclear phagocytes: fact, fancy and future, *J. Immunol.*, 121, 813, 1978.
38. **North, R. J.,** The concept of activated macrophages, *J. Immunol.*, 121, 806, 1978.
39. **Hamburger, J.,** "Macrophage activation". Imperfect terminology hiding imperfect knowledge, *Ann. Immunol. (Inst. Pasteur)*, 128, 731, 1977.
40. **Russell, S. E., Doe, W. F., and McIntosh, A. J.,** Functional characterization of a stable, noncytolytic stage of macrophage activation in tumors, *J. Exp. Med.*, 146, 1511, 1977.
41. **Nicola, N. A. and Metcalf, D.,** Specificity of action of colony-stimulating factors in the differentiation of granulocytes and macrophages, *Ciba Found. Symp.*, 118, 7, 1986.
42. **Metcalf, D.,** *The Hemopoietic Colony Stimulating Factors*, Elsevier, Amsterdam, 1984.
43. **Wing, E. J., Ampel, N. M., Waheed, A., and Shadduck, R. K.,** Macrophage colony-stimulating factor (M-CSF) enhances the capacity of murine macrophages to secrete oxygen reduction products, *J. Immunol.*, 135, 2052, 1985.
44. **Grabstein, K. H., Urdal, D. L., Tushinski, R. J., Mochizuki, D. Y., Price, V. L., Cantrell, M. A., Gillis, S., and Conlon, P. J.,** Induction of macrophage tumoricidal activity by granulocyte-macrophage colony-stimulating factor, *Science*, 232, 506, 1986.
45. **Grossberg, S. E. and Taylor, J. L.,** Interferon effects of cell differentiation, in *Interferon*, Vol. 3, Gresser, I., Ed., Elsevier, Amsterdam, 1985, 3.
46. **Moore, R. M., Pitruzzello, F. J., Deana, D. G., and Rouse, B. T.,** Endogenous regulation of macrophage proliferation and differentiation by E prostaglandins and interferon alpha/beta, *Lymphokine Res.*, 4, 43, 1985.
47. **Chen, B. D. M. and Cleark, C. R.,** Interleukin 3 regulates the in vitro proliferation of both blood monocytes and peritoneal exudate macrophages: synergism between a macrophage lineage-specific colony-stimulating factor (CSF-1) and IL-3, *J. Immunol.*, 137, 563, 1986.

48. **Broxmeyer, H. E., Williams, D. E., Boswell, H. S., Cooper, S., Shadduck, R. K., Gillis, S., Waheed, A., and Urdal, D. L.,** The effects in vivo of purified preparations of murine macrophage colony stimulating factor-1, recombinant murine granulocyte-macrophage colony stimulating factor and recombinant murine IL-3 with and without lactoferrin pretreatment, *Immunobiology,* 172, 168, 1986.
49. **Fisher, D. G. and Rubinstein, M.,** Human monocytes tumoricidal activity: the role of interferon-γ and bacterial lipopolysaccharide in its stimulation, preservation and decay, *Immunobiology,* 172, 110, 1986.
50. **Koike, K., Stanley, E. R., Ihle, J. N., and Ogawa, M.,** Macrophage colony formation supported by purified CSF-1 and/or interleukin 3 in serum-free culture: evidence for hierarchial difference in macrophage colony-forming cells, *Blood,* 67, 859, 1986.
51. **Tushinski, R. J., Oliver, I. T., Builbert, L. J., Tynan, P. W., Warner, J. R., and Stanley, E. R.,** Survival of mononuclear phagocytes depends on a lineage-specific growth factor that the differentiated cells selectively destroy, *Cell,* 28, 71, 1982.
52. **Walker, F., Nicola, N. A., Metcalf, D., and Burgess, A. W.,** Hierarchical down-modulation of hemopoietic growth factor receptors, *Cell,* 43, 269, 1985.
53. **Baserga, R.,** *The Biology of Cell Reproduction,* Harvard University Press, Cambridge, Mass., 1985.
54. **Wei, W. Z., Ratner, S., Fulton, A. M., and Heppner, G. H.,** Inflammatory infiltrates of experimental mouse mammary carcinomas, *Biochim. Biophys. Acta,* 865, 13, 1986.
55. **Volkman, A.,** The production of monocytes and related cells, *Haemetol. Lett.,* 10, 61, 1967.
56. **Volkman, A., Chang, N. C., Strausbauch, P. H., and Morahan, P. S.,** Differential effects of chronic monocyte depletion on macrophage populations, *Lab. Invest.,* 49, 291, 1983.
57. **Bouwens, L., Knook, D. L., and Wisse, E.,** Local proliferation and extrahepatic recruitment of liver macrophages (Kupffer cells) in partial-body irradiated rats, *J. Leukocyte Biol.,* 39, 687, 1986.
58. **Evans, M. J., Shami, S. G., and Martinez, L. A.,** Enhanced proliferation of pulmonary alveolar macrophages after carbon instillation in mice depleted of blood monocytes by strontium-89, *Lab. Invest.,* 54, 154, 1986.
59. **Van Furth, R. and Cohn, Z. A.,** The origin and kinetics of mononuclear phagocytes, *J. Exp. Med.,* 128, 415, 1968.
60. **Pelus, L. M., Broxmeyer, H. E., DeSousa, N., and Moore, M. A. S.,** Heterogeneity among resident murine peritoneal macrophages: separation and functional characterization of monocytoid cells producing granulocyte-macrophage colony-stimulating factor and responding to lactoferrin, *J. Immunol.,* 126, 1016, 1981.
61. **Lee, K. C., Wong, M., and McIntyre, D.,** Characterization of macrophage subpopulations responsive to activation by endotoxin and lymphokines, *J. Immunol.,* 126, 2474, 1981.
62. **Tabor, D. R. and Saluk, P. H.,** The functional heterogeneity of murine-resident macrophages to a chemotactic signal and induction of C3b-receptor mediated ingestion, *Immunol. Lett.,* 3, 371, 1981.
63. **Serio, C., Gandour, D. M., and Walker, W. S.,** Macrophage functional heterogeneity: evidence for different antibody-dependent effector cell activities and expression of Fc-receptors among macrophage subpopulations, *J. Reticuloendothel. Soc.,* 25, 197, 1979.
64. **Hopper, K. E. and Geczy, C. L.,** Characterization of guinea pig macrophage. I. Mobility and maturation of peritoneal cells following inflammatory stimuli, *Cell. Immunol.,* 56, 400, 1980.
65. **Kavai, M., Laczko, J., and Csaba, B.,** Functional heterogeneity of macrophages, *Immunology,* 36, 729, 1979.
66. **Lee, K. C.,** Regulation of T cell activation by macrophage subsets, *Lymphokines,* 6, 1, 1982.
67. **Reppun, T. S., Lin, H. S., and Kuhn, C.,** Isokinetic separation and characterization of mouse pulmonary alveolar colony-forming cells, *J. Reticuloendothel. Soc.,* 25, 379, 1979.
68. **Holian, A., Dauber, J. H., Diamond, M. S., and Daniele, R. P.,** Separation of bronchoalveolar cells from the guinea pig on continuous gradients of Percoll: functional properties of fractionated lung macrophage, *J. Reticuloendothel. Soc.,* 33, 157, 1983.
69. **Chandler, D. B., Fuller, W. C., Jackson, R. M., and Fulmer, J. D.,** Fractionation of rat alveolar macrophages by isopycnic centrifugation: morphological, cytochemical, biochemical, and functional properties, *J. Leukocyte Biol.,* 39, 371, 1986.
70. **Shellito, J. and Kaltreider, H. B.,** Heterogeneity of immunologic function among subfractions of normal rat alveolar macrophages, *Am. Rev. Respir. Dis.,* 131, 678, 1985.
71. **Noga, S. J., Normann, S. J., and Weiner, R. W.,** Differences in Fc receptor expression between small and large guinea pig monocytes, *J. Leukocyte Biol.,* 40, 737, 1986.
72. **Noga, S. J., Normann, S. J., and Weiner, R. W.,** Isolation of guinea pig monocytes and Kurloff cells: characterization of monocyte subsets by morphology, cytochemistry, and adherence, *Lab. Invest.,* 51, 244, 1984.
73. **Normann, S. J. and Noga, S. J.,** Population kinetic study on the origin of guinea pig monocyte heterogeneity, *Cell. Immunol.,* 99, 375, 1986.
74. **Miller, G. A., Morahan, P. S., White, S., and Jessee, E.,** Functional and biochemical heterogeneity among subpopulations of rat and mouse peritoneal macrophages, *J. Reticuoloendothel. Soc.,* 32, 111, 1982.

75. **Bellen, R. H. and Walker, W. S.,** Dynamics of cytochemically distinct subpopulations of macrophages in elicited rat peritoneal exudates, *Cell. Immunol.,* 82, 246, 1983.

76. **Morahan, P. S., Rozner, M. A., and Jessee, E. J.,** Effect of elicitation on peritoneal macrophage subpopulation: size distributions, ectoenzyme phenotypes and antitumor activity, *Int. J. Cancer,* 30, 787, 1982.

77. **Rice, S. G. and Fishman, M.,** Functional and morphological heterogeneity among rabbit peritoneal macrophages, *Cell. Immunol.,* 11, 130, 1974.

78. **Miller, G. A., Campbell, M. W., and Hudson, J. L.,** Separation of rat peritoneal macrophages into functionally distinct subclasses by centrifugal elutriation, *J. Reticuloendothel. Soc.,* 27, 167, 1980.

79. **Chapes, S. K. and Tompkins, W. A.,** Distribution of macrophage cytotoxic and macrophage helper functions of BSA discontinuous gradients, *J. Reticuloendothel. Soc.,* 30, 517, 1981.

80. **Drath, D. B.,** Enhanced superoxide release and tumoricidal activity by a postlavage, in situ pulmonary macrophage population in response to activation by mycobacterium bovis BCG exposure, *Infect. Immun.,* 49, 72, 1985.

81. **Moore, K. and McBride, W. H.,** Enhanced Fc receptor expression by a subpopulation of murine intra-tumor macrophages following intravenous *Corynebacterium parvum* therapy, *Br. J. Cancer,* 47, 797, 1983.

82. **Suga, M., Dannenberg, A. M., and Higuchi, S.,** Macrophage functional heterogeneity in vivo. Macrolocal and microlocal macrophage activation, identified by double-staining tissue sections of BCG granulomas for pairs of enzymes, *Am. J. Pathol.,* 99, 305, 1980.

83. **Metcalf, D. and MacDonald, H. R.,** Heterogeneity of in vitro colony- and cluster-forming cells in the mouse marrow segregation by velocity sedimentation, *Cell. Physiol.,* 85, 643, 1975.

84. **Caignard, A., Martin, M. S., Hammann, A., and Martin, F.,** Heterogeneity of the rat macrophage: antigenic specificity of resident peritoneal and pleural macrophages, *Cell. Mol. Biol.,* 31, 41, 1985.

85. **Lehnert, B. E., Valdez, Y. E., Fillak, D. A., Steinkamp, J. A., and Stewart, C. C.,** Flow cytometric characterization of alveolar macrophages, *J. Leukocyte Biol.,* 39, 285, 1986.

86. **Van der Brugge-Bamelkoorne, G. J., Dijkstra, C. D., and Sminia, T.,** Characterization of pulmonary macrophages and bronchus-associated lymphoid tissue (BALT) macrophages in the rat. An enzyme-cyto-chemical and immunocytochemical study, *Immunobiology,* 169, 553, 1985.

87. **Lakeya, M., Hsiao, L., and Takahashi, K.,** Three monoclonal antibodies TRPM-1, TRPM-2, and TEPM-3 recognize distinct macrophage subpopulations, *J. Leukocyte Biol.,* submitted.

88. **Dijkstra, C. D., Dopp, E. A., Jolling, P., and Kraael, G.,** The heterogeneity of mononuclear phagocytes in lymphoid organs: distinct macrophage subpopulations in rat recognized by monoclonal antibodies ED1, ED2, and ED3, *Adv. Exp. Med. Biol.,* 186, 409, 1985.

89. **Cowing, C., Schwartz, B. D., and Dickler, H. B.,** Macrophage Ia antigens. I. Macrophage populations differ in their expression of Ia antigens, *J. Immunol.,* 120, 378, 1978.

90. **Polman, C. H., Dijkstra, C. D., Sminia, T., and Koetsier, J. C.,** Immunohistological analysis of macrophages in the central nervous system of Lewis rats with acute experimental allergic encephalomyelitis, *J. Neuroimmunol.,* 11, 215, 1986.

91. **Bursuker, I. and Goldman, R.,** Distinct bone marrow precursors from mononuclear phagocytes expressing high and low 5'-nucleotidase activity, *J. Cell. Physiol.,* 112, 237, 1982.

92. **Baccarini, M., Bistoni, F., and Lohmann-Matthews, M. L.,** Organ-associated macrophage precursor activity: isolation of candidacidal and tumoricidal effectors from the spleens of cyclophosphamide-treated mice, *J. Immunol.,* 136, 837, 1986.

93. **Ju, S. and Dorf, M. E.,** Functional analysis of cloned macrophage hybridomas, *J. Immunol.,* 134, 3722, 1985.

94. **Hopper, K. E. and Cahill, J. M.,** Immunoregulation by macrophages. III. Separation of mouse peritoneal macrophages having tumoricidal and bactericidal activities and those secreting PGE and interleukin 1, *J. Reticuloendothel. Soc.,* 33, 443, 1983.

95. **Chapes, S. K. and Haskill, S.,** Role of *Corynebacterium parvum* in the activation of peritoneal macro-phages. II. Identification of distinguishable anti-tumor activities by macrophage subpopulations *Cell. Immunol.,* 76, 49, 1983.

96. **Takeda, Y., Woo, H. J., and Osawa, T.,** Mouse macrophage hybridomas secreting a cytotoxic factor and Interleukin 1, *Cell. Immunol.,* 90, 493, 1985.

97. **Roubin, R. and Zolla-Pazner, S.,** Markers of macrophage heterogeneity. I. Studies of macrophages from various organs of normal mice, *Eur. J. Immunol.,* 9, 972, 1979.

98. **Lee, K. C. and Guidos, C.,** Heterogeneity of macrophages and dendritic cells as accessory cells, *Immunobiology,* 168, 172, 1984.

99. **Grand-Perret, T., Petit, J. F., and Lemaire, G.,** Modifications induced by activation to tumor cytotoxicity in the protein secretory activity of macrophages, *J. Leukocyte Biol.,* 40, 1, 1986.

100. **Becker, S., Halme, J., and Haskill, S.,** Heterogeneity of human peritoneal macrophages: cytochemical and flow cytometric studies, *J. Reticuloendothel. Soc.,* 33, 127, 1983.

101. **Haskill, S. and Becker, S.,** Flow cytometric analysis of macrophage heterogeneity and differentiation: utilization of electronic cell volume and fluorescent substrates corresponding to common macrophage markers, *J. Reticuloendothel. Soc.,* 32, 273, 1982.

102. **Mottolese, M., Natali, P. G., Atlante, G., Cavallari, A., DiFilippo, F., and Ferrone, S.,** Antigenic profile and functional characterization of human peritoneal macrophages, *J. Immunol.,* 135, 200, 1985.

103. **Andreesen, R., Bross, K. J., Osterholz, J., and Emmrich, F.,** Human macrophage maturation and heterogeneity: analysis with a newly generated set of monoclonal antibodies to differentiation antigens, *Blood,* 67, 1257, 1986.

104. **Biondi, A., Rossing, T. H., Bennett, J., and Todd, R. F.,** Surface membrane heterogeneity among human mononuclear phagocytes, *J. Immunol.,* 132, 1237, 1984.

105. **Grant, V. A. and Hamblin, A. S.,** Human bronchoalveolar macrophage heterogeneity demonstrated by histochemistry, surface markers and phagocytosis, *Clin. Exp. Immunol.,* 60, 539, 1985.

106. **Hogg, N., Takacs, L., Palmer, D. G., Selvendran, Y., and Allen, C.,** The p150, 95 molecule is a marker of human mononuclear phagocytes: comparison with expression of Class II molecules, *Eur. J. Immunol.,* 16, 240, 1986.

107. **Steinmann, G., Broxmeyer, H. E., de Harven, E., and Moore, M. A. S.,** Immuno-electron microscopic tracing of lactoferrin, a regulator of myelopoiesis, into a subpopulation of human peripheral blood monocytes, *Br. J. Haematol.,* 50, 75, 1982.

108. **Akiyama, Y., Miller, P. J., Thurman, G. B., Neubauer, R. H., Oliver, C., Favilla, T., Beman, J. A., Oldham, R. K., and Stevenson, H. C.,** Characterization of a human blood monocyte subset with low peroxidase activity, *J. Clin. Invest.,* 72, 1093, 1983.

109. **Schriber, A. D., Kelley, M., Dziarski, A., and Levison, A. I.,** Human monocyte functional heterogeneity: monocyte fractionation by discontinuous albumin gradient centrifugation, *Immunology,* 49, 231, 1983.

110. **Tice, D. G., Goldberg, J., and Nelson, D. A.,** Functional properties of isopycnic fractions of human peripheral blood monocytes, *J. Reticuloendothel. Soc.,* 29, 459, 1981.

111. **Nunez, G., Giles, R. C., Ball, E. J., Hurley, C. K., Capra, J. D., and Stastny, P.,** Expression of HLA-DR, MB, MT and SB antigens of human mononuclear cells: identification of two phenotypically distinct monocyte populations, *J. Immunol.,* 133, 1300, 1984.

112. **Zembala, M., Uraca, W., Ruggiero, I., Mytar, B., and Pryjma, J.,** Isolation and functional characteristics of FcR + and FcR − human monocyte subsets, *J. Immunol.,* 133, 1293, 1984.

113. **Whisler, R. L., Newhouse, Y. G., and Lachman, L. B.** Heterogeneity of human monocyte subsets in the promotion of B cell colonies and the role of interleukin 1, *J. Immunol.,* 129, 455, 1982.

114. **Melewicz, F. M. and Spiegelberg, H. L.,** Fc receptors for IgE on a subpopulation of human peripheral blood monocytes, *J. Immunol.,* 125, 1026, 1980.

115. **Hofman, F. M., Lopez, D., Husmann, L., Meyer, P. R., and Taylor, C. R.,** Heterogeneity of macrophage populations in human lymphoid tissue and peripheral blood, *Cell. Immunol.,* 88, 61, 1984.

116. **Ettensohn, D. B. and Roberts, M. J.,** Influenza virus infection of human alveolar and blood-derived macrophages: differences in accessory cell function and interferon production, *J. Infect. Dis.,* 149, 942, 1984.

117. **Normann, S. J. and Weiner, R.,** Cytotoxicity of human peripheral blood monocytes, *Cell. Immunol.,* 81, 413, 1983.

118. **McLeod, R., Bensch, K., Smith, S., and Remington, J. S.,** Effects of human peripheral blood monocytes, monocyte-derived macrophages, and spleen mononuclear phagocytes on *Toxoplasma gondii, Cell. Immunol.,* 54, 330, 1980.

119. **Janossy, G., Bofill, M., Poultder, L. W., Rawlings, E., Burford, G. D., Navarret, C., Ziegler, A., and Kelemen, E.,** Separate ontogeny of two macrophage-like accessory cell populations in the human fetus, *J. Immunol.,* 136, 4354, 1986.

120. **Ferrero, D., Broxmeyer, H. E., Paglardi, G. L., Venuta, S., Lange, B., Pessano, S., and Rovera, G.,** Antigenically distinct subpopulations of myeloid progenitor cells (CFU-GM) in human peripheral blood and marrow, *Proc. Natl. Acad. Sci. U.S.A.,* 80, 4114, 1983.

121. **Chiu, K. M., McPherson, L. H., Harris, J. E., and Braun, D. P.,** The separation of cytotoxic human peripheral blood monocytes into high and low phagocytic subsets by centrifugal elutriation, *J. Leukocyte Biol.,* 36, 729, 1984.

122. **Thompson, J. and Van Furth, R.,** The effect of glucocorticosteroids on the kinetics of mononuclear phagocytes, *J. Exp. Med.,* 131, 429, 1970.

123. **Sawyer, R.,** The cytokinetic behavior of pulmonary alveolar macrophages in monocytopenic mice, *J. Leukocyte Biol.,* 39, 89, 1986.

124. **Alblas, A. and Van Furth, R.,** Kinetics and characteristics of pulmonary macrophages in the normal steady state, *J. Exp. Med.,* 149, 1504, 1979.

125. **Volkman, A.,** The unsteady state of the Kupffer cell, in *International Kupffer Cell Symposium,* Wisse, E. and Knook, D. L., Eds., Elsevier/North-Holland, Amsterdam, 1977.

126. **Till, J. E. and McCulloch, E. A.**, A direct measurement of the radiation sensitivity of normal mouse bone marrow cells, *Radiat. Res.*, 14, 213, 1961.
127. **Till, J. E. and McCulloch, E. A.**, Hemopoietic stem cell differentiation, *Biochim. Biophys. Acta*, 605, 431, 1980.
128. **Cleaver, J. E.**, *Thymidine Metabolism and Cell Kinetics*, North-Holland, Amsterdam, 1967.
129. **Van Furth, R. and Diesselhoff-denDulk, M. M. C.**, Dual origin of mouse spleen macrophages, *J. Exp. Med.*, 160, 1273, 1984.
130. **Austyn, J. M. and Gordon, S.**, F4/80, a monoclonal antibody directed specifically against the mouse macrophage, *Eur. J. Immunol.*, 11, 805, 1981.
131. **Metchnikoff, E.**, Ueber die Phagocytare Rolle der Tuberkelriesenzellen, *Virchows Arch. Pathol. Anat. Physiol.*, 113, 63, 1888.
132. **Lewis, W. H.**, The transformation of mononuclear blood cells into macrophages, epithelioid cells and giant cells, *Harvey Lect.*, 21, 77, 1926.
133. **Ebert, R. H. and Florey, H. W.**, The extravascular development of the monocyte observed in vivo, *Br. J. Exp. Pathol.*, 20, 342, 1939.
134. **Hughes, W. L., Bond, V. P., Brecher, G., Cronkite, E. P., Painter, R. B., Quastler, H., and Sherman, F. G.**, Cellular proliferation in the mouse as revealed by autoradiography with tritiated thymidine, *Proc. Natl. Acad. Sci.*, 44, 476, 1958.
135. **Volkman, A. and Gowans, J. L.**, The production of macrophages in the rat, *Br. J. Exp. Pathol.*, 46, 50, 1965.
136. **Volkman, A. and Gowans, J. L.**, The origin of macrophages from bone marrow in the rat, *Br. J. Exp. Pathol.*, 46, 62, 1965.
137. **Van Furth, R., Hirsh, J. G., and Fedorkao, M. E.**, Morphology and peroxidase cytochemistry of mouse promonocytes, monocytes, and macrophages, in *Promonocyte Morphology*, 1970, 794.
138. **Metcalf, D.**, Transformation of granulocytes to macrophages in bone marrow colonies in vitro, *Cell. Physiol.*, 77, 277, 1971.
139. **Moore, M. A. S. and Owen, J. J. T.**, Stem cell migration in developing myeloid and lymphoid systems, *Lancet*, 1, 658, 1967.
140. **Moore, M. A. S. and Owen, J. J. T.**, Chromosome marker studies on the development of the haemopoietic system in the chick embryo, *Nature (London)*, 208, 956, 1965.
141. **Metcalf, D.**, Granulocyte-macrophage colony stimulating factors, *Science*, 229, 16, 1985.
142. **Oehmichen, M.**, *Phagocytes in the Central Nervous System*, Springer-Verlag, Berlin, 1978, 1.
143. **Schleper, R. L. and Adrian, E. K.**, Monocytes become macrophages: they do not become microglia: a light and electron microscopic autoradiographic study using 125-iododeoxyuridine, *J. Neuropathol. Exp. Neurol.*, 45, 1, 1986.
144. **Takahashi, K., Naito, M., Yamamura, F., and Takeya, M.**, Ontogeny of macrophages in the yolk sac of murine fetuses, *XVth Int. Congr. Int. Acad. Pathol.*, 1986.
145. **Takahashi, K., Takahashi, H., Naito, M., Saito, T., and Kojima, M.**, Ultrastructural and functional development of macrophages in the dermal tissue of rat fetuses, *Cell Tissue Res.*, 232, 539, 1983.
146. **Naito, M., Takahashi, K., Takahashi, H., and Kojima, M.**, Ontogenic development of Kupffer cells, in *Sinusoidal Liver Cells*, Elsevier, Amsterdam, 1982, 155.
147. **Breathnach, A. S.**, Development and differentiation of dermal cells of man, *J. Invest. Dermatol.*, 71, 2, 1978.
148. **Dawd, D. S. and Hinchcliff, J. R.**, Cell death is the "opaque path" in the central mesenchyme of the developing chick limb: a cytological, cytochemical, and electron microscope analysis, *J. Embryol. Exp. Morphol.*, 26, 401, 1971.
149. **Daems, W. T., Koernten, H. K., and Soranzo, M. R.**, On the differences between monocyte-derived and tissue macrophages.
150. **Daems, W. T. and Brederoo, P.**, The fine structure and peroxidase activity of resident and exudate peritoneal macrophages in the guinea pig, in *The Reticuloendothelial System and Immune Phenomena*, Vol. 13, DiLuzio, N. R., Ed., Plenum Press, New York, 1971, 19.
151. **Bodel, P. T., Nichols, B. A., and Bainton, D. F.**, Appearance of peroxidase reactivity within the rough endoplasmic reticulum of blood monocytes after surface adherence, *J. Exp. Med.*, 145, 264, 1977.
152. **Diemann, W. and Fahimi, H. D.**, The ontogeny of mononuclear phagocytes in fetal rat liver using endogenous peroxidase as a marker, in *Kupffer Cells and Other Liver Sinusoidal Cells*, Wisse, E. and Knook, D. L., Eds., Elsevier/North-Holland, Amsterdam, 1977, 487.
153. **Stewart, C. C., Walker, E. G., Warner, N. L., and Walker, W. S.**, Mononuclear phagocyte proliferation and differentiation, in *Mononuclear Phagocyte Biology*, Volkman, A., Ed., Marcel Dekker, New York, 1985, 403.
154. **Goodman, J. W.**, Transplantation of peritoneal fluid cells, *Transplantation*, 3, 334, 1963.
155. **Goodman, J. W.**, The use of isoimmune sera for identification of hemopoietic cells from blood-infected radiation chimera, *Ann. N.Y. Acad. Sci.*, 97, 95, 1962.

156. **Cappel, D. F.,** Intravitam and supravital staining. IV. The cellular reactions following mild irritation of the peritoneum in normal and vitally stained animals with special reference to the origin and nature of the mononuclear cells, *J. Pathol. Bacteriol.,* 33, 429, 1930.

157. **Mims, C. A.,** The peritoneal macrophages of mice, *Br. J. Exp. Pathol.,* 45, 37, 1963.

158. **DeBakker, J. M., deWit, A. W., Onderwater, J. J. M., Ginsfel, L. A., and Daems, W. T.,** On the origin of peritoneal resident macrophages. I. DNA synthesis in mouse peritoneal resident macrophages, *J. Submicrosc. Cytol.,* 17, 133, 1985.

159. **DeBakker, J. M., deWit, A. W., Onderwater, J. J. M., Ginsfel, L. A., and Daems, W. T.,** On the origin of peritoneal resident macrophages. II. Recovery of the resident macrophage population in the peritoneal cavity and in the milky spots after peritoneal cell depletion, *J. Submicrosc. Cytol.,* 17, 141, 1985.

160. **DeBakker, J. M., deWit, A. W., Onderwater, J. J. M., Ginsfel, L. A., and Daems, W. T.,** On the origin of peritoneal resident macrophages. III. EM-immunocytochemical studies on the origin of mouse peritoneal resident macrophages, *J. Submicrosc. Cytol.,* 17, 153, 1985.

161. **Sawyer, R. T., Strausbauch, P. H., and Volkman, A.,** Resident macrophage proliferation in mice depleted of blood monocytes by strontium-89, *Lab. Invest.,* 46, 165, 1982.

162. **Lee, K. C. and Berry, D.,** Functional heterogeneity in macrophages activated by *C. parvum:* characteristics of subpopulations with different activities in promoting immune responses and suppressing tumor cell growth, *J. Immunol.,* 118, 1530, 1977.

163. **Normann, S. and Noga, S.,** Population kinetics study of guinea pigs monocytes and their subsets during acute inflammation, *Cell. Immunol.,* 102, 1, 1986.

164. **Murphy, M. and Herscowitz, H.,** Heterogeneity among alveolar macrophages in humoral and cell mediated immune responses: separation of functional subpopulations by density gradient centrifugation on Percoll, *J. Leukocyte Biol.,* 35, 317, 1984.

165. **Athers, J. W., Raab, S. Q., Hwab, O. P., Mauer, A. M., Aschenbrocher, H., Cartwright, G. E., and Wintrole, M. M.,** Leukokinetic studies. III. The distribution of granulocytes in the blood of normal subjects, *J. Clin. Invest.,* 40, 159, 1961.

166. **Athers, J. W., Mauer, A. M., Aschenbrucker, H., Cartwright, G. E., and Wintrole, M. M.,** Leukokinetic studies. I. A method for labeling leukocytes with diisopropylfluorophosphates, *Blood,* 4, 303, 1959.

167. **Meuret, G., Rau, M., Kasten, G., and Hoffman, G.,** Kinetics of monocytopoiesis and blood monocytes in man, *Verh. Dtsch. Ges. Inn. Med.,* 77, 377, 1971.

168. **Van Furth, R. and Sluiter, W.,** Distribution of blood monocytes between a marginating and a circulating pool, *J. Exp. Med.,* 163, 474, 1986.

169. **Van Furth, R. and Sluiter, W.,** Current views on the ontogeny of macrophages and the humoral regulation of monocytopoiesis, *Trans. R. Soc. Trop. Med. Hyg.,* 77, 614, 1983.

170. **Volkman, A.,** Disparity in origin of mononuclear phagocyte populations, *J. Reticuloendothel. Soc.,* 19, 249, 1976.

171. **Parawaresch, M. and Walker, H.,** Origin and kinetics of resident tissue macrophages and radiolabelled leukocytes, *Cell Tissue Kinet.,* 17, 25, 1983.

172. **Volkman, A., Change, N-C. A., Strausbauch, P. H., and Morahan, P. S.,** Maintenance of resident macrophage populations in monocyte-depleted mice, in *Mononuclear Phagocyte Biology,* Volkman, A., Ed., Marcel Dekker, New York, 1984, 419.

173. **DeFelici, M., Heasman, J., Wylie, C. C., and McLaren, A.,** Macrophages in the urogenital ridge of the mid-gestation mouse fetus, *Cell Differ.,* 18, 119, 1986.

174. **Bowmens, L., Baekeland, M., and Wisse, E.,** Cytokinetic analysis of the expanding Kupffer-cell population in rat liver, *Cell Tissue Kinet.,* 19, 217, 1986.

175. **Decker, T., Lohmann-Matthes, M. L., and Baccarini, M.,** Heterogeneous activity of immature and mature cells of the murine monocyte-macrophage lineage derived from different anatomical districts against yeast phase *Candida albicans, Infect. Immun.,* 54, 477, 1986.

176. **Shibata, Y. and Volkman, A.,** The effect of hemopoietic microenvironment on splenic suppressor macrophages in congenitally anemic mice of genotype Sl/Sldl, *J. Immunol.,* 135, 3905, 1985.

177. **Foot, N. C.,** Studies of endothelial reactions; origins of pulmonary, *Am. J. Pathol.,* 3, 413, 1927.

178. **Robertson, O. H. and Ohley, C. G.,** Changes occurring in the macrophage system of the lungs in pneumococcus lobar pneumonia, *J. Clin. Invest.,* 15, 115, 1936.

179. **Adams, D. O. and Snydermann, R.,** Do macrophages destroy nascent tumors?, *J. Natl. Cancer Inst.,* 62, 1341, 1979.

180. **Evans, R., Duffy, T., and Cullen, R. T.,** Tumor associated macrophages stimulate the proliferation of murine tumor cells surviving treatment with the oncolytic cyclophosphamide analog asta Z-7557: in vivo implications, *Int. J. Cancer,* 34, 883, 1984.

181. **Evans, R., Blake, S. S., and Saffer, M. D.,** Expression of class II MHC antigens by tumor associated and peritoneal macrophages: systemic induction during tumor growth and tumor rejection, *J. Leukocyte Biol.,* 40, 499, 1986.

182. **Yui, S. and Yamazaki, M.,** Induction of macrophage growth by effete cells, *J. Leukocyte Biol.,* 39, 489, 1986.

183. **Hopper, K. E. and Nelson, D. S.,** Specific triggering of macrophage accumulation at the site of secondary tumor challenge in mice with concomitant tumor immunity, *Cell. Immunol.,* 47, 163, 1979.

184. **Bugelski, P. J.,** Sequential histochemical staining for resident and recruited macrophages, *J. Leukocyte Biol.,* 38, 687, 1985.

185. **Bugelski, P. J., Kirsh, R., Buscarino, C., Corwin, S. P., and Poste, G.,** Recruitment of exogenous macrophages into metastases at different stages of tumor growth, *Cancer Immunol. Immunother.,* 24, 93, 1987.

186. **Jackson, R. A., Kill, P. H., and Gangemi, J. D.,** Role of pulmonary macrophages in resistance to experimental metastasis, *J. Leukocyte Biol.,* 40, 575, 1986.

187. **Bursuker, I. and Goldman, R.,** On the origin of macrophage heterogeneity: a hypothesis, *J. Reticuloen-dothel. Soc.,* 33, 207, 1983.

188. **Dexter, T. M.,** The regulation of haemopoietic stem cells, progenitor cells and macrophage development, *R. Soc. Trop. Med. Hyg.,* 77, 597, 1983.

189. **Esiri, M. M. and McGee, J. O.,** Monoclonal antibody to macrophages (EMB/11) labels macrophages and microglial cells in human brain, *J. Clin. Pathol.,* 39, 615, 1986.

190. **Mahoney, K. H., Fulton, A. M., and Heppner, G. H.** Tumor-associated macrophages of mouse mammary tumors. II. Differential distribution of macrophages from metastatic and nonmetastatic tumors, *J. Immunol.,* 131, 2079, 1983.

191. **Urban, J. L. and Schreibner, H.,** Selection of macrophage resistant progressor tumor variants by the normal host, *J. Exp. Med.,* 157, 642, 1983.

192. **Miner, K. M. and Nicolson, G. L.,** Differences in the sensitivities of murine metastatic lymphoma/lymphosarcoma variants to macrophage mediated cytolysis and/or cytostatis, *Cancer Res.,* 43, 2063, 1983.

193. **Takeo, S., Yasumoto, K., Nagashima, A., Nakahashi, H., Sugimachi, K., and Nomoto, K.,** Role of tumor-associated macrophages in lung cancer, *Cancer Res.,* 46, 3179, 1986.

194. **Chapes, S. K. and Gooding, L. R.,** Evidence of the involvement of cytolytic macrophages in rejection of SV40 induced tumors, *J. Immunol.,* 135, 2192, 1985.

195. **Haskill, J. S.,** Adriamycin activated macrophages as tumor growth inhibitors, *Cancer Res.,* 41, 3852, 1981.

196. **Young, M. R. and Newby, M.,** Enhancement of Lewis lung carcinoma cell migration by prostaglandin E2 produced by macrophages, *Cancer Res.,* 46, 160, 1986.

197. **Nelson, M. and Nelson, D. S.,** Stimulation of proliferation in mixed cultures of mouse tumor cells and nonimmune peritoneal cells. II. Stimulation of tumor cells by MO and of lymphocytes by a tumor cells product, *J. Natl. Cancer Inst.,* 74, 637, 1985.

198. **Gabizon, A., Leibovich, S. J., and Goldman, R.,** Contrasting effects of activated and nonactivated macrophages and macrophages from tumor bearing mice on tumor growth in vivo, *J. Natl. Cancer Inst.,* 65, 913, 1980.

199. **Mantovani, A.,** Effects of in vitro tumor growth of murine macrophages isolated from sarcoma lines differing in immunogeneity and metastasizing capacity, *Int. J. Cancer,* 22, 741, 1978.

200. **Evans, T.,** Macrophage requirement for growth of a murine fibrosarcoma, *Br. J. Cancer,* 37, 1086, 1978.

201. **Yamashima, K., Miller, B. E., and Heppner, G. H.,** Macrophage mediated induction of drug resistant variants in a mouse mammary tumor cell line, *Cancer Res.,* 46, 2396, 1986.

202. **Kuhn, T. S.,** *The Structure of Scientific Revolution,* University of Chicago Press, Chicago, Ill., 1962, 1.

203. **Raup, D. A.,** New ideas are "guilty until proven innocent", *Scientist,* 1, 18, 1986.

204. **Orme, I. M. and Collins, F. M.,** Immune response to atypical mycobacteria, *Infect. Immun.,* 43, 32, 1984.

205. **Baird, L. G. and Kaplan, A. M.,** Macrophage regulation of mitogen-induced blastogenesis, *Cell. Immunol.,* 28, 22, 1977.

206. **Deodhar, S. D. and Barna, B. P.,** Macrophage activation, potential for cancer therapy, *Cleveland Clin. Q.,* 53, 223, 1986.

207. **Lee, J. C., Gibson, C. W., and Eisenstein, T. K.,** Macrophages mediated mitogenic suppression induced in mice of the C3H lineage by a vaccine strain of *Salmonella typhimurium, Cell. Immunol.,* 91, 75, 1985.

208. **Bloom, E. T., Babbitt, J. T., and Kawakami, K.,** Monocyte-mediated augmentation of human natural killer cell activity: conditions, monocyte and effector cell characteristics, *J. Immunol.,* 137, 172, 1986.

209. **Douvas, G. S., Looker, D. L., Vatter, A. E., and Crowle, A. J.,** Gamma interferon activates human monocytes to become tumoricidal and leishmanicidal but enhances replication of monocyte associated mycobacteria, *Infect. Immun.,* 58, 1, 1985.

210. **Holden, H. T., Haskill, J. S., Kirchner, H., and Herberman, R. B.,** Two functionally distinct antitumor effector cells isolated from primary murine sarcoma virus induced tumors, *J. Immunol.,* 117, 440, 1976.

211. **Morahan, P. S., Dempsey, W. L., Volkman, A., and Connor, J.,** Antimicrobicidal activity of various immunomodulators: independence from normal levels of circulating monocytes and natural killer cells, *Infect. Immun.,* 51, 87, 1986.

212. **Morahan, P. S. and Murasko, D. M.,** *Natural Immunity to Virus Infection,* in press, 1987.

213. **Weinberg, J. B., Blinder, R. A., and Coleman, R. E.,** In vitro function of indium-111 oxine labeled monocytes, *J. Immunol. Methods,* in press.

214. **Baumbach, W. R., Keath, E. J., and Cole, M. D.,** A mouse c-myc retrovirus transforms established fibroblast lines in vitro and induces monocyte-macrophage tumors in vivo, *J. Virol.,* 59, 276, 1986.

215. **McBride, W. H.,** Phenotype and functions of intratumoral macrophages, *Biochim. Biophys. Acta,* 865, 27, 1986.

216. **Heidl, G., Davaris, P., Zwaldo, G., Jagoda, M. S., Duchting, S., Biefhoff, E., Gruter, T., Krieg, V., Sorg, C., and Grundmann, E.,** Association of macrophages detected with monoclonal antibody 25 F9 with progressive and pathobiological classification of gastric carcinoma, *J. Cancer Res. Clin. Oncol.,* 113, 567, 1987.

217. **Woolford, J., Rothwell, V., and Rohrschneider, L.,** Characterization of the human c-fms gene product and its expression in cells of the monocyte-macrophage lineage, *Mol. Cell. Biochem.,* 5, 3458, 1985.

218. **Todd, R. F., Bury, M. J., Alvarez, P. A., Brott, D. A., and Liu, D. Y.,** Regulation of human monocyte surface antigen expression. I. Up-modulation of Mo3e antigen expression on U-937 and HL-60 cells stimulated by pharmacological activators of protein kinase C, *Blood,* 68, 1154, 1986.

219. **Treves, A. J.,** Human monocytes and macrophages: establishment and analysis of cloned populations and functional cell lines, *Crit. Rev. Immunol.,* 5, 371, 1985.

220. **Franklin, W. A., Mason, D. Y., Pulford, K., Falini, B., Bliss, E., Gatter, K. C., Stein, H., Clarke, L. C., and McGee, J. O.,** Immunohistological analysis of human mononuclear phagocytes and dendritic cells by using monoclonal antibodies, *Lab. Invest.,* 54, 322, 1986.

221. **Elias, J. A., Schreiber, A. D., Gustilo, K., Chien, P., Rossman, M. D., Lammie, P. J., and Daniele, R. P.,** Differential interleukin 1 elaboration by unfractionated and density fractionated human alveolar macrophages and blood monocytes: relationship to cell maturity, *J. Immunol.,* 135, 3198, 1985.

222. **Gorelik, E., Wiltrout, R. H., Brunda, M. J., Bere, W. E., and Herberman, R. B.,** Influence of adoptively transferred thioglycollate stimulated peritoneal macrophages on metastasis formation in mice with depressed or stimulated NK cell activity, *Clin. Exp. Metastasis,* 3, 111, 1985.

223. **Jo, M. K. and Springer, T. A.,** Preparation and use of monoclonal antimacrophage antibodies, *Methods Enzymol.,* 108, 313, 1984.

224. **Hopper, K. E.,** Kinetics of macrophage recruitment and turnover in peritoneal inflammatory exudates induced by salmonella or thioglycholate broth, *J. Leukocyte Biol.,* 39, 435, 1986.

225. **Kawasaki, H., Martin, C. A., Uchida, T., Usui, M., Noma, T., Minami, M., and Dorf, M. E.,** Functional analysis of cloned macrophage hybridomas. V. Induction of suppressor T cell responses, *J. Immunol.,* 137, 2145, 1986.

226. **Lee, K. C. and La Posta, V. J.,** Differential expression of tumor target binding and cytolytic activities by bone marrow culture-derived macrophages, *J. Natl. Cancer Inst.,* 77, 1287, 1986.

227. **Mitchell, R. L., Zokas, L., Schreibner, R. D., and Verman, I. M.,** Rapid induction of the expression of prot-oncogene fos during human monocyte differentiation, *Cell,* 40, 209, 1985.

228. **Moore, T. A., Joshi, J. G., Deana, D. G., Pitruzzello, F. J., Llorohov, D. W., and Rouse, B. T.,** Characterization of a two-signal-dependent Ia+ mononuclear phagocyte progenitor subpopulation that is sensitive to inhibition by ferritin, *J. Immunol.,* 136, 1605, 1986.

229. **Pullman, W., Hanna, R., Sullivan, P., Booth, J. A., Lomas, F., and Doe, W. F.,** Technetium-99 autologous phagocyte scanning: a new imaging technique for inflammatory bowel disease, *Br. Med. J.,* 293, 171, 1986.

230. **Robinson, A. P., White, T. M., and Mason, D. W.,** Macrophage heterogeneity in the rat as delineated by two monoclonal antibodies MCR OX-41 and MRC OX-42, the latter recognizing complement receptor type 3, *Immunology,* 57, 239, 1986.

231. **Russell, S. W., Witz, I. P., and Herberman, R. B.,** A review of data problems and open questions pertaining to *in situ* tumor immunity, *Contemp. Top. Immunobiol.,* 10, 1, 1980.

232. **Simmons, B. M., Stahl, P. D., and Russell, J. H.,** Mannose receptor-mediated uptake of ricin toxin and ricin A chain by macrophages, *J. Biol. Chem.,* 261, 7912, 1986.

233. **Classen, E., Kors, N., and Van Rooigen, N.,** Influence of carriers on the development and localization of anti-2,4,6-trinotrophenyl (TNP) antibody-forming cells in the murine spleen. II. Suppressed antibody response to TNP-Ficoll after elimination of marginal zone cells, *Eur. J. Immunol.,* 16, 492, 1986.

234. **Meddens, M. J. M., Thompson, J., Bauer, W. C., and Van Firth, R.,** Role of granulocytes and monocytes in experimental *Escherichia coli* endocarditis, *Infect. Immun.,* 43, 491, 1984.

235. **Sawyer, R. T.,** The significance of local resident pulmonary alveolar macrophage proliferation to population renewal, *J. Leukocyte Biol.,* 39, 77, 1986.
236. **Sawyer, R. T.,** The cytokinetic behavior of pulmonary alveolar macrophages in monocytopenic mice, *J. Leukocyte Biol.,* 39, 89, 1986.
237. **Coggle, J. E. and Tarling, J. D.,** The proliferation kinetics of pulmonary alveolar macrophages, *J. Leukocyte Biol.,* 35, 317, 1984.
238. **Golde, D. W., Finley, T. N., and Cline, M. J.,** The pulmonary macrophage in acute leukemia, *N. Engl. J. Med.,* 290, 875, 1974.
239. **Kaminski, N. E., Roberts, J. F., and Guthrie, F. E.,** Target ricin by coupling to an anti-macrophage monoclonal antibody, *J. Immunopharmacol.,* 8, 15, 1986.
240. **Friedlander, A. M.,** Macrophages are sensitive to anthrax lethal toxin through an acid-dependent process, *J. Biol. Chem.,* 261, 7123, 1986.
241. **Sitar, G., Masheretti, P. M., Pesce, G., Fornasari, P., and Peveri, G.,** Isolation of human monocytes according to volume and density, *Eur. J. Cell Biol.,* 40, 251, 1986.
242. **Yasumizu, R., Onoe, K., Iwabuchi, K., Ogawawara, M., Fujita, M., Okuyama, H., Good, R. A., and Morikawa, K.,** Characteristics of macrophages in irradiation chimeras in mice reconstituted with allogenic bone marrow cells, *J. Leukocyte Biol.,* 38, 305, 1985.
243. **Zwaldo, G., Schlegel, R., and Sorg, C.,** A monoclonal antibody to a subset of human monocytes found only in the peripheral blood and inflammatory tissues, *J. Immunol.,* 137, 512, 1986.
244. **Gillian,** personal communication.
245. **Melnicoff, M. J., Morahan, P. S., Jensen, B. D., Breslin, E. W., and Horan, P. K.,** In vivo labeling of resident peritoneal macrophages, *J. Leukocyte Biol.,* 1988, in press.
246. **Sorokin, S. P., Hoyt, R. F., and Grant, M. M.,** Development of macrophages in the lungs of fetal rabbits, rats, and hamsters, *Anat. Record,* 208, 103, 1984.

Chapter 2

ACTIVATION OF MACROPHAGES FOR TUMOR CELL KILL: EFFECTOR MECHANISMS AND REGULATION

Dolph O. Adams and Thomas A. Hamilton

TABLE OF CONTENTS

I. INTRODUCTION

Over the past decade and a half, considerable emphasis and interest have been placed on the role of mononuclear phagocytes in host protection against the emergence and spread of neoplasia. Although the intriguing proposition that mononuclear phagocytes participate in immune surveillance against nascent tumors remains neither proven nor disproven,[1] considerable evidence does indicate that mononuclear phagocytes can participate in the destruction of established neoplasms (for reviews see Chapters 7, 9, and 10 and References 2 to 4). Specifically, studies on various experimental models of immunotherapy employing either nonspecific stimulants such as Bacillus Calmette-Guerin (BCG) or specific antibodies directed against tumor cells have shown that mononuclear phagocytes may be major and final effectors of the tumor destruction observed in such settings.[2-5] The successes achieved in such experimental models have not, unfortunately, been mirrored in clinical settings where effective immune-mediated therapy of established tumors remains elusive. These mixed successes in human trials have focused attention on increasing understanding of the fundamental biology of macrophage-mediated destruction of tumor cells and how it is regulated.

Observations relating mononuclear phagocytes to the destruction of tumor cells date at least to the 1950s. Peter Gorer and Bernard Amos, examining the antibody-mediated rejection of histoincompatible tumors in the peritoneal cavity of mice, found that a major cellular participant was the macrophage.[6,7] Almost concomitantly, Old, Clark, and Bennaceraf observed that the nonspecific stimulant, BCG, produced nonspecific resistance to tumors.[8] In the early 1970s, Peter Alexander and Bob Evans, and then John Hibbs and Jack Remington found that nonspecifically activated macrophages could destroy neoplastic cells without the aid of antibodies.[9,10] For many years, macrophages were believed able to destroy antibody-coated erythrocytes but not tumor cells in vitro,[5] but work from our laboratories and from that of Carl Nathan showed that macrophages, when activated appropriately, could destroy tumor cells in the presence of antibodies.[11-13] The destructive interaction between macrophages and tumor cells has subsequently been investigated in many laboratories and from these studies, the effector mechanisms and the regulation of macrophage activation for tumor cell kill have been brought into focus.

Mononuclear phagocytes, it is now clear, lyse tumor cells in at least three distinct circumstances (Table 1).[5,14-19] Although these three forms of lysis can be clearly distinguished from one another, all require that the macrophages be activated in some way; the precise form of activation for each form of lysis is distinct. Furthermore, regulation of these three forms of kill is governed, in part, by lymphokines such as macrophage activating factor (MAF) and by the potent immunoregulatory signal lipopolysaccharide (LPS). Emphasis in this laboratory is currently being placed on how a purified MAF (i.e., Interferon-gamma, IFN_γ) and LPS act, in molecular terms, to alter the fundamental physiology and hence, functional behavior of mononuclear phagocytes. The analysis of various forms of kill and their physiological requirements on the part of the macrophages have been a necessary prelude to these studies.

II. MECHANISMS OF KILL BY MACROPHAGES

A. Macrophage-Mediated Tumor Cytotoxicity

Mononuclear phagocytes obtained from sites of infection with chronic intracellular parasites such as BCG, can selectively lyse tumor cells in vitro.[3,17] Lysis, which is relatively slow and requires 1 to 3 days for completion, is contact-dependent, nonphagocytic, and independent of antibody.[17] A remarkable feature of macrophage-mediated tumor cytotoxicity (MTC) is that lytic macrophages clearly distinguish between neoplastically-transformed cells and their untransformed counterparts. Another striking feature is that the macrophages must

Table 1

THREE BASIC MODES OF LYSIS OF TUMOR CELLS BY MACROPHAGES[5]

Characteristic	MTC	Rapid ADCC	Slow ADCC
Stages of target injury	Binding and lysis	Binding and lysis	Binding and lysis
Contact dependent	Yes	Yes	Yes
Activation of macrophage necessary	Yes	Yes	Yes
Stage of effector activation where macrophage most effective	Fully activated	Responsive, primed, and fully activated	Responsive or primed (selected preparations)
Target selectivity	Cells neoplastically transformed	Antibody-dependent	Antibody-dependent
Mediator(s)	CP TNF	H_2O_2 Other?	H_2O_2 Other?
Recognition system	Binding site for tumor cells	FcR's	FcR's
Time for completion	24—48 hr	4—6 hr	24—48 hr

be appropriately activated for such lysis to occur. The interaction between activated macrophages and tumor cells, when observed by cinemicroscopy, involves approach of macrophages to the target, long periods of active and intimate contact between the two cells, and ultimate lysis of the neoplastic cells. This interaction can be experimentally divided into two fundamental components: (1) avid binding of targets by macrophages to form stable cell-cell aggregates and (2) target attack which involves secretion of lytic mediators from the macrophages. Subsequently, target injury progresses culminating in explosive cytolysis of targets.

The initial step in MTC is the selective formation of cell pairs between activated macrophages and tumor cells.[18] The strength of such cell pairs can be quantified by a recently devised technique.[20] Macrophages, whether activated or unactivated, form weak cell-cell bonds with targets, whether these be neoplastic or nonneoplastic. Only in the selected case of activated macrophages and neoplastic targets, the weak cell-cell bonds develop into much stronger bonds, such that the forces required to disrupt the cell pair are increased more than 20-fold (from ~ 12 dyn to > 250 dyn). The development of strong cell-cell bonds is an active metabolic process on the part of the macrophage, though not of the tumor cell, and appears to be a multistep event.[18] The development of strong cell-cell bonds appears to include the participation of lymphocyte function associated antigen 1 (LFA-1) molecules and a cytoskeleton-mediated arrangement of surface recognition structures on the macrophages.[20-23] The precise molecular basis of this cell-cell recognition remains to be elucidated. The binding of various targets can be both homologously and heterologously inhibited by plasma membranes prepared from a variety of tumor cells, though not by membranes from untransformed cells, implying that common recognition structures on neoplastic cells but not non-neoplastic cells may be involved.[24] Several lines of evidence, including the fact that the binding of tumor cells or membranes to activated macrophages initiates active secretion of lytic effectors, have been put forth to suggest that the capture may be mediated by a receptor on the macrophages.[14,18]

The second or lytic step in MTC appears to involve active secretion of lytic effector molecules from the macrophages.[14-19] One substance, identified in this laboratory, is a cytolytic principal (CP) which selectively lyses tumor cells in the absence of serum. This material is extremely active, since its ED_{50} (effective dose 50%) is ~ 10^{-9} M. Although the active CP has not been purified to homogeneity, considerable progress has been made.[25] CP is active on a wide variety of murine tumor cells (though not normal) including carcinomas, melanomas, sarcomas, lymphomas, and leukemias. Several lines of evidence suggest that the material is a trypsin-like serine protease of $M_r \sim 38,000$ daltons. Of interest, protease inhibitors which block the lytic and proteolytic activities of isolated CP also inhibit the contact-mediated lysis of tumor cells by activated macrophages. Additional lines of evidence strongly suggest that release of this lytic principal is involved in cytolysis of tumor cells. It should be emphasized, however, that it has not been determined whether this material directly causes the destruction of tumor cells, cooperates with other molecules to produce injury, or acts with or on other molecules to produce a final toxic substance or substances that effect target injury. Another molecule which has received considerable emphasis is tumor necrosis factor (TNF), first described by Old and colleagues.[26,27] Several lines of recent evidence suggest that TNF can participate in the macrophage-mediated lysis of certain tumor cells.[28-30] It should be emphasized that multiple mediators may cooperate in the destruction of tumor cells. Precedent for this was set with the observation that CP and hydrogen peroxide (H_2O_2) can cooperate synergistically in a strictly controlled fashion to promote lysis of tumor cells.[31] Recently, IFN_γ and TNF have been noted to work cooperatively in destructive effects upon tumor cells.[28] The catalog of substances secreted by macrophages which are toxic to tumor cells is long and has been recently reviewed.[32] At present, it seems reasonable to conclude that multiple toxic mediators from macrophages may participate in the destruction of tumor cells.

The final endpoint of target destruction in MTC ultimately depends upon close inter-relationship and interaction between target binding and the release of cytolytic factors.[14-19] Binding appears to serve several roles which include target recognition, provision of a protective space between macrophages and targets, and enhanced and more rapid secretion of cytolytic materials.

B. Antibody-Dependent Cellular Cytotoxicity (ADCC)

Macrophages are well established to effect lysis of antibody-coated red cells over 1 to 2 hr.[33,34] Several years ago, macrophages, which had been activated in vivo by BCG, were found to lyse a variety of nonadherent, lymphoid tumor cells coated with specific polyclonal antisera over 4 to 6 hr.[11-13] Other macrophages were not capable of effecting such lysis. When this reaction was subsequently dissected, it was found that competence for this rapid form of ADCC and for MTC were closely related but clearly distinguishable.[33] Macrophages, which are activated for rapid ADCC, can be characterized biochemically as macrophages which can mount a large respiratory burst in response to stimulation by phorbol diesters.[34]

The rapid ADCC reaction is divisible into two steps: (1) an initial antibody-mediated binding of the antibody-coated targets and (2) target lysis.[35] Target binding, which is dependent on the presence of Fc receptors on the macrophages and antibody on the targets, occurs over 10 to 20 min and proceeds at temperatures ranging from 4 to 37°C. Recent studies in this laboratory indicate that there are no metabolic requirements for the binding, but that the binding can be slowed by incubation at 2.5°C, presumably by impairing the lateral mobility of Fc receptors in the plane of the plasma membrane of the macrophages.[36] This binding begins with weak cell-cell bonds which are subsequently converted to strong cell-cell bonds. The lytic step, which requires 2 to 6 hr for completion, is entirely dependent on incubation at 37°C and can also be shut off either by inhibitors of the respiratory burst or nonspecific scavengers of H_2O_2.[35] Nathan and colleagues have studied this meticulously and provided strong evidence that reactive oxygen intermediates, such as H_2O_2, represent a major lytic mediator mechanism in the rapid form of ADCC.[34] The role of other potential mediators of ADCC remains controversial.[32]

Over the past 3 years, our laboratory and those of several collaborators have been interested in the rejection of established tumors by the systemic administration of monoclonal antibodies.[37-39] In our studies of these reactions, we have delineated a distinct form of the ADCC reaction which requires 1 to 2 days for completion.[40] This form of lysis may be of considerable biological importance for we have found that the vast majority of tumor targets in our laboratory are lysed slowly. The slow version of ADCC, like the rapid, comprises two steps: binding and lysis. The binding step, based on the evidence available to date, closely resembles or is identical with that seen in the rapid form. By contrast, the lytic step requires 1 to 2 days rather than 2 to 6 hr for completion. The lytic step does, however, involve secretion of reactive oxygen intermediates as a major mediator; no evidence for involvement of cytolytic proteases has been adduced. The particularly striking feature of slow ADCC is that only selected populations of macrophages are capable of mediating such lysis and these are not activated for MTC or rapid ADCC. Although we have not been able to characterize these activated macrophages precisely in biochemical terms, current evidence suggests that there may be macrophages which are capable of sustained release of H_2O_2 in response to immune complexes over many hours. The role of other lytic substances in such lysis remains to be established.

Our current interpretation is that the rapid and slow forms of ADCC represent basic variants on the same fundamental biological process.[5] We have hypothesized that the rapid ADCC reaction takes place between macrophages which are capable of mounting a rapid and strong respiratory burst, and targets which are relatively susceptible to lysis by reactive oxygen intermediates. The slow variant represents an interaction between macrophages which secrete reactive oxygen intermediates (ROI) slowly and which may secrete other mediators as well, and targets which are relatively resistant to lysis by H_2O_2. This remains to be tested critically.

C. Macrophage Activation

The delineation of macrophage-mediated destruction into at least three forms of kill has both practical and theoretical implications. On the practical side, the type of effector function macrophages express and the type of activation required must be considered in immunotherapy trials. In experimental models which are presumed to depend upon MTC, all appropriate signals for inducing that form of activation would obviously be required. On the other hand, immunotherapeutic trials involving antibodies might actually be hampered by administration of inappropriate immune modifiers since certain combinations of signals (see below) can suppress the slow form of ADCC.

These observations also have implications for our understanding of the fundamental concept of macrophage activation. Macrophage activation, dating to the earliest observations of Metchnikoff, has frequently been defined as acquiring enhanced competence to destroy microbes. This definition has subsequently been broadened by some to include destruction of tumor cells as well. Macrophage activation has thus been viewed as linear development, progressing toward more and more complex functions.[17] From the foregoing, it is now clear that macrophages can be activated to kill tumor cells in at least three distinct ways. Whatever formal definition of macrophage activation one wishes to employ, these observations change our fundamental understanding of activation. Macrophages must now be viewed as multipotential cells which can gain competence to mediate a wide variety of diverse functions.[15] Acquisition of competence for each of these diverse functions is often distinct and, in some cases, mutually exclusive. Macrophage activation can, therefore, usefully be defined as gaining competence to mediate a complex function, such as one form of destruction of tumor cells, presentation of antigen to T cells, regulation of hematopoiesis, etc.[15,17] Tissue macrophages may thus be viewed as multipotential cells which can be activated in a wide variety of diverse and disparate directions.[15,17]

III. REGULATION OF ACTIVATION

The activation of mononuclear phagocytes for antibody-independent MTC has been thoroughly dissected in the laboratories of Hibbs et al., Meltzer et al., and Russell et al.[41-43]

This development of competence results from a complex and closely controlled set of interactions. In brief, young, responsive mononuclear phagocytes must first interact with a macrophage-activating factor such as IFN_γ, and then and only then receive a second signal such as LPS, maleylated proteins, heat-killed *Listeria monocytogenes* (HKLM), or supernatants from tumor cells. These various stages of development can now be characterized by a large library of objective, quantifiable markers.[15,44] Of note, the two requirements for destruction of tumor cells in MTC (i.e., competence for binding of tumor cells and competence for secretion of CP) are closely regulated by these signals. Specifically, competence for tumor cell binding is induced solely by MAF or IFN_γ.[44] Competence for release of CP, by contrast, is induced first by application of IFN_γ, but actual secretion of the molecule is triggered by application of LPS to IFN_γ-treated macrophages.[44]

The signals which regulate competence for ADCC in vitro have not been so well defined. The Fc receptors of macrophages can, depending on the particular receptor, be up- and down-regulated in a complex fashion by a variety of signals including lymphokines and endotoxins.[45] Lymphokines are further known to induce enhanced competence for rapid oxidative bursts in response to phorbol myristate acetate (PMA) after several days of culture.[46] Macrophages can be stimulated to lyse tumor cells over 20 hr by LPS, PMA, preparations containing lymphokines, and crude supernatants containing colony-stimulating factors.[47] The application of lymphokines plus endotoxin to macrophages, however, suppresses competence for the slow ADCC reaction.[48]

IV. MOLECULAR MECHANISMS OF SIGNAL TRANSDUCTION IN MACROPHAGE ACTIVATION

Numerous forms of macrophage activation are regulated in whole or in part by IFN_γ, LPS, or a combination of these two agents.[5,15] For example, activation for MTC requires both signals, while competence for slow ADCC is shut off by both signals. Identification of the molecular mechanisms of signal transduction induced by IFN_γ and LPS is thus a potential strategy for developing effective pharmacologic agents to modulate the mononuclear phagocyte system. Over the past few years, we have examined these responses and have begun to develop a general picture of how these signals act and interact to regulate macrophage function.[49] Our resulting observations can be categorized temporally into three rather artificial time groupings: (1) immediate events, occurring over 10 sec to 5 min; (2) intermediate events, occurring over 5 min to 4 hr; and (3) late events, occurring over 4 to 24 hr.

The molecular mechanisms by which interferons signal cells are, in general, still quite elusive.[50,51] Surface receptors for these molecules have been identified, and subsequent events in terms of antiviral activity include activation of a kinase that phosphorylates initiation factor eIF-2, and of the enzyme $2',5'$-oligo(a)synthetase after several hours. Of interest, genomic effects induced by α- and β-interferon occur much more rapidly (i.e., over 30 min than those induced by IFN_γ, i.e., over several hours).[51] The signal transduction mechanisms in other cells linking surface perception of interferon via its receptor to nuclear events remain to be established.[50,51] Macrophages possess a distinct surface receptor for IFN_γ.[52] Ligation of this receptor on macrophages initiates two events in the intermediate time frame. First, intracellular levels of calcium are raised over 10 to 15 min and remain elevated for several hours.[53] Second, interferon induces a modification in protein kinase C (PKc), such that phosphorylation is not induced but that the degree of phosphorylation, when PKc is appropriately stimulated, is enhanced four- to sixfold.[54-56]

The molecular mechanism by which LPS acts on cells also remains elusive.[57] Current models of its action emphasize adherence of the molecule to cells and then a subsequent melting or intercalation of the lipid A portion of LPS into the lipid bilayer of the plasma membrane to initiate signaling responses.[57] In macrophages, LPS and lipid A initiate in the early time frame a rapid (observable at 10 sec) breakdown of phosphatidylinositol-4,5-bisphosphate (PIP_2) into inositol-triphosphate and diacylglycerol.[58] The predominant isomer of IP_3 formed is $I_{1,4,5}P_3$. Subsequently, lipid A, presumably acting via the generation of $I_{1,4,5}P_3$, causes rapid and extensive intracellular fluxes of Ca^{++} (i.e., rises from basal levels of 80 nM to ~ 600 nM Ca^{++} at 30 sec). LPS and lipid A also initiate enhanced phosphorylation of a characteristic set of phosphoproteins which are first detectable within 15 min after LPS is applied to macrophages.[58,59] Several lines of evidence imply that these proteins are phosphorylated via protein kinase C.[59] LPS initiates, in the intermediate time frame, synthesis of a defined set of new proteins.[60] These proteins, when detected by autoradiography of SDS gels prepared from ^{35}S-methionine-labeled macrophages, appear rapidly (at 1 to 2 hr), are synthesized for brief periods of time (i.e., 2 to 4 hr), and can have quite short half-lives (i.e., T1/2 = 3 hr). Platelet-derived growth factor (PDGF) stimulates in fibroblasts a set of early gene products which have been termed competence genes.[61,62] LPS initiates enhanced expression in macrophages of messages for at least four members of this family of competence genes including c-myc, c-fos, JE, and KC.[63-65] Several lines of evidence imply that some members of this family of early genes, as defined by analysis of specific cytoplasmic mRNA, are induced in response to the breakdown of PIP_2, but that other members of this family are induced by a signal transduction mechanism which does not involve the breakdown of PIP_2.[60,63,65]

Our current understanding of molecular mechanisms of macrophage activation thus indicates that there are apparently three distinct pathways of early and intermediate events initiated by IFN_γ and LPS (Figure 1).[49] The first pathway, initiated by IFN_γ, regulates both of the second pathways. Phosphorylation initiated by LPS is markedly enhanced in macrophages previously exposed to IFN_γ, consistent with the observation that IFN_γ raises the potential activity of PKc.[59] The amount of LPS required to initiate synthesis of some early proteins is lowered ~100-fold by pretreatment of the cells with IFN_γ.[60]

Several lines of evidence indicate that all three of these events are probably necessary for the full biological effects of IFN_γ and LPS on macrophages. First, inhibitors of calcium fluxes and of protein synthesis respectively block the effects of IFN_γ and LPS.[53,55] Second, the physiologic effects of both IFN_γ and/or LPS can be mimicked, in part, pharmacologically by providing a known source of calcium fluxes (i.e., the ionophore A23187 in the presence of extracellular calcium), and/or a potent pharmacologic stimulant of PKc (i.e., phorbol myristate acetate).[53,63,66,67] Third, inbred strains of mice provide useful examples of deficiencies in signal transduction mechanisms. A/J mice, which are lymphokine unresponsive but which have receptors comparable for IFN_γ comparable in number and affinity to those on control mice, do not initiate the intermediate events observed in control mice in response to IFN_γ.[68] Pharmacologic restoration of these events, by ionophore plus PMA, effectively restores the response to IFN_γ. In a similar vein, mice of the C3H/HeJ strain are deficient in functional responses to LPS. Macrophages from C3H/HeJ mice do not initiate protein phosphorylation or protein synthesis in response to LPS.[5,59] When function is restored to these macrophages by providing them an alternate second signal such as HKLM, protein synthesis and protein phosphorylation are also restored by that signal.[5,59]

The ultimate alterations in macrophage function induced by various regulatory signals must finally depend upon alterations in existing protein function or by synthesis of new proteins. Activation of macrophages for presentation of antigen to T cells provides a useful example of such remodeling since macrophage activation for this function is acquired (in part) when macrophages express class II histocompatibility molecules (i.e., Ia antigens) on their surface.[69] Surface expression of Ia molecules, which is closely regulated by a variety of signals, is induced in macrophages by IFN_γ.[69] The effects of IFN_γ on Ia can be pharmacologically mimicked by PMA or A23187, and the effects of native IFN_γ can be blocked

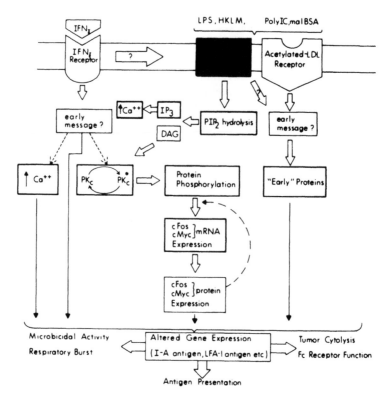

FIGURE 1.   A schematic model of signal transduction events in macrophage activation.[49] Poly IC — polyinosinic cytidilic acid; mal BSA—maleylated BSA; acetylated LDL — acetylated low density lipoprotein; IFN$_\gamma$ — interferon gamma; PK$_c$ — protein kinase C; LPS — bacterial lipopolysaccharide; IP$_3$ — inositol triphosphate; DAG — diacylglycerol; PIP$_2$ — phosphatidylinositol 4'5' bisphosphate; I-A — the I-A *determinant* of immune associated antigens (Ia); LFA — leukocyte function antigen-1.

by chelators of calcium, implying that the intermediate signaling events induced by IFN$_\gamma$ lead, in part, to surface expression of Ia molecules.[67,70] In macrophages treated with IFN$_\gamma$, surface expression of Ia requires both transcription and translation.[70] Consistent with this finding, IFN$_\gamma$ induces heightened levels of mRNA encoding for Ia molecules.[71] LPS, furthermore, can down-regulate surface expression of Ia induced by IFN$_\gamma$.[72] LPS does so, at least in part, by substantially reducing the amount of mRNA accumulated in response to IFN$_\gamma$.[71] Of interest, the suppressive effects of LPS can be blocked by cycloheximide, implying that one or more of the early proteins may act to suppress accumulation of message for Ia.[73]

These observations can be summarized in an integrated model of the signal transduction effects of IFN$_\gamma$ and LPS on mononuclear phagocytes.[49] Cardinal features of the model, identified to date, are the intermediate frame events induced by IFN$_\gamma$; the immediate events initiated by LPS (i.e., PIP$_2$ hydrolysis and the consequence of such hydrolysis); the distinct pathway of new protein synthesis also initiated by LPS; the regulation of these latter two pathways by IFN$_\gamma$; and the emerging information as to how these pathways regulate gene function. Obviously, far more information is required to understand how this model works in detail. Evidence has, however, already accumulated that the three early signaling pathways may all be important to macrophage activation.

V. CODA

The analysis of tumor cell destruction effected by macrophages has defined at least three distinct forms of kill and some of the mechanisms of recognition and destruction operative in each. Though clearly distinct, these types of destruction do have certain features in common, including a requirement for macrophage activation. From these observations have come different views on defining activation of macrophages and understanding the development potential of members of the mononuclear phagocyte system (MPS).

Perhaps the most important outcome of studies of tumor cell destruction by macrophages has been the development of markers that define macrophages in the various stages of development. These markers and the availability of purified regulatory signals have permitted analysis, in molecular terms, of the signal transduction mechanisms that govern macrophage activation. Although these studies are still in progress, a clearer picture of how the stringently regulated developmental process termed macrophage activation works should emerge within the next several years.

ACKNOWLEDGMENTS

Supported in part by USPHS Grants CA29589, CA16784, CA39621, ES02922, Grant #1733 from the Council for Tobacco Research U.S.A. Inc., and a grant from R. J. Reynolds/Nabisco Inc. Submitted for publication in October 1986.

REFERENCES

1. **Adams, D. O. and Snyderman, R.,** Do macrophages destroy nascent tumors?, *J. Natl. Cancer Inst.,* 16, 1341, 1979.
2. **Nelson, D. S., Hopper, K. E., and Nelson, M.,** Role of the macrophage in resistance to cancer, in *Handbook of Cancer Immunology,* Vol. 1, Waters, H., Ed., Garland Publ., New York, 1978, 107.
3. **Hibbs, J. B., Remington, J. S., and Stewart, C. C.,** Modulation of immunity and host resistance by micro-organisms, *Pharmacol. Ther. Dent.,* 8, 37, 1980.
4. **Haskill, S., Ed.,** *Tumor Immunity in Prognosis. The Role of Mononuclear Cell Infiltration,* Marcel Dekker, New York, 1982.
5. **Adams, D. O. and Hamilton, T. A.,** Destruction of tumor cells by mononuclear phagocytes: models for analyzing effector mechanisms and regulation of macrophage activation, in *Basic Mechanisms of Host Resistance to Infectious Agents, Tumors, and Allografts,* North, R. J. and Steinman, R. M., Eds., Rockefeller University Press, New York, 1986, 185.
6. **Gorer, P. A.,** Some reactions of H-2 antibodies *in vitro* and *in vivo, Ann. N.Y. Acad. Sci.,* 73, 707, 1958.
7. **Amos, D. B.,** Possible relationship between cytotoxic effects of isoantibody and host cell function, *Ann. N.Y. Acad. Sci.,* 87, 273, 1960.
8. **Old, L. J., Clark, D. A., and Bennaceraf, B.,** Effect of Bacillus Calmette-Guerin infection on transplanted tumors in the macrophages, *Nature (London),* 184, 291, 1959.
9. **Alexander, P. and Evans, R.,** Endotoxin and double stranded RNA render macrophages cytotoxic, *Nature (London) New Biol.,* 232, 76, 1971.
10. **Hibbs, J. B., Lambert, L. H., and Remington, J. S.,** Possible role of macrophage mediated nonspecific cytotoxicity in tumor resistance, *Nature (London) New Biol.,* 235, 48, 1972.
11. **Adams, D. O. and Koren, H. S.,** BCG-activated macrophages: comparison as effectors in direct tumor-cell cytotoxicity and antibody dependent cell-mediated cytotoxicity, *Adv. Exp. Med. Biol.,* 121B, 195, 1979.
12. **Nathan, C. F., Brukner, L. H., Kaplan, G., Unkeless, J., and Cohn, Z. A.,** Role of activated macrophages in antibody-dependent lysis of tumor cells, *J. Exp. Med.,* 152, 183, 1980.
13. **Koren, H. S., Anderson, S. J., and Adams, D. O.,** Studies on the antibody-dependent cell-mediated cytotoxicity (ADCC) of thioglycollate-stimulated and BCG-activated peritoneal macrophages, *Cell. Immunol.,* 57, 51, 1981.
14. **Adams, D. O., Johnson, W., and Marino, P. A.,** Mechanisms of target recognition and destruction in macrophage-mediated tumor cytotoxicity, *Fed. Proc. Fed. Am. Soc. Exp. Biol.,* 41, 115, 1982.
15. **Adams, D. O. and Hamilton, T. A.,** The cell biology of macrophage activation, *Ann. Rev. Immunol.,* 2, 283, 1984.

16. **Adams, D. O., Lewis, J. G., and Johnson, W. J.,** Multiple modes of cellular injury by macrophages: requirement for different forms of effector activation, in *Progress in Immunology,* Vol. 5, Yamamura, T., Ed., Academic Press, New York, 1984, 1009.

17. **Adams, D. O. and Marino, P.,** Activation of mononuclear phagocytes for destruction of tumor cells as model for study of macrophage development, in *Contemporary Topics in Hematology-Oncology,* Vol. 3, Gordon, A. S., Silber, R., and LoBue, J., Eds., Plenum Press, New York, 1984, 69.

18. **Somers, S. D., Johnson, W. J., and Adams, D. O.,** Destruction of tumor cells by macrophages: mechanisms of recognition and lysis and their regulation, in *Cancer Immunology: Innovative Approaches to Therapy,* Herberman, R., Ed., Martinus Nishoff, The Hague, 1986, 69.

19. **Johnson, W. J., Somers, S. D., and Adams, D. O.,** Expression and development of macrophage activation for tumor cytotoxicity, *Contemp. Top. Immunobiol.,* 13, 127, 1984.

20. **Somers, S. D., Whisnant, C. C., and Adams, D. O.,** Quantification of the strength of cell-cell adhesion: the capture of tumor cells by activated murine macrophages proceeds through two distinct stages, *J. Immunol.,* 136, 1490, 1986.

21. **Somers, S. D., Yuli, I., Snyderman, R., and Adams, D. O.,** Activation of murine macrophages for cytotoxicity results in enhanced membrane fluidity: studies with anisotropic polarization, *Cell. Immunol.,* 104, 232, 1986.

22. **Somers, S. D. and Adams, D. O.,** Enhancement of selective tumor cell binding by activated murine macrophages in response to phorbol myristate acetate, *J. Immunol.,* 136, 2323, 1986.

23. **Strassmann, G., Springer, T. A., Somers, S. D., and Adams, D. O.,** Mechanisms of tumor cell capture by activated macrophage. Evidence for involvement of anti-lymphocyte function associated antigen (LFA-1)-1, *J. Immunol.,* 136, 4328, 1986.

24. **Marino, P. A., Whisnant, C. C., and Adams, D. O.,** The binding of BCG-activated macrophages to tumor targets: selective inhibition by membrane preparations from homologous and heterologous neoplastic cells, *J. Exp. Med.,* 154, 77, 1981.

25. **Johnson, W. J., Goldfarb, R. H., and Adams, D. O.,** Secretion of a novel cytolytic protease by activated murine macrophages: its properties and role in tumor cytolysis, in *Lymphokines,* Vol. 11, Mizell, S. and Pick, E., Eds., Academic Press, New York, 1986, 157.

26. **Old, L. J.,** Tumor necrosis factor, *Science,* 230, 630, 1985.

27. **Beutler, B. and Cerami, A.,** Cachectin and tumor necrosis factor as two sides of the same biological coin, *Nature (London),* 325, 84, 1986.

28. **Urban, J. L., Shepherd, H. M., Watchstein, J. L., Sugarman, B. J., and Schreiber, H.,** Tumor necrosis factor: a potent effector molecule for tumor cell killing by activated macrophages, *Proc. Natl. Acad. Sci. U.S.A.,* 83, 5233, 1986.

29. **Phillip, R. and Epstein, L. B.,** Tumor necrosis factor as immunomodulator and mediator of monocyte cytotoxicity induced by itself. Interferon-γ and interleukin-1, *Nature (London),* 323, 86, 1986.

30. **Kornbluth, R. S. and Edgington, T. S.,** Tumor necrosis factor production by human monocytes as a regulated event: induction of TNFα-mediate cellular cytotoxicity by endotoxin, *J. Immunol.,* 137, 2585, 1986.

31. **Adams, D. O., Johnson, W. J., Fiorito, E., and Nathan, C. F.,** H_2O_2 and CF can interact synergistically in effecting cytolysis of neoplastic targets, *J. Immunol.,* 127, 1973, 1981.

32. **Adams, D. O. and Nathan, C. F.,** Molecular mechanisms operative in cytolysis of tumor cells by activated macrophages, *Immunol. Today,* 4, 166, 1983.

33. **Adams, D. O., Cohen, M., and Koren, H. S.,** Activation of mononuclear phagocytes for cytolysis: parallels and contrast between activation for tumor cytotoxicity and for ADCC, in *Macrophage-Mediated Antibody Dependent Cellular Cytotoxicity,* Koren, H. S., Ed., Marcel Dekker, New York, 1983, 43.

34. **Nathan, C. F.,** Reactive oxygen intermediates in lysis of antibody coated tumor cells, in *Macrophage-Mediated Antibody Dependent Cellular Cytotoxicity,* Koren, H. S., Ed. Plenum Press, New York, 1982, 199.

35. **Johnson, W. J., Bolognesi, D., and Adams, D. O.,** Antibody dependent cytolysis (ADCC) of tumor cells by activated murine macrophages is a two step process: quantification of target binding and subsequent target lysis, *Cell. Immunol.,* 83, 170, 1984.

36. **Fan, S. and Adams, D. O.,** Development of binding strength in antibody-dependent macrophage-tumor cell capture, (abstr.) 27th Annu. Meet. Am. Soc. Cell Biol., St. Louis, MO, November 16, 1987.

37. **Langlois, A. J., Matthews, T. J., Roloson, G. J., Thiel, H.-J., Collins, J. J., and Bolognesi, D. P.,** Immunologic control of the ascites form of murine adenocarcinoma 755. V. Antibody-directed macrophages mediate tumor cell destruction, *J. Immunol.,* 126, 2337, 1981.

38. **Herlyn, D. and Koprowski, H.,** Ig2a monoclonal antibody inhibits human tumor cell growth through interaction with effector cells, *Proc. Natl. Acad. Sci. U.S.A.,* 79, 4761, 1982.

39. **Adams, D. O., Hall, T., Steplewski, Z., and Koprowski, H.,** Tumors undergoing rejection induced by monoclonal antibodies of the IgG_{2a} isotype contain increased numbers of macrophages activated for a distinctive form of antibody-dependent cytolysis, *Proc. Natl. Acad. Sci. U.S.A.,* 81, 3506, 1984.

40. **Johnson, W. J., Steplewski, Z., Matthews, T. J., Hamilton, T. A., Koprowski, H., and Adams, D. O.**, Cytolytic interaction between murine macrophages, tumor cells, and monoclonal antibodies: characterization of lytic conditions and requirements for effector activation, *J. Immunol.*, 136, 4704, 1986.

41. **Hibbs, J. B., Taintor, R. R., Chapman, H. A., and Weinberg, J. B.**, Macrophage tumor killing: influence of the local environment, *Science*, 197, 279, 1977.

42. **Meltzer, M. S., Ruco, L. P., Boraschi, D., and Nacy, C. A.**, Macrophage activation for tumor cytotoxicity: analysis of intermediary reactions, *J. Reticuloendothel. Soc.*, 26, 403, 1979.

43. **Russell, S. W., Doe, W. F., and McIntosh, A. J.**, Functional characterization of a stable, noncytolytic stage of macrophage activation in tumors, *J. Exp. Med.*, 146, 1511, 1977.

44. **Johnson, W. J., Marino, P. A., Schreiber, R. D., and Adams, D. O.**, Sequential activation of murine mononuclear phagocytes for tumor cytolysis: differential expression of markers by macrophages in the several stages of development, *J. Immunol.*, 131, 1038, 1983.

45. **Vogel, S. N. and Friedman, R.**, Interferon and macrophages: activation and cell surface changes, in *Interferon*, Vol. 2, Vilcek, J. and deMacyer, E., Eds., Elsevier, Amsterdam, 1984, 35.

46. **Nathan, C. F., Murray, H. W., Wiebe, M. E., and Rubin, B. Y.**, Identification of interferon-gamma as the lymphokine that activates macrophage oxidative metabolism in antimicrobial activity, *J. Exp. Med.*, 158, 670, 1983.

47. **Ralph, P., Williams, N., Nakoinz, I., Jackson, H., and Watson, J. D.**, Distinct signals for antibody-dependent and nonspecific killing of tumor targets mediated by macrophages, *J. Immunol.*, 129, 427, 1982.

48. **Johnston, P. A., Adams, D. O., and Hamilton, T. A.**, Regulation of Fc-mediated respiratory burst: treatment of primed murine macrophages with LPS selectively inhibits H_2O_2 secretion, *J. Immunol.*, 135, 513, 1985.

49. **Hamilton, T. A. and Adams, D. O.**, Molecular mechanisms of signal transduction in macrophage activation, *Immunol. Today*, 8(5), 151, 1987.

50. **Lengyel, P.**, The mechanism of action of interferon, *Annu. Rev. Biochem.*, 51, 251, 1982.

51. **Revel, M. and Cheboth, J.**, Interferon activated genes, *Trends in Biochem. Sci.*, 11, 166, 1986.

52. **Celada, A., Gray, P. W., Rinderknecht, E., and Schreiber, R. D.**, Evidence for a γ-interferon receptor that regulates macrophage tumoricidal activity, *J. Exp. Med.*, 160, 55, 1984.

53. **Somers, S. D., Weiel, J. E., Hamilton, T. A., and Adams, D. O.**, Phorbol esters and calcium ionophore can prime murine peritoneal macrophages for tumor cell destruction, *J. Immunol.*, 136, 4199, 1986.

54. **Becton, D. L., Hamilton, T. A., and Adams, D. O.**, Characterization of protein kinase C activity in interferon-gamma treated murine peritoneal macrophages, *J. Cell. Physiol.*, 125, 485, 1985.

55. **Hamilton, T. A., Rigsbee, J. A., Scott, W. A., and Adams, D. O.**, Gamma interferon enhances the secretion of arachidonic acid metabolites from murine peritoneal macrophages stimulated with phorbol derivatives, *J. Immunol.*, 134, 2631, 1985.

56. **Hamilton, T. A., Becton, D. L., Somers, S. D., Gray, P. W., and Adams, D. O.**, Interferon-gamma modulates protein kinase C activity in murine peritoneal macrophages, *J. Biol. Chem.*, 260, 1378, 1985.

57. **Morrison, D. C. and Rudbach, J. A.**, Endotoxin-cell membrane interactions leading to transmembrane signalling, *Contemp. Top. Mol. Immunol.*, 8, 187, 1981.

58. **Prpic, V., Weiel, J. E., Somers, S. D., DiGuiseppi, J., Gonias, S. D., Pizzo, S. V., Hamilton, T. A., Herman, B., and Adams, D. O.**, Effects of bacterial lipopolysaccharide on the hydrolysis of phosphatidylinositol 4,5-bis phosphate in murine peritoneal macrophages, *J. Immunol.*, 139, 526, 1987.

59. **Weiel, J., Hamilton, T., and Adams, D. O.**, LPS induces altered phosphate labeling of proteins in murine peritoneal macrophages, *J. Immunol.*, 136, 3012, 1986.

60. **Hamilton, T. A., Jansen, M. J., Somers, S. D. and Adams, D. O.**, Effect of bacterial lipopolysaccharide on protein synthesis in murine peritoneal macrophages: relationship to activation for macrophage tumoricidal function, *J. Cell Physiol.*, 128, 9, 1986.

61. **Stiles, C. D.**, The molecular biology of platelet-derived growth factor, *Cell*, 33, 653, 1983.

62. **Cohran, B. H.**, The molecular action of platelet-derived growth factor, *Cancer Res.*, 45, 183, 1985.

63. **Introna, M., Hamilton, T. A., Kaufman, R. E., Adams, D. O., and Bast, R. C., Jr.**, Treatment of murine peritoneal macrophages with bacterial lipopolysaccharide alters expression of c-Fos and c-Myc oncogenes, *J. Immunol.*, 137, 2711, 1986.

64. **Introna, M., Bast, R. C., Jr., Johnston, P. A., Adams, D. O., and Hamilton, T. A.**, Homologous and heterologous desensitization of protooncogene c-Fos expression in murine peritoneal macrophages, *J. Cell Physiol.*, 131, 36, 1987.

65. **Introna, M., Bast, R. C., Jr., Tannenbaum, C., Hamilton, T. A., and Adams, D. O.**, The effect of LPS on expression of the "early" competence genes JE and KC in murine peritoneal macrophages, *J. Immunol.*, 138, 3891, 1987.

66. **Weiel, J., Adams, D. O., and Hamilton, T.**, Biochemical models of γ-interferon activation: altered expression of transferrin receptors on murine peritoneal macrophages following treatment in vitro with PMA or A23187, *J. Immunol.*, 134, 293, 1985.

67. **Strassmann, G., Somers, S. D., Springer, T. A., Adams, D. O., and Hamilton, T. A.,** Biochemical models of interferonγ mediated macrophage activation. Independent regulation of lymphocyte function associated antigen (LFA)-1 and I-A antigen on murine peritoneal macrophages, *Cell. Immunol.,* 97, 110, 1986.

68. **Hamilton, T. A., Somers, S. D., Becton, D. L., Celada, A., Schreiber, R. D., and Adams, D. O.,** Analysis of deficiencies in IFNγ-mediated priming for tumor cytotoxicity in peritoneal macrophages from A/J mice, *J. Immunol.,* 137(3), 3367, 1986.

69. **Unanue, E. R.,** Antigen presenting function of the macrophage, *Annu. Rev. Immunol.,* 2, 395, 1984.

70. **Hamilton, T. A.,** unpublished observations, 1986.

71. **Koerner, T. J., Hamilton, T. A., and Adams, D. O.,** Suppressed expression of surface I-A$_\beta$ on macrophages by lipopolysaccharide: evidence for regulation at the level of accumulation of mRNA, *J. Immunol.,* 139, 239, 1987.

72. **Steeg, P. S., Johnson, H. M., and Oppenheim, J. J.,** Regulation of murine macrophage I-A antigen expression by an immune interferon-like lymphokine: inhibitory effect of endotoxin, *J. Immunol.,* 129, 2402, 1984.

73. **Hamilton, T. A., Gainey, P. V., Jr., and Adams, D. O.,** Maleylated BSA suppresses IFN$_\gamma$-mediated Ia expression in murine peritoneal macrophages, *J. Immunol.,* 138, 4063, 1987.

Chapter 3

EFFECTOR MECHANISMS FOR MACROPHAGE-INDUCED CYTOSTASIS AND CYTOLYSIS OF TUMOR CELLS

Carleton C. Stewart, Anita P. Stevenson, and John Hibbs

TABLE OF CONTENTS

I. INTRODUCTION

Since Hibbs et al. first observed that macrophages from mice infected with obligate and facultative intracellular organisms could kill tumor cells,[1-4] there has been an effort to understand the mechanisms involved in the activation of macrophages to the tumoricidal state,[5-32] how macrophages distinguish normal and neoplastic cells,[32-34] and how macrophages kill tumor cells.[35-47] We will review the kinetics of macrophage interaction with tumor cells and the schemes that have evolved to describe the mechanism of induction of cytostasis and cytolysis. Recently, evidence for the likely biochemical pathways involved in macrophage-induced cytostasis and death of tumor cells has been described.[43-47] We will provide an interpretation of the current literature that shows recognition may actually be susceptible to killing. This will be accomplished by correlating the kinetics of macrophage interaction with normal and neoplastic cells with the identification of the likely biochemical pathways that are interrupted by macrophages. From this information, a likely mechanism by which macrophages kill neoplastic cells and microbes but not normal cells will evolve.

II. KINETICS OF MACROPHAGE CYTOTOXICITY

Macrophages are not tumoricidal unless they are first fully activated. The mechanisms involved in macrophage activation will not be discussed here, but they have been described in Chapter 2. We define activated macrophages as those that exhibit tumoricidal activity or are microbicidal for facultative intracellular pathogens. Macrophages elicited with sterile phlogogenic agents like starch, peptone, or thioglycollate medium are *not* activated macrophages but are termed stimulated or inflammatory macrophages. Stimulated or inflammatory macrophages do not cause cytolysis or cytostasis of tumor cells. These cells can be activated in vitro with interferon-gamma (IFN-γ) and nanogram quantities of lipopolysaccharide. Activated macrophages are obtained from the peritoneal cavity of mice infected with certain microbes or from mice treated with agents such as *Corynebacterium parvum* or pyran copolymer. In contrast to stimulated macrophages, activated macrophages cause cytostasis and cytolysis of tumor cells following exposure to nanogram or picogram amounts of lipopolysaccharides during in vitro culture. The details of the macrophage activation process have been recently summarized.[45] Stimulated or inflammatory macrophages can be activated by several regimens described in Chapter 2.

A. Kinetics of Death

Unlike cytotoxic lymphocytes and natural killer (NK) cells that cause rapid target cell cytolysis, tumor cell death induced by activated macrophages requires many hours to be expressed. This phenomenon is conceptually shown in Figure 1, where the frequency of cell death is plotted vs. time. The data for this figure were obtained from time-lapse movies.* In this study activated macrophages were cultured with EMT6 tumor cells. The time at which each tumor cell died was recorded. For EMT6 tumor cells, the greatest frequency of cell death was at 30 hr. For other tumor cells this time may be earlier or later.

At a recent workshop,[48] two separate P815 lineages were used because one was susceptible and the other was resistant to macrophage killing based on an 18 to 24 hr assay. It was found at this workshop that the "resistant" ones actually took 30 to 40 hr to die, but because cell death had been previously assayed at 24 hr, they were thought to be resistant to macrophage lysis. They weren't resistant at all; they just took longer to die.

These results illustrate two important points: (1) cell death occurs at different times for

---

* These movies (or videotapes) are available from one of the authors, Dr. Carleton C. Stewart.

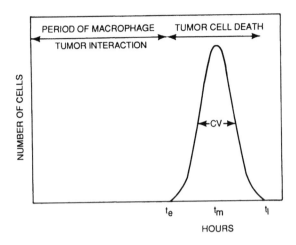

FIGURE 1. Death of target cells. This plot of the frequency of EMT6 tumor-cell death vs. the length of exposure to activated macrophages illustrates that individual tumor cells die over a broad range of time. Cell death begins at t_e = 16 hr and ends at t_l = 42 hr, the highest frequency of cell death occurs at t_m = 30 hr. These data were obtained from time-lapse movies. The coefficient of variation (CV) describes the heterogeneity of cell death. Such plots are not available for other types of tumor cells, but it is likely that the overall shape is similar although t_e, t_m, t_l may differ.

different type tumor cells, and (2) there is a heterogeneity of individual lysis times within a particular tumor cell population.

The heterogeneity in lysis times for various tumor cells and the basis for it have not been studied and represent a deficiency in our understanding. It is important because some tumor cells ultimately escape the cytolytic effects of macrophages. We will explore some of the reasons for this escape which represents a failure on the part of macrophages to completely prevent tumor cell regrowth.

B. Macrophage Density

Activated macrophages must remain in contact with a susceptible tumor cell for a sufficient length of time in order to kill it. Factors that affect contact include ratio of macrophages to tumor cells, macrophage density, and proximity of macrophage to targets. Our time-lapse movies clearly show that macrophages do not have to remain in contact with the tumor cell the entire time between initial contact and its eventual death. Since contact is important, there must be enough macrophages per centimeter squared (or cubic centimeter in a solid tumor) to ensure contact with the tumor cell. We refer to this as cell density, and it is totally independent of the ratio of macrophages to tumor cells. For example, in Figure 2A there are ten macrophages for each tumor cell, but they are so far apart they never come in contact with a tumor cell. In contrast, Figure 2B shows the same ratio of macrophages to tumor cells but at a sufficient cell density for contact to occur.

At a sufficiently high cell density, macrophages effectively kill tumor cells. In our studies with EMT6 tumor cells, we found that 10^5 macrophages per centimeter squared was the minimum cell density for maximum lysis to occur. As the density of macrophages was reduced below this level, even though the ratio was not changed, increasing numbers of tumor cells survived and proliferated. Our time-lapse movies of these cultures revealed that tumor cells too far away from macrophages proliferated normally, while tumor cells with macrophages attached exhibited cytostasis usually followed by cytolysis. Surprisingly, we

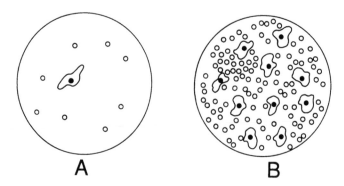

FIGURE 2.   Effect of macrophage density on likelihood of contact. Both (A) and (B) depict the same ratio of macrophages to tumor cells, but in (A) the macrophage (and tumor-cell) density is so low that the likelihood of contact is small. However, at the greater density shown in (B), the likelihood of contact is increased. For the EMT6 tumor, we have found that the minimum macrophage density for optimal killing of EMT6 tumor cells is about $10^5/cm^2$. At a density of $10^4/cm^2$ no tumor-cell death was detected.

found no evidence to suggest that macrophages actively migrated toward tumor cells no matter how close they were to them, but when actual contact was made, by chance, they remained attached to them. While occasionally a macrophage would become detached, most stayed in contact with the tumor cell until it died. In contrast, nonactivated macrophages tended to remain attached to tumor cells for very short periods of time (several minutes to a few hours).

When the macrophage density was high, most tumor cells had macrophages attached to them. As the density was decreased, there was sufficient space between macrophages and tumor cells so that increasing numbers of macrophages had no initial contact with tumor cells. These results point out that under most circumstances contact is necessary for macrophages to exert their cytostatic and cytolytic effect on tumor cells.

C. Macrophage-to-Target Cell Ratio

We have also studied the effect of the ratio of macrophages to tumor cells on tumoricidal activity. In addition to cell density, which affects the likelihood of interaction due to random migration on the surface of a dish or within a tumor, there must also be enough macrophages so that there is at least one per tumor cell. Thus, if the ratio is less than one, as might be the case within a progressing tumor, some tumor cells will have no macrophages attached while others will have one or more attached. The extent to which this simple model can be applied to in vivo tumors is unknown. Distribution of chemotactic factors within the tumor mass has not been adequately determined. Indeed, their role in the tumor is still not understood and represents an area for further investigation.

Since the attachment of a macrophage to a tumor cell is a random event, we can apply Poisson statistics to estimate the number of free tumor cells there would be at a given ratio of macrophages to tumor cells. This possible effect of macrophage-to-tumor cell ratio, where density is not limiting, is shown in Figure 3. At a ratio of 1 macrophage per tumor cell, 37% of tumor cells have one macrophage attached, 18% have 2, and 8% have more than 2, i.e., 63% have 1 or more macrophages attached; but, most important, 37% have no macrophages attached and these would escape killing and proliferate to eventually repopulate the culture (or in vivo tumor). Figure 3 also shows that a ratio of 4 macrophages per tumor cell is necessary to ensure that 98% of the tumor cells would have at least one macrophage attached. While this model has not been adequately tested, our own results suggest that the

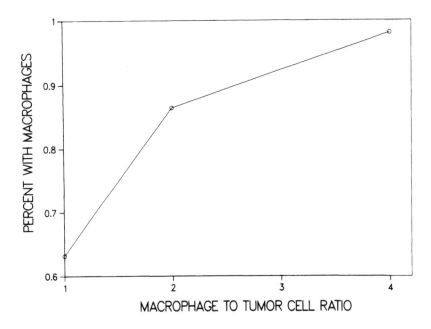

FIGURE 3.   Effect of macrophage-to-tumor cell ratio. This plot of the percentage of tumor
cells with at least one macrophage attached vs. ratio was obtained by assuming that contact
is a random event and that the probability (P_k) of contact to a tumor cell by k macrophages
(k = 0, 1, 2, ...) is described by the Poisson distribution: $P_k = c^{-\mu}\mu^k/k!$.

tumoricidal effect of macrophages is maximal at ratios above 4.[49] However, the most efficient
killing of tumor cells we have ever found is 80%. Clearly, other factors not defined by this
simple model of contact are important. Furthermore, we have never found any progressing
murine or human tumors with a ratio of macrophages to tumor cells > 1.[111] Thus, one
possible reason why macrophages are not able to control tumor growth is that there just
aren't enough of them in the tumor.

D. Decay of Tumoricidal Activity

As mentioned above, macrophages exhibit random migration at low density; they do not
migrate to a tumor cell. With time, activated macrophages lose their ability to kill tumor
cells,[50,51] presumably because, once acquired, the activated state decays when the activating
factors are removed. The mechanism for this inactivation is unclear, although prostaglandins
may be involved.[52,53] In order to better define the decay in tumoricidal activity, we incubated
activated macrophages for various lengths of time before culturing them for 40 hr with
EMT6 tumor cells. The number of surviving tumor cells was then determined using a flow-
cytometric method[49,54] described in Figure 4. The data, summarized in Figure 5, show that
the ability of macrophages to kill tumor cells continuously decreases with incubation time
and that those macrophages incubated for 17 hr prior to addition of tumor cells were unable
to kill them. Thus, tumoricidal activity is a completely reversible function. We know of no
current effort to determine the biochemical basis for this loss of tumoricidal activity.

E. A Minimum Lethal Exposure Time

As mentioned above, the macrophage-induced death of tumor cells requires considerable
time. Must the tumor cells be exposed to the macrophages for all that time or for a lesser
interaction time during which they suffer some eventually lethal damage? The latter seems
reasonable since the data presented in Figures 1 and 5 indicate that EMT6 tumor cells begin
to die only *after* the macrophages have lost their ability to kill them.

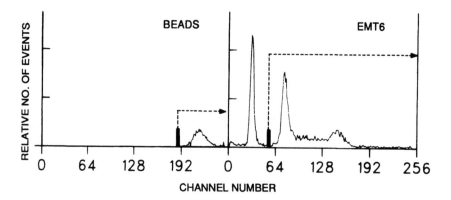

FIGURE 4.   Flow-cytometric assay of surviving EMT6 tumor cells. Cells were fixed in 70% ethanol for at least 1 hr, and then centrifuged. The cell pellet was resuspended in 1 mℓ of phosphate-buffered saline containing 20 μg/mℓ of the DNA dye propidium iodide and 20,000 10-μm superbright fluorescent microspheres.[49]   The beads and propidium iodide were excited with an argon laser operating at 488 nm. The bead fluorescence (BEADS) was measured with a narrow band-pass filter (530 ± 15 nm), and the propidium iodide fluorescence (EMT6) was measured above 580 nm. The tetraploid EMT6 tumor cells (right of dotted line) and the diploid macrophages removed by the trypsinization procedure (left of dotted line) were well resolved. Since both the concentration of beads in the sample and the number of beads counted are known, it is possible to calculate the concentration of tumor cells in the sample from the equation

$$\text{Tumor-cell concentration} = \frac{\text{Number of tumor cells counted}}{\text{Beads counted}} \times \text{Bead concentration}$$

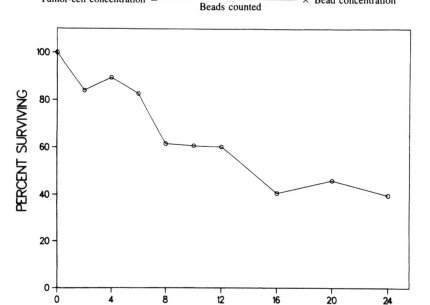

FIGURE 5.   Decay of tumoricidal activity of macrophages. To quantify this phenomenon, EMT6 tumor cells (at a density of $2 \times 10^4/\text{cm}^2$) were added to macrophages ($2 \times 10^5/\text{cm}^2$) immediately after their activation or at various later times. The number of tumor cells surviving after a 48-hr coculture was then determined by flow cytometry. The graph displays the number of surviving tumor cells (as a percentage of those surviving in a control culture of EMT6 tumor cells only) vs. the time lapse between activation of the macrophages and addition of the tumor cells. The macrophages used in this study were elicited by thioglycolate medium and activated with *Escherichia coli* LPS (1 μg/mℓ) and supernatant medium from a 24-hr culture of rat spleen cells ($10^6/\text{mℓ}$) stimulated with concanavalin A (6 μg/mℓ).

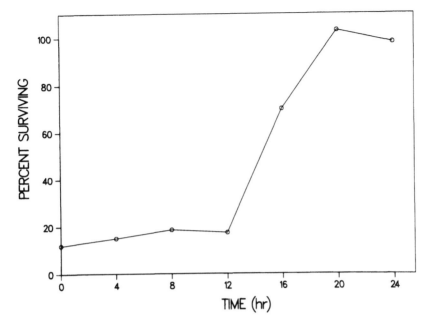

FIGURE 6. Minimum lethal exposure time. To determine this parameter, EMT6 tumor cells (at a density of $2 \times 10^4/cm^2$) were added to macrophages immediately after their activation. At various later times tumor cells were removed by trypsinization, vigorously pipetted to remove attached macrophages, diluted to $10^3/m\ell$, and replated at a density of about $200/cm^2$. (Microscopic examination showed that less than 5% of the tumor cells had macrophages attached.) A variable number of macrophages contaminated the suspension, but the low plating density ensured that these would not contact the tumor cells. After a 40-hr culture the number of surviving tumor cells was determined by flow cytometry. The graph displays the number of surviving tumor cells, as a percentage of those surviving in a control culture of tumor cells not exposed to the macrophages versus exposure time. The macrophages used in this study were those described in Figure 5.

To determine the minimum lethal exposure time, we incubated activated macrophages with EMT6 tumor cells, removed the tumor cells by trypsinization after various incubation times, replated them in new dishes at a density of 200 cells per centimeter squared, and 40 hr later determined the number of surviving tumor cells per plate by flow cytometry. As shown in Figure 6, an exposure time of at least 10 hr was required for maximal cell death. Those tumor cells removed after a lesser interaction time escaped death, although perhaps not cytostasis. Although the flow-cytometric assay can distinguish cytostasis and cytolysis when several measurements are taken at frequent intervals, our single assay time point at 40 hr could not. Further experiments will be required to determine the minimum exposure times for these two processes. Thus, regardless of the means by which macrophages induce cytostasis and cytolysis in tumor cells, they do so in the first 12 hr of exposure, even though the tumor cells may not die until considerably later.

F. Summary

Our studies have revealed several important features of the macrophage-induced death of tumor cells.

- Physical contact between tumor cells and macrophages is required.
- To ensure contact, the ratio of the number of macrophages to the number of tumor cells must be sufficiently high (>4).
- To ensure contact, the macrophage density must be sufficiently high (>$10^5/cm^2$).

- The tumor cells must be exposed to the macrophages for a minimum length of time.
- The time required for cell death is long.
- The time required for cell death varies from one type of target cell to another, and within a population of a given type, from one cell to another.
- Macrophages lose their tumoricidal activity with time.

III. CYTOSTASIS

In the previous section we discussed the kinetics of cytolysis. Prior to cell death, however, activated macrophages induce tumor cell cytostasis. In addition, some tumor cell phenotypes may not progress to cytolysis after developing cytostasis.[36] A major question, which has eluded an answer, is whether cytostasis is concomitant with, independent of, or a prerequisite for cell death. Current dogma also holds that macrophages kill neoplastic and transformed cells but spare normal cells. In a review of the literature, we were unable to find any reports on whether macrophages caused cytostasis in normal cells. Accordingly, we designed experiments to determine if macrophages inhibit the progression through the cell cycle of normal fibroblasts even though they do not kill them.[49]

In order to measure cytostasis in several different cell types, we used the flow-cytometric approach shown in Figure 7. Briefly, target cells were incubated for 1 hr with 10 μM BrdU (bromodeoxyuridine) to pulse label all cells in DNA synthesis at that time. This created a cohort of viable cells whose position in cell cycle just prior to their addition to macrophages was known and could be followed. The labeled target cells were then added to activated macrophages. The target cells were removed at various times by trypsinization and stained with propidium iodide to reveal the DNA distribution of cells at the time of assay and with a fluoresceinated antibody to BrdU to label the cohort of cells that were in S phase at time 0 hr. As conceptually shown in Figure 7, if the cells progress through the cell cycle, the labeled cohort will be found first coincident with cells in S phase, as revealed by the propidium iodide staining, then with cells in G_2/M, then with cells in G_1, and then back with cells in S phase again at progressively later assay times. If the cells are blocked in a specific phase of the cell cycle, (e.g., G_2/M), the BrdU-labeled cells accumulate in that phase and progress no further. If they are stopped uniformly in all phases of the cell cycle, the labeled cohort will not progress out of S phase nor will the unlabeled cells progress into S phase.

Figure 8 shows results of our studies for normal fibroblasts, a transformed nontumorigenic cell line, and a neoplastic cell line. All three cell types are stopped uniformly in every phase of cell cycle. Normal low-passage fibroblasts were as effectively stopped as were the most neoplastic cells. These same results were obtained using five other cell lines.[54] Thus, whatever macrophages do to cells to inhibit cell cycle progression, they do it to normal as well as neoplastic cells. Either cytostasis is independent of cell death or normal cells tolerate cytostasis better than tumor cells.

IV. MECHANISMS OF CYTOTOXICITY

We have just considered the kinetics of macrophage-induced cytostasis and cytolysis but these studies do not reveal the biochemical pathways involved in these processes. What do macrophages actually do to target cells that (1) is an early event that induces cytostasis in both normal and neoplastic cells and does not require continuous macrophage contact, and (2) results in death at some later time in some neoplastic but not normal cells? Must cytostasis precede death? In the last 15 years several mechanisms have been proposed to explain tumor-cell killing by macrophages. The following is a brief review of these proposed mechanisms.

A. Lysosome Exocytosis
In this earliest hypothesis an exocytosis and transfer of lysosomes from the macrophage

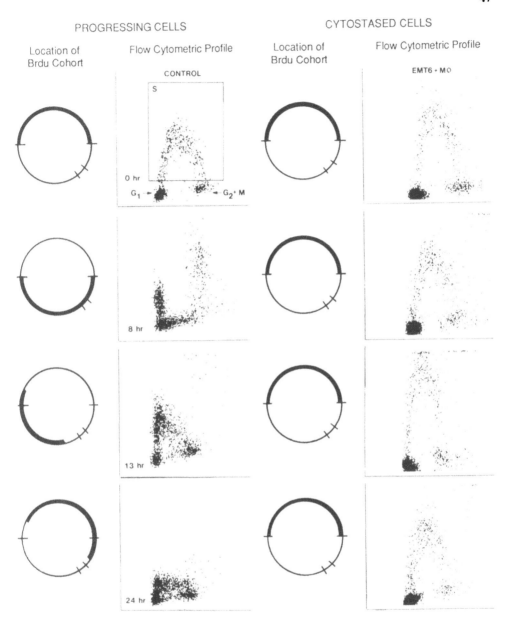

PROGRESSING CELLS

Location of Brdu Cohort | Flow Cytometric Profile

CYTOSTASED CELLS

Location of Brdu Cohort | Flow Cytometric Profile

CONTROL

EMT6 + MO

S

0 hr

G₁ →

→ G₂⁺ M

8 hr

13 hr

24 hr

FIGURE 7. Analysis of cytostasis. Target cells were incubated with 10 μM BrdU for 1 hr, washed, and then added to activated macrophages. Control cultures contained target cells only. At selected times target cells were removed with trypsin, washed, and fixed in ethanol (see Figure 4). When all the samples had been collected, the cells were centrifuged and resuspended in 4 N HCl for 30 min to hydrolyze the DNA and expose the incorporated BrdU. After being centrifuged, the cells were resuspended in 50 μℓ of diluted fluoresceinated anti-BrdU (B-D) for 15 min, washed once, and resuspended in 2 mℓ of PBS containing 20 μg/mℓ propidium iodide and 100 μg/mℓ RNAse. The flow-cytometric analysis was performed as described in Figure 4. Columns 1 and 3 show the position in the cell cycle of the BrdU-labeled cohort for progressing and cytostased cells respectively. Columns 2 and 4 show the flow cytometric profiles for normal EMT6 cells and EMT6 cells cultured with activated macrophages, respectively.

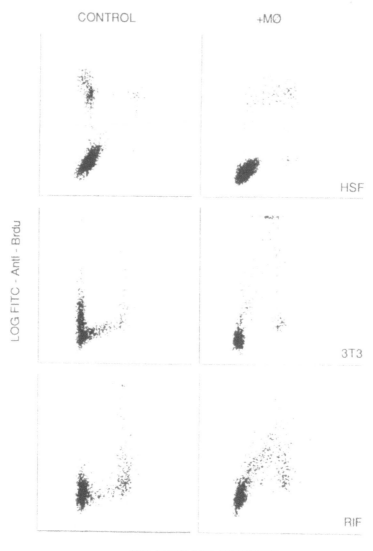

FIGURE 8. Cytostasis of target cells. Human skin fibroblasts after their second in vitro passage (HSF), nontumorigenic 3T3 murine fibroblasts (3T3), and a neoplastic radiation-induced murine fibrosarcoma (RIF) were labeled for 1 hr with 10 μM BrdU, washed, and cultured without (control) or with activated macrophages (+ Mϕ) for 12 hr. Cells were then analyzed by flow cytometry as described in Figure 7.

to the tumor cell was proposed. When macrophage lysosomes were prelabeled with dextran sulfate and then incubated with tumor cells, there was an accumulation of dextran sulfate in the tumor cells.[55] This suggested that lysosomal material from activated macrophages was transferred to the cytoplasm of tumor cells. Bucana et al.[56,57] also provided electron microscopic evidence for lysosomal transfer from activated macrophages to tumor cells. While transfer of activated macrophage-derived lysosomal material to target cells appears to occur, the cause and effect relationship of this transfer to development of cytotoxic changes in target cells is uncertain.

B. Superoxide Anion and Hydrogen Peroxide

Macrophages are a potent source of superoxide anion and hydrogen peroxide, the generation of which is known to be an important means by which macrophages (and granulocytes) kill bacteria intracellularly. Some tumor cells, notably leukemic, may be susceptible to being killed by hydrogen peroxide and superoxide anion.[58-64] It has also been shown that superoxide anion can synergize with neutral protease in the killing process.[64] The time course of killing by superoxide anion of leukemic target cells, however, was only 6 hr rather than the 18 to 40 hr noted for most tumor cells co-cultivated with activated macrophages. Furthermore, only a limited number of tumor cells, primarily those of hematopoietic origin, were susceptible to lysis by this mechanism. To our knowledge no target cells of solid-tumor origin have been shown to be susceptible to lysis by superoxide anion. The importance of this mechanism to macrophage-induced killing is not clear. While it may contribute to lysis for some tumor cells, it probably does not represent the major pathway of cytostasis and cytolysis.

C. Interleukin 1

Many biological activities have been associated with the monokine interleukin 1, and these have been extensively reviewed recently.[65] One possible role is in both the activation of macrophages and as an effector molecule in cytotoxicity.[66] Before any definitive statements can be made about the role of this molecule in tumor-cell killing, much more work needs to be done.

D. Arginase

Currie[67] and Currie and Basham[68,69] proposed that the effector molecule might be arginase. He showed that the V79 Chinese hamster lung cells failed to form colonies when co-cultured with activated macrophages that produced arginase or with 24- or 48-hr supernatants obtained from them. When arginase was added to the tumor cells, they were lysed; when arginase was fractionated from the conditioned supernatant medium, it was the lytic fraction. He envisioned that macrophages at the site of the tumor might produce high local concentrations of arginase and thereby deprive the tumor cells of required arginine. Such a deprivation could account for the time required for cytolysis to develop. While many leukemic cell lines require arginine for cell survival, most solid tumors, which are equally sensitive to the tumoricidal activity of macrophages, do not require arginine. This inconsistency makes it unlikely that arginase is of major importance in macrophage-mediated tumoricidal activity.

E. Neutral Proteases

Adams et al. isolated a serine protease from a tissue-culture medium of activated macrophages in the process of killing tumor cells. In a series of publications,[70-87] this group described several features of the macrophage-tumor cell interaction that supported a role for this neutral protease in cytolysis of tumor cells.

They found that activated macrophages bound more strongly to neoplastic cells than to normal cells, while unactivated cells bound poorly to both. Plasma membranes from a variety of transformed cells inhibited this binding, but those from untransformed cells did not. They proposed that a specific receptor for neoplastic cells was induced by activated macrophages.

Only activated macrophages secreted the neutral protease and this secretion was enhanced after binding of a macrophage to a tumor cell. They found that macrophages from A/J mice, which respond poorly to macrophage-activation regimens but respond normally to endotoxin, secreted normal amounts of protease when endotoxin was added to them. These same cells, however, bound very poorly to target cells. In contrast, when macrophages from C3H/HeJ mice, which do not respond to endotoxin, were activated, they bound strongly to target cells but did not secrete any protease. They concluded from these studies that the role of activation factors was to induce binding and that endotoxin was required for production and secretion of neutral protease.

They also studied the direct effect of a semipurified neutral protease on tumor cells in the absence of macrophages. They found that the protease induced cytostasis and that the time course of cytotoxicity was similar to that observed when macrophages were present. Protease inhibitors blocked this activity.

These observations prompted Adams to suggest a two-step mechanism for cytolysis. In the first step, macrophages, whether activated or not, interact with target cells for short periods of time. Activated macrophages, however, firmly bind to tumor cells for prolonged time periods because their receptor density for binding is high. This binding receptor is apparently up-regulated by the priming signal produced by the activation regimens, but no cytostasis or cytolysis results. When lipopolysaccharide (LPS) is added, however, the lytic phase is initiated as the cytolytic protease is synthesized and released into the target cell. The latter process takes several hours to become expressed as cytolysis of the tumor cell.

While the biochemical pathways interrupted by the neutral protease have not yet been defined, it produces the phenotypic changes and kinetic events in the target cells ascribed to macrophages themselves. Further work needs to be done to define its mode of action in tumor cells.

F. Tumor Necrosis Factor

In 1975, Old et al.[88,89] described an activity in serum from Bacillus Calmette-Guerin (BCG) and endotoxin treated mice which would cause tumors to become necrotic. They called this activity tumor necrosis factor (TNF). Since that time, it has been shown that this factor is produced by activated macrophages,[88-92] and has been purified, cloned, and sequenced.[93-95] TNF is synthesized when macrophages are activated and it is cytostatic and cytocidal for a variety of neoplastic cells.[88,89,91,93] Recently, Urban et al.[96] showed that neoplastic cells that were susceptible to killing by activated macrophages were also susceptible to killing by recombinant TNF (rTNF) and that cells resistant to killing by activated macrophages were also resistant to killing by rTNF. They also showed that an antibody to rTNF inhibited the tumoricidal activity of activated macrophages.

In addition to its tumoricidal activity, TNF also causes lung fibroblasts and endothelial cells to release granulocyte-macrophage colony-stimulating factor (GM-CSF) in vitro.[97] It can also act as a growth factor for normal fibroblasts[98,99] and as a differentiation factor for myelomonocytic cells.[100] It is not clear how these two different kinds of activity — killing tumor cells vs. proliferation and differentiation of normal cells — fit together.

Generally, TNF activity is assayed in vitro using mouse L929 cells, a transformed fibroblast line. Several groups[101-103] have also shown that L-929 cells have receptors for TNF. Recently, it was shown that TNF-resistant L-929 cells lack cell surface receptors for TNF.[104] It is not known, however, if all transformed cell populations susceptible to TNF lysis have receptors and if those that are resistant lack them. Furthermore, it is currently not known if normal cells have receptors for TNF.

Kirstein et al.[105] have shown that L929 cells were growth inhibited by TNF but did not actually die until they approached a high density. This study is most informative because it suggests that nutrient depletion may be an important component for the expression of cell death. The importance of this possibility will become clearer later.

It was noted above that activated macrophages lose their ability to kill tumor cells. This loss of tumoricidal activity could be caused by a decay in the level of their activation. Prostaglandin E$_2$ (PGE$_2$) has been implicated in this loss of tumoricidal activity. Kunkel et al.[106] have shown that PGE$_2$ inhibits the production of TNF. This may be an important autocrine regulation. Activated macrophages produce high levels of TNF and low levels of PGE$_2$. As activation decays, PGE$_2$ levels increase causing TNF production to decrease.

The mechanism by which TNF acts to induce cytostasis and cytotoxicity is not known. Virtually all current reports are concerned with its production and effects on normal and transformed cells because of its importance as a biological response modifier in cancer therapy. While it is a major mediator of the antitumor cell activity exerted by activated macrophages, it appears that it is not a protease and its activity is not blocked by catalase.[107] An important area of future research will be the elucidation of the mechanism of TNF action on neoplastic and normal cells.

G. L-Arginine-Dependent Effector Mechanism

In 1980 the first of a series of studies by Hibbs and co-workers led to an understanding of a number of the biochemical changes induced in target cells by activated macrophages.[36,38,39] They found that when L1210 leukemia cells were co-cultivated with activated macrophages for 24 hr, in medium with high glucose, the leukemia cells did not lyse. When these cells were added to a culture medium that contained all components except glucose, they rapidly lysed. These observations led to the discovery that activated macrophages induced inhibition of mitochondrial respiration in L1210 cells and in other target cells. This explained the requirement for glucose for maintenance of viability of injured target cells. Consumption of glucose via the glycolytic pathway is the only ATP (adenosine triphosphate) generating pathway available to injured target cells following inhibition of mitochondrial ATP formation induced by activated macrophages. Such injured target cells rapidly undergo lysis when cultured in medium without glucose because the absence of activity of both ATP synthesizing pathways, mitochondrial oxidative phosphorylation, and glycolysis results in depletion of energy stores. Normal control target cells or target cells that were co-cultivated with normal or stimulated macrophages remain viable when cultured in medium without glucose. Glycolysis is not active in these cells in the glucose-free medium but ATP continues to be synthesized in their normally functioning mitochondria.

Granger and Lehninger subsequently described the enzymatic basis for activated macrophage-induced inhibition of mitochondrial respiration in target cells.[37] They demonstrated that the proximal two oxidoreductases of the mitochondrial electron transport chain complex I [NADH (nicotinamide-adenine dinucleotide): ubiquinone oxidoreductase] and complex II (succinate: ubiquinone oxidoreductase) were inhibited by the activated macrophage cytotoxic effect while the more distal portion of the mitochondrial electron transport chain remained functional. Hibbs et al. then observed that activated macrophages induce a marked loss of intracellular iron from viable target cells.[39,42] Complex I and complex II contain most of the iron-sulfur clusters of the mitochondrial electron transport system. To test the hypothesis that the activated macrophage cytotoxic mechanism induces iron loss from enzymes containing iron-sulfur prosthetic groups more readily than heme-containing enzymes, Drapier and Hibbs examined the citric acid cycle enzyme aconitase which contains an iron-sulfur cluster essential for its catalytic activity.[41,43,44] The results showed that activated macrophages cause rapid inhibition of aconitase in target cells. Furthermore, they demonstrated that removal of iron from the iron-sulfur prosthetic group was causally related to aconitase inhibition. Removal of iron from iron-sulfur prosthetic groups of complex I and complex II by the activated macrophage cytotoxic effector mechanism could explain the pattern of enzymatic inhibition which occurs in the mitochondrial electron transport system.

Activated macrophages cause inhibition of DNA replication[108,109] in target cells in addition to causing iron loss, inhibition of complex I, inhibition of complex II, and inhibition of aconitase. It is significant that ribonucleotide reductase, the rate limiting enzyme in DNA replication, contains two nonheme iron molecules that are essential for its catalytic activity. Removal of iron from ribonucleotide reductase could explain activated macrophage-induced inhibition of DNA replication. However, no data are currently available proving or disproving this possibility.

Recently, Hibbs et al. discovered a biochemical pathway synthesizing L-citrulline and nitrite in the presence of L-arginine but not D-arginine.[46,47] This pathway is coupled to the activated macrophage effector mechanism causing inhibition of mitochondrial respiration, aconitase activity, and DNA replication. L-Citrulline and nitrite biosynthesis by activated

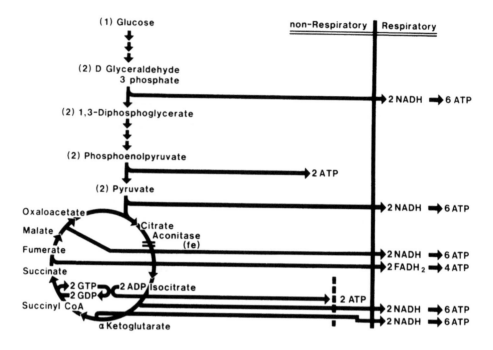

FIGURE 9.   Glycolysis and production of ATP from glucose.

macrophages are inhibited by N^G-monomethyl-L-arginine which also inhibits this cytotoxic effector mechanism. The experiments demonstrated that the activated macrophage cytotoxic effector mechanism is associated with L-arginine deiminase activity and that the imino nitrogen removed from the guanido group of L-arginine by the deiminase reaction subsequently undergoes oxidation to nitrite. Recent experiments show that the activated macrophage L-arginine-dependent effector mechanism synthesizes L-citrulline:nitrite:nitrate from L-arginine with a stoichiometry of 1:1/2:1/2.[110] The actual mechanism of metabolic inhibition by products of the L-arginine-dependent effector mechanism remains to be defined. However, nitrite or oxygenated nitrogen intermediates in the pathway of nitrite and nitrate synthesis could participate in causing iron loss from aconitase and other enzymes containing iron-sulfur clusters in target cells of activated macrophages in addition to inducing other intracellular effects.

V. CONCLUSION

Activated macrophages induce iron release from mammalian and microbial target cells. Iron loss appears to be caused by the activated macrophage L-arginine-dependent effector system which synthesizes oxygenated nitrogen derivates from imino nitrogen derived from the guanido group of L-arginine. This effector mechanism inhibits certain iron-containing enzymes, particularly enzymes containing iron-sulfur prosthetic groups. Complex I, complex II, and aconitase, all of which have iron-sulfur prosthetic groups essential for catalytic activity, have been shown to be inhibited by the activated macrophage cytotoxic effector mechanism. All three enzymes are involved in mitochondrial bioenergetic activity. In Figure 9 the metabolism of glucose by the glycolytic pathway, the citric acid cycle, and the mitochondrial electron transport system are depicted schematically. We would like to advance the following testable hypothesis which may explain, in part at least, the response of target cells to the activated macrophage cytotoxic reaction. There are 38 ATP molecules generated by the oxidative metabolism of 1 molecule of glucose. However, the production of only a

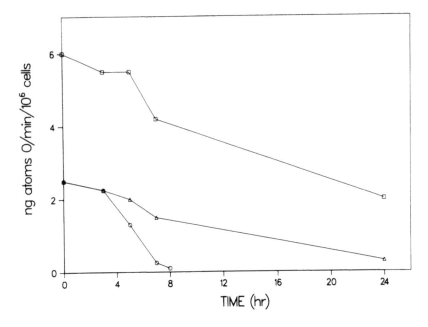

FIGURE 10. Kinetics of aconitase and complexes I and II Inhibition. L10 cells, cultured with activated macrophages, were analyzed at various times over a 24-hr period for aconitase (O) complex I (△), and complex II (□) activity. Control cells exhibited no appreciable change from the time zero measurement over the 24-hr culture period.[44]

net two ATP molecules occurs via the glycolytic pathway functioning independently of mitochondrial oxidative phosphorylation. The synthesis of two ATP molecules by the glycolytic pathway functioning independently does not require the participation of iron-containing enzymes. It is possible that the decreased energy production, which occurs when mitochondrial respiration is inhibited in target cells of activated macrophages, is sufficient to inhibit their progression through the cell cycle. Alternatively, inhibition of ribonucleotide reductase, the rate-limiting enzyme in DNA synthesis, may be responsible for the target cell cytostasis observed.

As shown in Figure 10, aconitase was inhibited prior to inhibition of complex I and complex II of the mitochondrial electron-transport system. However, inhibition of aconitase activity may not have a significant effect on mitochondrial respiration and ATP synthesis. As shown in Table 1, aconitase activity was completely inhibited in target cells that had been co-cultivated with activated macrophages for 6 hr, but endogenous coupled and uncoupled respiration was unchanged from that measured in control target cells.[44] These results suggest that a citric acid cycle block at the level of aconitase, which occurs early in the co-cultivation period, does not inhibit mitochondrial respiration and that as long as complex I and complex II are still functional, endogenous substrates are able to circumvent the aconitase block. However, after 24 hr of co-cultivation of target cells, both endogenous coupled and uncoupled respiration was markedly inhibited. In addition, when complex I and complex II becomes inhibited, the cell loses 95% of its energy production potential. This would lead to cell death unless compensated for by increased glycolysis and the presence of high glucose in the medium. We propose that the observed variation in time to the expression of death is a function of how long the cell can survive on this severely limited energy production and its ability to restore respiratory function (or initiate glycolysis) when macrophages can no longer produce the appropriate effector molecules resulting in iron release.

This model is consistent with the finding that when L1210 cells were cultured in high glucose they produced sufficient energy through glycolysis to survive. L10 cells, on the

Table 1

**EXOGENOUS CITRATE-DEPENDENT STATE 3
RESPIRATION AND ENDOGENOUS RESPIRATION IN
CONTROL L10 CELLS AND L10 CELLS CO-CULTIVATED
WITH CYTOTOXIC ACTIVATED MACROPHAGES[44]**

	Oxygen consumption[a]			
	6 hr		22 hr	
	L10 cells alone	L10 cells + cytotoxic activated macrophages	L10 cells alone	L10 cells + cytotoxic activated macrophages
Citrate-dependent respiration	14	0	N.D.[b]	N.D.
Endogenous respiration + 100 μM 2,4-dinitrophenol	19 26	16 24	14 33	2 2

Note: L10 cells were cultured alone or co-cultivated with cytotoxic activated macrophages for the time interval indicated before respiration measurements were made. There was 5 mM citrate present in the respiration medium for measurement of citrate-dependent O_2 consumption in digitonin permeabilized L10 cells. Endogenous respiration was measured in parallel experiments in nonpermeabilized L10 cells in the presence or absence of 2,4-dinitrophenol.

[a]   Units, ng atoms O · min^{-1} · 10^{-6} L10 cells.
[b]   N.D., not done.

other hand, were not able to adapt to this energy depletion. One would predict that cells conditioned for survival in hypoxic conditions would be less susceptible to macrophage killing than those more dependent on aerobic glycolysis. Thus, the survival or death of a cell does not depend on whether it is normal or neoplastic or whether macrophages recognize it or not but rather whether it is susceptible to irreversible metabolic disorganization when ATP synthesis is limited to the glycolytic pathway.

Taken together we would propose that activated macrophages synthesize molecules, perhaps oxygenated derivatives of nitrogen, which cause iron release. This results in the inhibition of the iron-containing respiratory enzymes and ribonucleotide reductase. The ability of the target cell to survive this inhibition in energy production will define its susceptibility to lysis. Thus, macrophages do not recognize or distinguish between normal and neoplastic cells. Rather, cells having higher metabolic requirements such as neoplastic cells are more susceptible to lysis by activated macrophages than are normal, more differentiated, cells. Since the inhibition of iron metabolism is totally reversible, the loss of the activated state of macrophages would provide for a means by which normal cells could recover. It is this delicate balance that determines whether or not a particular cell is killed by macrophages not whether it is neoplastic or normal.

While the accumulated evidence over the past 15 years supports the above hypothesis, the greatest challenge will be to prove or disprove the general features of the model, to identify explicitly the macrophage-derived effector molecules, and to understand the true role of the macrophage in controlling neoplasia in vivo, not in vitro.

REFERENCES

1. **Hibbs, J. B., Jr., Lambert, L. H., Jr., and Remington, J. S.,** Resistance to murine tumors conferred by chronic infection with intracellular protozoa, *Toxoplasma gondii* and *Besnoitia jellisoni, J. Infect. Dis.,* 124, 587, 1971.
2. **Hibbs, J. B., Jr., Lambert, L. H., Jr., and Remington, J. S.,** Possible role of macrophage mediated nonspecific cytotoxicity in tumor resistance, *Nature (London),* 235, 48, 1972.
3. **Hibbs, J. B., Jr.,** Heterocytolysis by macrophages activated by Bacillus Calmette-Guerin: lysosome exocytosis into tumor cells, *Science,* 184, 468, 1974.
4. **Hibbs, J. B., Jr.,** Discrimination between neoplastic and non-neoplastic cells in vitro by activated macrophages, *J. Natl. Cancer Inst.,* 531, 487, 1974.
5. **Churchill, W. H., Jr., Piessens, W. F., Sulis, C. A., and David, J. R.,** Macrophages activated as suspension cultures with lymphocyte mediators devoid of antigen become cytotoxic for tumor cells, *J. Immunol.,* 115, 781, 1975.
6. **Piessens, W. F., Churchill, W. H., Jr., and David, J. R.,** Macrophages activated in vitro with lymphocyte mediators kill neoplastic but not normal cells, *J. Immunol.,* 114, 293, 1975.
7. **Fidler, I. J., Darnell, J. H., and Budmen, M. B.,** In vitro activation of mouse macrophages by rat lymphocyte mediators, *J. Immunol.,* 117, 666, 1976.
8. **Ruco, L. P. and Meltzer, M. S.,** Macrophage activation for tumor cytotoxicity: induction of tumoricidal macrophages by supernatants of PPD-stimulated Bacillus Calmette-Guerin-immune spleen cell cultures, *J. Immunol.,* 119, 889, 1977.
9. **Schultz, R. M., Papamatheakis, J. D., and Chirigos, M. A.,** Interferon: an inducer of macrophage activation by polyanions, *Science,* 197, 674, 1977.
10. **Weinberg, J. B., Chapman, H. A., Jr., and Hibbs, J. B., Jr.,** Characterization of the effects of endotoxin on macrophage tumor cell killing, *J. Immunol.,* 121, 72, 1978.
11. **Ruco, L. P. and Meltzer, M. S.,** Macrophage activation for tumor cytotoxicity: development of macrophage cytotoxic activity requires completion of a sequence of short-lived intermediary reactions, *J. Immunol.,* 121, 2035, 1978.
12. **Ruco, L. P. and Meltzer, M. S.,** Macrophage activation for tumor cytotoxicity: increased lymphokine responsiveness of peritoneal macrophage during acute inflammation, *J. Immunol.,* 120, 1054, 1978.
13. **Leonard, E. J., Ruco, L. P., and Meltzer, M. S.,** Characterization of macrophage activation factor, a lymphokine that causes macrophages to become cytotoxic for tumor cells, *Cell. Immunol.,* 41, 347, 1978.
14. **Weinberg, J. B. and Hibbs, J. B., Jr.,** In vitro modulation of macrophage tumoricidal activity: partial characterization of a macrophage-activating factor(s) in supernatants of NaIO$_4$-treated peritoneal cells, *J. Reticuloendothel. Soc.,* 26, 283, 1979.
15. **Schultz, R. M.,** Macrophage activation by interferons, *Lymphokine Rep.,* 1, 63, 1980.
16. **Pace, J. L., Taffet, S. M., and Russell, S. W.,** The effect of endotoxin in eliciting agents on the activation of mouse macrophages for tumor cell killing, *J. Reticuloendothel. Soc.,* 30, 15, 1981.
17. **Fleishmann, W. R., Jr., Kleyn, K. M., and Baron, S.,** Potentiation of antitumor effect of virus-induced interferon by mouse immune interferon preparations, *J. Natl. Cancer Inst.,* 65, 963, 1980.
18. **Pace, J. L. and Russell, S. W.,** Activation of mouse macrophages for tumor cell killing. I. Quantitative analysis of interactions between lymphokine and lipopolysaccharide, *J. Immunol.,* 126, 1863, 1981.
19. **Boraschi, D. and Tagliabue, A.,** Interferon-induced enhancement of macrophage tumor cytolysis and its difference from activation by lymphokines, *Eur. J. Immunol.,* 11, 110, 1981.
20. **Roberts, W. K. and Vasil, A.,** Evidence for the identity of murine gamma interferon and macrophage activating factor, *J. Interferon Res.,* 2, 519, 1982.
21. **Schultz, R. M.,** Synergistic activation of macrophages by lymphokine and lipopolysaccharide: evidence for lymphokine as the primer and interferon as the trigger, *J. Interferon Res.,* 2, 459, 1982.
22. **Ortaldo, J. R., Mantovani, A., Hobbs, D., Rubinstein, M., Pestka, S., and Herberman, R. B.,** Effects of several species of human leukocyte interferon on cytotoxic activity of NK cells and monocytes, *Int. J. Cancer,* 31, 285, 1983.
23. **Pace, J. L., Russell, S. W., Schreiber, R. D., Altman, A., and Katz, D. H.,** Macrophage activation: priming activity from a T-cell hybridoma is attributable to interferon-γ, *Proc. Natl. Acad. Sci. U.S.A.,* 80, 3782, 1983.
24. **Pace, J. L., Russell, S. W., Torres, B. A., Johnson, H. M., and Gray, P. W.,** Recombinant mouse γ-interferon induces the priming step in macrophage activation for tumor cell killing, *J. Immunol.,* 130, 2011, 1983.
25. **Schreiber, R. D., Pace, J. L., Russell, S. W., Altman, A., and Katz, D. H.,** Macrophage-activating factor produced by a T cell hybridoma: physicochemical and biosynthetic resemblance to γ-interferon, *J. Immunol.,* 131, 826, 1983.
26. **Schultz, R. M. and Kleinschmidt, W. J.,** Functional identity between murine γ interferon and macrophage activating factor, *Nature (London),* 305, 239, 1983.

27. **Varesio, L., Blasi, E., Gray, P., Herberman, R. B., and Wiltrout, R. H.,** Activation of cytotoxic macrophages by cloned murine gamma interferon (γ-IFN), *Fed. Proc. Fed. Am. Soc. Exp. Biol.,* 42, 1076, 1983.

28. **Weigent, D. A., Langford, M. P., Fleischmann, W. R., Jr., and Stanton, G. J.,** Potentiation of lymphocyte natural killing by mixtures of alpha or beta interferon with recombinant gamma interferon, *Infect. Immun.,* 40, 35, 1983.

29. **Svedersky, L. P., Benton, C. V., Berger, W. H., Rinderknecht, E., Harkins, R. N., and Palladino, M. A.,** Biological and antigenic similarities of murine interferon-γ and macrophage-activating factor, *J. Exp. Med.,* 159, 812, 1984.

30. **Pace, J. L., Russell, S. W., LeBlanc, P. A., and Morasho, D. M.,** Comparative effects of various classes of mouse interferons on macrophage activation for tumor cell killing, *J. Immunol.,* 134, 977, 1985.

31. **Sharma, S. D. and Piessens, W. F.,** Tumor cell killing by macrophages activated in vitro with lymphocyte mediators, *Cell. Immunol.,* 47, 106, 1979.

32. **Puvion, F., Fray, A., and Halpern, B.,** A cytochemical study of the in vitro interaction between normal and activated mouse peritoneal macrophages and tumor cells, *J. Ultrastruct. Res.,* 54, 95, 1976.

33. **Keller, R.,** Cytostatic and cytocidal effects of activated macrophages, in *Immunobiology of the Macrophage,* Nelson, D. S., Ed., Academic Press, New York, 1976, 487.

34. **Fidler, I. J.,** Recognition and destruction of target cells by tumoricidal macrophages, *Isr. J. Med. Sci.,* 14, 177, 1978.

35. **Weinberg, J. B. and Hibbs, J. B., Jr.,** Endocytosis of red blood cells or hemoglobin by activated macrophages inhibits their tumoricidal effect, *Nature (London),* 269, 245, 1977.

36. **Granger, D. L., Taintor, R. R., Cook, J. L., and Hibbs, J. B., Jr.,** Injury of neoplastic cells by murine macrophages leads to inhibition of mitochondrial respiration, *J. Clin. Invest.,* 65, 357, 1980.

37. **Granger, D. L. and Lehninger, L.,** Sites of inhibition of mitochondrial electron transport in macrophage-injured neoplastic cells, *J. Cell Biol.,* 95, 527, 1982.

38. **Hibbs, J. B., Jr. and Granger, D. L.,** Activated macrophage-induced cytostasis and inhibition of aerobic energy metabolism in transformed cells: evaluation of lytic and nonlytic target cell responses, in *Self-Defense Mechanisms: Role of Macrophages,* Mizuno, D., Cohn, Z. A., Takeya, K., and Ishida, N., Eds., University of Tokyo Press, Tokyo, 1982, 319.

39. **Hibbs, J. B., Jr., Taintor, R. R., and Vavrin, Z.,** Iron depletion: possible cause of tumor cell cytotoxicity induced by activated macrophages, *Biochem. Biophys. Res. Commun.,* 123(2), 716, 1984.

40. **Kilbourn, R. G., Klostergaard, J., and Lopez-Berestein, G.,** Activated macrophages secrete a soluble factor that inhibits mitochondrial respiration of tumor cells, *J. Immunol.,* 133, 2577, 1984.

41. **Hibbs, J. B., Jr. and Drapier, J. C.,** Activated macrophage mediated iron removal from enzymes with iron-sulfur clusters in tumor target cells: a possible mechanism for selective inhibition of metabolic pathways, in *Leukocytes and Host Defense,* Oppenheim, J. J. and Jacobs, D. M., Eds., Alan R. Liss, New York, 1986, 261.

42. **Hibbs, J. B., Jr., Taintor, R. R., and Vavrin, Z.,** Possible role of iron depletion as cause of tumor cell cytotoxicity induced by activated macrophages, in *Immunity to Cancer,* Reif, A. and Mitchell, M., Eds., Academic Press, N.Y., 1985, 309.

43. **Drapier, J. C. and Hibbs, J. B., Jr.,** Aconitase, a Krebs cycle enzyme with an iron-sulfur center, is inhibited in tumor target cells after cocultivation with cytotoxic activated macrophages, in *Leukocytes and Host Defense,* Oppenheim, J. J. and Jacobs, D. M., Eds., Alan R. Liss, New York, 1986, 269.

44. **Drapier, J. C. and Hibbs, J. B., Jr.,** Murine cytotoxic activated macrophages inhibit aconitase in tumor cells. Inhibition involves the iron-sulfur prosthetic group and is reversible, *J. Clin. Invest.,* 78, 790, 1986.

45. **Hibbs, J. B., Jr. and Taintor, R. R.,** Activated macrophage mediated cytotoxicity: use of the in vitro cytotoxicity assay for study of bioenergetic and biochemical changes that develop in tumor target cells, *Methods Enzymol.,* 132, 508, 1986.

46. **Hibbs, J. B., Jr., Vavrin, Z., and Taintor, R. R.,** L-Arginine is required for expression of the activated macrophage effector mechanism causing selective metabolic inhibition in target cells, *J. Immunol.,* 138, 550, 1987.

47. **Hibbs, J. B., Jr., Taintor, R. R., and Vavrin, Z.,** Macrophage cytotoxicity: role for L-arginine deiminase and imino nitrogen oxidation to nitrite, *Science,* 235, 473, 1987.

48. **Stewart, C. C., Stevenson, A. P., and Steinkamp, J. S.,** Characterization of self populations in tumors by multiparameter flow cytometry, in *Applications of Fluorescence in the Biomedical Sciences,* Taylor, D. L., Waggoner, A. S., Murphy, R. F., Lanni, F., and Birge, R. R., Eds., Alan R. Liss, New York, 1986, 585.

49. **Stevenson, A. P., Martin, J. C., and Stewart, C. C.,** Simultaneous measurements of macrophage-induced cytostasis and cytotoxicity of EMT6 cells by flow cytometry, *Cancer Res.,* 46, 99, 1986.

50. **Poste, G. and Kirsh, R.,** Rapid decay of tumoricidal activity and loss of responsiveness to lymphokines inflammatory macrophages, *Cancer Res.,* 39, 2582, 1979.

51. **Thomasson, D. L. and Stewart, C. C.**, Macrophage tumoricidal activity: activation and killing kinetics, in *Mediation of Cellular Immunity in Cancer by Immune Modifiers*, Chirigos, M. A., et al., Eds., Raven Press, New York, 1981, 1.

52. **Taffet, S. M. and Russell, S. W.**, Macrophage-mediated tumor cell killing: regulation of expression of cytolytic activity by prostaglandin E, *J. Immunol.*, 126, 424, 1981.

53. **Russell, S. W. and Pace, J. L.**, Both the kind and magnitude of stimulus are important to overcoming the negative regulation of macrophage activation by PGE_2, *J. Leukocyte Biol.*, 35, 291, 1984.

54. **Stevenson, A. P., Crissman, H. A., and Stewart, C. C.**, Macrophage-induced cytostasis: kinetic analysis of bromodeoxyuridine-pulsed cells, *Cytometry*, 6, 578, 1985.

55. **Hibbs, J. B., Jr.**, Activated macrophages as cytotoxic effector cells. I. Inhibition of specific and nonspecific tumor resistance by trypan blue, *Transplantation*, 19, 77, 1975.

56. **Bucana, C., Hoyer, L. C., Hobbs, B., Breesman, S., McDaniel, M., and Hanna, M. G., Jr.**, Morphological evidence for the translocation of lysosomal organelles from cytotoxic macrophages into the cytoplasm of tumor target cells, *Cancer Res.*, 36, 4444, 1976.

57. **Bucana, C. D., Hoyer, L. C., Schroit, A. J., Kleinerman, E., and Fidler, I. J.**, Ultrastructural studies of the interaction between liposome-activated human blood monocytes and allogeneic tumor cells in vitro, *Am. J. Pathol.*, 112, 101, 1983.

58. **Johnston, R. B., Jr., Godzik, C. A., and Cohn, Z. A.**, Increased superoxide anion production by immunologically activated and chemically elicited macrophages, *J. Exp. Med.*, 115, 127, 1978.

59. **Nathan, C. F., Bruker, L. H., Silverstein, S. C., and Cohn, A. Z.**, Extracellular cytolysis by activated macrophages and granulocytes. I. Pharmacologic triggering of effector cells and the release of hydrogen peroxide, *J. Exp. Med.*, 149, 84, 1979.

60. **Nathan, C. F., Silverstein, S. C., Brukner, L. H., and Cohn, Z. A.**, Extracellular cytolysis by activated macrophages and granulocytes. II. Hydrogen peroxide as a mediator of cytotoxicity, *J. Exp. Med.*, 149, 1979, 1979.

61. **Nathan, C. F.**, Reactive oxygen intermediates in lysis of tumor cells, in *Macrophage-Mediated Antibody-Dependent Cellular Cytotoxicity*, Vol. 21, (Immunology Series), Koren, H. S., Ed., Marcel Dekker, New York, 1983, 199.

62. **Weiss, S. J. and Slivka, A.**, Monocyte and granulocyte-mediated tumor cell destruction. A role for the hydrogen peroxide-myeloperoxidase chloride system, *J. Clin. Invest.*, 69, 255, 1982.

63. **Mavier, P. and Edgington, T. S.**, Human monocyte-mediated tumor cytotoxicity. I. Demonstration of an oxygen-dependent myeloperoxidase-independent mechanism, *J. Immunol.*, 132, 1980, 1984.

64. **Adams, D. O., Johnson, W. J., Fiorito, E., and Nathan, C. F.**, Hydrogen peroxide and cytolytic factor can interact synergistically in effecting cytolysis of neoplastic targets, *J. Immunol.*, 127, 1973, 1981.

65. **Matsushima, K., Onozaki, K., Benczur, M., and Oppenheim, J. J., Eds.**, Studies of the production of interleukin 1 (IL1) and potential antitumor activity of IL1, in *The Physiologic, Metabolic and Immunologic Actions of Interleukin 1*, (Progress in Leukocyte Biology Series), Alan R. Liss, New York, 1985, 253.

66. **Matsushima, K., Onozaki, K., Benczur, M., and Oppenheim, J. J.**, Studies of the production of interleukin 1 (IL1) and potential antitumor activity of IL1, *Prog. Leukocyte Biol.*, 2, 253, 1985.

67. **Currie, G. A.**, Activated macrophages kill tumor cells by releasing arginase, *Nature (London)*, 273, 758, 1978.

68. **Currie, G. A. and Basham, C.**, Differential arginine dependence and the selective cytotoxic effects of activated macrophages for malignant cells in vitro, *Br. J. Cancer*, 38, 653, 1978.

69. **Currie, G. A. and Basham, C.**, Activated macrophages release a factor which lyses malignant cells, but not normal cells, *J. Exp. Med.*, 142, 1600, 1975.

70. **Adams, D. O. and Marino, P. A.**, Evidence for a multistep mechanism of cytolysis by BCG-activated macrophages: the interrelationship between the capacity for cytolysis, target binding, and secretion of cytolytic factor, *J. Immunol.*, 126, 981, 1981.

71. **Adams, D. O.**, Effector mechanisms of cytolytically activated macrophages. I. Secretion of neutral proteases and effect of protease inhibitors, *J. Immunol.*, 124, 286, 1980.

72. **Adams, D. O., Kao, K. J., Fark, R., and Pizzo, S. W.**, Effector mechanisms of cytolytically activated macrophages. II. Secretion of a cytolytic factor by activated macrophages and its relationship to secreted neutral proteases, *J. Immunol.*, 124, 293, 1980.

73. **Marino, P. A. and Adams, D. O.**, Interaction of Bacillus Calmette-Guerin-activated macrophages and neoplastic cells in vitro. I. Conditions of binding and its selectivity, *Cell. Immunol.*, 54, 11, 1980.

74. **Marino, P. A. and Adams, D. O.**, Interaction of Bacillus Calmette-Guerin-activated macrophages and neoplastic cells in vitro. II. The relationship of selective binding to cytolysis, *Cell. Immunol.*, 54, 26, 1980.

75. **Adams, D. O. and Marino, P.**, Activation of mononuclear phagocytes for destruction of tumor cells as a model for study of macrophage development, *Contemp. Hematol. Oncol.*, 3, 69, 1984.

76. **Johnson, W. J., Somers, S. D., and Adams, D. O.**, Activation of macrophages for tumor cytotoxicity, *Contemp. Top. Immunobiol.*, 14, 127, 1984.

77. **Adams, D. O., Johnson, W., and Marino, P. A.,** Mechanisms of target recognition and destruction in macrophage-mediated tumor cytotoxicity, *Fed. Proc. Fed. Am. Soc. Exp. Biol.,* 41, 2212, 1982.
78. **Somers, D. S., Whisnant, C. C., and Adams, D. O.,** Quantification of the strength of cell-cell adhesion: The capture of tumor cells by activated murine macrophages proceeds through two direct stages, *J. Immunol.,* 136(4), 1490, 1986.
79. **Johnson, W. J., Goldfarb, R. H., and Adams, D. O.,** Secretion of a novel cytolytic protease by activated murine macrophages: its properties and role in tumor cytolysis, in *Lymphokines,* Mizell, S. and Pick, E., Eds., Academic Press, New York, 11, 157, 1986.
80. **Adams, D. O., Marino, P. A., and Meltzer, M. S.,** Characterization of genetic deficits in macrophage tumoricidal capacity: identification of murine strains with abnormalities in secretion of cytolytic factor and ability to bind neoplasic targets, *J. Immunol.,* 126, 1843, 1981.
81. **Johnson, W. J., Pizzo, S. V., Imber, M. J., and Adams, D. O.,** Receptors for maleylated proteins regulate the secretion of neutral proteases by murine macrophages, *Science,* 218, 574, 1982.
82. **Adams, D. O., Cohen, M. S., and Koren, H. S.,** Activation of mononuclear phagocytes for cytolysis: parallels and contrasts between activation for tumor cytotoxicity and for ADCC, in *Macrophage-Mediated Antibody-Dependent Cellular Cytotoxicity,* Koren, H. S., Ed., Marcel Dekker, New York, 1983, 43.
83. **Johnson, W. J., Marino, P. A., Schreiber, R. D., and Adams, D. O.,** Sequential activation of murine mononuclear phagocytes for tumor cytolysis: differential expression of markers by macrophages in the several stages of development, *J. Immunol.,* 131, 1083, 1983.
84. **Johnson, W. J., Bolognesi, D., and Adams, D. O.,** Antibody-dependent cytolysis (ADCC) of tumor cells by activated murine macrophages is a two-step process: quantification of target binding and subsequent target lysis, *Cell. Immunol.,* 83, 170, 1984.
85. **Adams, D. O. and Nathan, C. F.,** Molecular mechanisms operative in cytolysis of tumor cells by activated macrophages, *Immunol. Today,* 4, 166, 1983.
86. **Adams, D. O. and Hamilton, T. A.,** Destruction of tumor cells by mononuclear phagocytes: models for analyzing effector mechanisms and regulation of macrophage activation, in *Basic Mechanisms of Host Resistance to Infectious Agents, Tumors, and Allografts,* North, R. J. and Steinman, R. M., Eds., Rockefeller University Press, New York, 1986, 185.
87. **Adams, D. O. and Hamilton, T. A.,** The cell biology of macrophage activation, *Annu. Rev. Immunol.,* 2, 283, 1984.
88. **Carswell, E. A., Old, L. J., Kassel, R. L., Green, S., Fiore, N., and Williamson, B.,** An endotoxin-induced serum factor that causes necrosis of tumors, *Proc. Natl. Acad. Sci. U.S.A.,* 72, 3666, 1975.
89. **Old, L. J.,** Tumor necrosis factor (TNF), *Science,* 230, 630, 1985.
90. **Mannel, D. H., Moore, R. H., and Mergenhagen, S. E.,** Macrophages as a source of tumoricidal activity (tumor-necrotizing factor), *Infect. Immun.,* 30, 523, 1980.
91. **Matthews, N.,** Tumor necrosis factor from the rabbit. II. Production by monocytes, *Br. J. Cancer,* 38, 310, 1978.
92. **Matthews, N.,** Production of an anti-tumor cytotoxin by human monocytes, *Immunology,* 44, 135, 1981.
93. **Gray, P. W., Aggarwal, B. B., Benton, C. V., Bringman, T. S., Henzel, W. J., Jarrett, J. A., Lung, D. W., Moffat, B., Ng, P., Svedersky, L. P., Palladino, M. A., and Nedwin, G. E.,** Cloning and expression of cDNA for human lymphotoxin, a lymphokine with tumor necrosis activity, *Nature (London),* 312, 721, 1984.
94. **Pennica, D., Nedwin, G. E., Hayflick, J. S., Seeburg, P. H., Derynck, S. R., Palladino, M. A., Kowr, W. J., Aggarwal, B. B., and Goeddel, D. V.,** Human tumor necrosis factor: precursor structure, expression, and homology to lymphotoxin, *Nature (London),* 312, 724, 1984.
95. **Wang, A. M., Creasy, A. A., Ladner, M. B., Lin, L. S., Strickler, J., Van Arsdell, J. N., Yamamoto, R., and Mark, D. F.,** Molecular cloning of the complementary DNA for human tumor necrosis factor, *Science,* 228, 149, 1985.
96. **Urban, J. L., Shepard, H. M., Rothstein, J. L., Sugarman, B. J., and Schreiber, H.,** Tumor necrosis factor: a potent effector molecule for tumor cell killing by activated macrophages, *Proc. Natl. Acad. Sci. U.S.A.,* 83, 5233, 1986.
97. **Munker, R., Gasson, J., Ogawa, M., and Koeffler, H. P.,** Recombinant human TNF induces production of granulocyte-monocyte colony-stimulating factor, *Nature (London),* 323, 79, 1986.
98. **Sugarman, B. J., Aggarwal, B. B., Hass, P. E., Figari, I. S., Palladino, M. A., and Shepard, H. M.,** Recombinant human tumor necrosis factor-α: effects on proliferation of normal and transformed cells in vitro, *Science,* 230, 943, 1985.
99. **Vilcek, J., Palombella, V. J., Henriksen-Destefano, D., Swenson, C., Feinman, R., Hirai, M., and Tsujmoto, M.,** Fibroblast growth enhancing activity of tumor necrosis factor and its relationship to other polypeptide growth factors, *J. Exp. Med.,* 163, 632, 1986.
100. **Trinchieri, G., Kobayashi, M., Rosen, M., London, R., Murphy, M., and Periassia, B.,** Tumor necrosis factor and lymphotoxin induce differentiation of human myeloid cell lines in synergy with immune interferon, *J. Exp. Med.,* 164, 1206, 1986.

101. **Rubin, B. Y., Anderson, S. L., Sullivan, S. A., Williamson, B. D., Carswell, E. A., and Old, L. J.**, High affinity binding of ^{125}I-labelled human tumor necrosis factor (LukII) to specific cell surface receptors, *J. Exp. Med.*, 162, 1099, 1985.

102. **Kull, F. C., Jacobs, S., and Cuatrecasas, P.**, Cellular receptor for ^{125}I labeled tumor necrosis factor: specific binding, affinity labeling, and relationship to sensitivity, *Proc. Natl. Acad. Sci. U.S.A.*, 82, 5756, 1985.

103. **Hass, P. E., Hotchkiss, A., Mohler, M., and Aggarwal, B. B.**, Characterization of specific high affinity receptors for human tumor necrosis factor on mouse fibroblasts, *J. Biol. Chem.*, 260, 1214, 1985.

104. **Rubin, B. Y., Anderson, S. L., Sullivan, S. A., Williamson, B. D., Carswell, E. A., and Old, L. J.**, Nonhematopoietic cells selected for resistance to tumor necrosis factor produce tumor necrosis factor, *J. Exp. Med.*, 164, 1305, 1986.

105. **Kirstein, M., Fiers, W., and Baglioni, C.**, Growth inhibition and cytotoxicity of tumor necrosis factor in L929 cells is enhanced by high cell density and inhibition of mRNA synthesis, *J. Immunol.*, 137, 2277, 1986.

106. **Kunkel, S. L., Wiggins, R. C., Chensue, S. W., and Larrick, J.**, Regulation of macrophage tumor necrosis factor production by prostaglandin E2, *Biochem. Biophys. Res. Commun.*, 137, 404, 1986.

107. **Zacharchuk, C. M., Drysdale, B. E., Mayer, M. M., and Shin, H. S.**, Macrophage-mediated cytotoxicity: role of a soluble macrophage cytotoxic factor similar to lymphotoxin and tumor necrosis factor, *Proc. Natl. Acad. Sci. U.S.A.*, 80, 6341, 1983.

108. **Krahenbuhl, J. L. and Remington, J. S.**, The role of activated macrophages in specific and nonspecific cytostasis of tumor cells, *J. Immunol.*, 113, 507, 1974.

109. **Keller, R.**, Cytostatic elimination of syngeneic rat tumor cells in vitro by nonspecifically activated macrophages, *J. Exp. Med.*, 138, 625, 1973.

110. **Hibbs, J. B. et al.**, unpublished observations.

111. **Stewart, C. C.**, unpublished data.

Chapter 4

PROSTAGLANDIN REGULATION OF MACROPHAGE FUNCTION

Bruce S. Zwilling and Louis B. Justement

TABLE OF CONTENTS

I. INTRODUCTION

Prostaglandins act as important mediators of inflammation by regulating the function of the cells that participate in inflammatory and immune responses. Macrophages produce prostaglandins and are also affected by them. There is a complex relationship between the inflammatory (stimulatory) and anti-inflammatory (inhibitory) effects of prostaglandins and how macrophages respond to the binding of these products to specific receptors on the cell membrane. Prostaglandins appear to stimulate resting macrophages and to inhibit activated cells. Although in some cases the effects of prostaglandins on macrophage function may be mediated by as yet undefined mechanisms, most of their effects appear to be mediated by increases in intracellular cyclic AMP. Here, we review the effects of agents that stimulate adenylate cyclase and result in an increase in intracellular cAMP, as well as the effects of cAMP itself on macrophage function. Most of the effects of cAMP occur by the activation of a set of cAMP-dependent protein kinases (A-kinases). Although very little information is available concerning the role of these A-kinases in macrophages, the evidence indicates that changes in the ratio of the two isozymes may be important in regulating macrophage differentiation.

II. PROSTAGLANDIN SYNTHESIS AND RELEASE BY MACROPHAGES

Prostaglandins are locally acting lipid hormones. They are derived from arachidonic acid which is cleaved from membrane phospholipids by phospholipase enzymes in the cell membrane. The phospholipases are activated by substances that disturb the cell membrane. Free arachidonic acid is oxygenated by one of two enzyme pathways: cyclooxygenase which results in the production of the prostaglandins, or the lipoxygenase enzymes which catalyze the production of the leukotrienes (Figure 1). Which final fatty acid metabolites are formed depends upon the cell and its environment. Thus, a cell may have the synthetic capacity for any or all of the oxygenation products, but only one of the pathways may be activated. This may account for some of the confusion in the literature concerning the major prostaglandins that are produced by macrophages. Although the leukotrienes also affect macrophage function, we will limit our discussion to the effects of the prostaglandins. The prostaglandins produced by macrophages are PGE_1, PGE_2, $PGF_{2\alpha}$, prostacyclin (PGI_2, detected as 6-keto-$PGF_{1\alpha}$), and thromboxane A_2 (detected as TXB_2).

A variety of stimuli result in the activation of phospholipase and the cleavage of arachidonic acid. Lipopolysaccharide[1] (LPS), calcium ionophore,[2] zymosan,[3] phorbol acetate,[4,5] complement components,[6] interferon,[6,7] and immune complexes[9,10] are among the stimuli that will activate the phospholipase enzymes. Two enzymes have been identified that cleave arachidonic acid from membrane phosphatidylcholine, phosphatidylethanolamine, or phosphatidylinositol.[4] One, phospholipase C, has a pH optimum of 4.5 and is Ca^{2+} independent; the second, phospholipase A_2, has a pH optimum of 8.5 and requires Ca^{2+}.

Once cleaved, arachidonic acid is converted to prostaglandins by cyclooxygenase enzymes. A recent report indicates that arachidonic acid may be transported, by an as yet unidentified mechanism, to the endoplasmic reticulum for this conversion. Darte and Beaufay[11] examined the subcellular localization of the enzymes that convert arachidonic acid to PGE_2. Using homogenates from unstimulated macrophages, they found that PGE_2 synthesis was associated with sedimentable elements derived from the endoplasmic reticulum. The density distribution in the linear sucrose gradient indicated that PGE_2 synthesis behaved like sulfatase C, an enzyme that is used as a reference for endoplasmic reticulum. The optimum pH of the cyclooxygenase enzymes was 6.5 to 7.5.

Most of the studies that have determined the type and amount of prostaglandin produced by macrophages have utilized cells purified by adherence and then cultured for at least 16

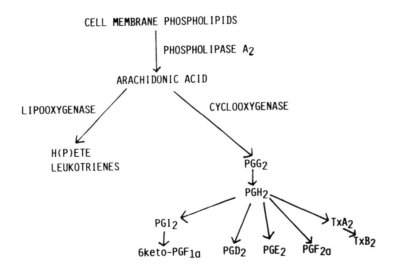

FIGURE 1. Arachidonic acid oxygenation products. Activation of membrane phospholipase A_2 cleaves arachidonic acid from phosphatidylcholine or phosphatidylethanolamine. The arachidonic acid is oxygenated by cyclooxygenase enzymes to PGG_2 which is converted to prostaglandins, thromboxane, or protacyclin (PGI_2). The lipoxygenase enzymes oxygenate arachidonic acid to hydroperoxyeicosatetraenoic acids (H(P)ETES) or leukotrienes.

hr in the presence of fetal bovine serum.[2-4,12-19] Since it is likely that the fetal bovine serum used in these studies contained amounts of bacterial LPS sufficient to provide some stimulus to the cells, definitive information concerning the endogenous production of prostaglandins is unavailable nor does there appear to be a consensus concerning which of the prostaglandins is the likely predominant product of unstimulated cells. PGE_2, prostacyclin, and thromboxane B_2 have all been reported to be the predominant arachidonic acid metabolite produced by resident mouse peritoneal macrophages. There is a general consensus, however, that PGE_2 is the major prostaglandin produced in response to inflammatory stimuli such as zymosan or immune complexes. Interestingly, macrophages elicited by thioglycollate, protease peptone, and *Corynebacterium parvum* produce less PGE_2 than do resident cells.[19,20] The release of arachidonic acid from thioglycollate-elicited cells is only 20% of that released by the resident macrophages and could account for the decrease in cyclooxygenase products.

The amount of arachidonic acid oxygenation products released by macrophages does not appear to correlate with macrophage activation.[19-21] Although LPS-treated macrophages and macrophages from Bacillus Calmette Guerin (BCG)- and pyran-injected mice release high levels of PGE_2, those from *C. parvum*-injected animals release low levels of PGE_2. Lymphokine treatment has been reported to result in increases and decreases in the level of PGE_2 released by the cells. A study by Snider et al. compared the prostaglandin production by operationally defined macrophage subsets (Table 1).[19] They found that PGE_2 was the major arachidonic acid metabolite produced by activated cells; PGE_2 and PGI_2 were produced in equal amounts by resident cells, and peptone and thioglycollate-elicited cells produced even lower amounts.

Synthesis and release of prostaglandins were initially thought to be a direct and immediate consequence of phagocytosis. Studies by Rouzer et al.,[9] however, showed that binding to the Fc receptor was a sufficient stimulus. Although ingestion of particles did stimulate prostaglandin synthesis, inhibition of phagosome-lysosome fusion with dextran sulfate or inhibition of membrane internalization with cytochalasin D did not block prostaglandin synthesis. In this regard Suzuki et al.[10] has shown that binding of $Fc\gamma_{2b}$ receptors by immune

Table 1

**PROSTAGLANDINS PRODUCED BY
OPERATIONALLY DEFINED MACROPHAGE
POPULATIONS[19]**

Macrophage	Prostaglandins produced[a]			
	PGE$_2$	TXB$_2$	6-keto-PGE$_{1\alpha}$	PGF$_{2\alpha}$
Resident	602	120	600	10
Thioglycollate	300	180	130	24
Peptone	0	120	50	0
Pyran activated	750	375	200	125
BCG activated	1146	510	200	180

Note: The concentrations of PGs were determined by radioimmunoassay. Macrophages were incubated for 24 hr in McCoy's 5A medium containing 10% fetal bovine serum. The amount of PG released into the supernatant fluid was determined.

[a]   Picograms per 10^6 cells.

Table 2

**EFFECT OF PGE$_2$ ON MACROPHAGE
FUNCTIONAL CAPACITY**

Function	Effect	Ref.
Phagocytosis	Stimulates	23, 24, 25
	Inhibits	22
Collagenase production	Stimulates	30, 31, 84
Protease production	Stimulates?	32
	Inhibits	82, 83
Antitumor activity	Stimulates	34, 35, 36, 37
	Inhibits	44, 45, 46, 47
Ia expression	Inhibits	38, 39, 41
Chemotactic response	Inhibits	48
CSF-1 response	Inhibits	49, 50
MIF response	Inhibits	51
IL-production	Inhibits	52

complexes activates phospholipase A$_2$ activity, freeing arachidonic acid for conversion to prostaglandins.

Even as macrophages are stimulated to produce prostaglandins, the effect of these endogenous products can have important consequences on macrophage function. Prostaglandins, mostly PGE$_2$, have been reported to stimulate as well as to inhibit the functional activity of the mononuclear phagocyte (Table 2).

III. PROSTAGLANDINS AND MACROPHAGE FUNCTION

A. Prostaglandins Affect Phagocytosis

Initial reports indicated that prostaglandins of the E series inhibited phagocytosis of inert particles.[22] Studies by Razin et al.,[23] however, demonstrated that low concentrations of PGE could stimulate phagocytosis of opsonized sheep red blood cells (RBC). Further studies showed that indomethacin, a potent cyclooxygenase inhibitor, decreased the phagocytic activity of murine peritoneal exudate macrophages. Activity could be restored by the addition of PGE_2. Addition of PGE_2 to untreated cells also enhanced phagocytosis of opsonized sheep RBC. These studies were later confirmed and extended by Vogel et al.,[24] who showed that agents, such as PGE_2, that stimulated an increase in intracellular cAMP, restored a defect in Fc-receptor-mediated phagocytosis by macrophages from LPS-unresponsive C3H/HeJ mice. Similarly, Schneck et al.[25] showed that Fc-receptor-mediated phagocytosis by defective variants of the J774.2 macrophage cell line could be restored by the addition of cAMP. It was concluded that cAMP enhanced the number of Fc receptors expressed by the cells and increased Fc-receptor-mediated phagocytosis. It was further suggested that the phagocytosis mediated by IgG_{2a} and IgG_{2b} was different and that the effect of cAMP on phagocytosis mediated by the two IgG receptors was also different.

In addition to the ability of PGE_2 and other agents that increase intracellular cAMP to stimulate phagocytosis of opsonized particles per se, the binding of these particles to the macrophage Fcγ receptors also results in increased synthesis of PGE_2 (with a concomitant increase in intracellular cAMP). Studies by Suzuki and co-workers[10,26-28] have shown that the Fcγ_{2b} receptor isolated from the murine macrophage cell line P388D1 possesses an intrinsic phospholipase A_2 activity, whereas the Fc$\gamma_{2\alpha}$ receptor lacks this activity. Since phospholipase A_2 results in an increase in free arachidonic acid, binding of the Fcγ_{2b} receptor by immune complexes results in an increase in prostaglandin release, whereas binding of immune complexes to the Fcγ_{2a} receptor does not. Binding of both receptors, however, induces an increase in intracellular cAMP, albeit by different pathways, and leads to enhanced phagocytosis. The prostaglandins produced in response to Fc receptor binding also affect other functional activities of the macrophage.[29]

B. Prostaglandins Stimulate Enzyme Production

Binding of immune complexes has been shown to stimulate collagenase production by both guinea pigs and murine macrophages.[30,31] This stimulation is dependent on the production of PGE_2, in that the addition of indomethacin to cultures of LPS-stimulated macrophages inhibited both PGE_2 synthesis and production of collagenase and that the addition of PGE_2 to the indomethacin treated cultures restored collagenase production. The possibility that the secretion of other macrophage enzymes may be stimulated by PGE_2 is raised by a recent report by Takemura and Webb.[32] Although the involvement of prostaglandins was not directly tested, these workers reported that binding of Fc receptors resulted in an increase in neutral protease secretion. The authors discounted the possibility that PGE_2 played a role because they observed a stimulatory effect with both IgG_{2a} and IgG_{2b} immune complexes, although only IgG_{2b} resulted in an increase in PGE_2. However, as described above, both types of Fc receptors stimulate an increase in cAMP. Procoagulant activity of rabbit alveolar macrophages has also been reported to be stimulated by PGE_2.[33]

C. Stimulation of Antitumor Activity

The stimulation of macrophage-tumoricidal activity by prostaglandins has been reported. The cytotoxic activity of LPS-activated macrophages was shown to be inhibited by the presence of indomethacin or aspirin in cultures of macrophages and tumor cells. The addition of PGE_2 to these cultures restored antitumor activity.[34-37] It has been suggested that prostaglandins may affect tumoricidal activity differently depending upon the state of macrophage activation; PGE_2 stimulated resident macrophages but inhibited the antitumor activity of activated macrophages.[35,36] However, most reports concerning the effect of prostaglandins on macrophage function indicate that PGE_2 is inhibitory.[43-47]

IV. PROSTAGLANDIN INHIBITION OF MACROPHAGE FUNCTION

A. Ia Expression

PGE_2 inhibits the lymphokine-induced maintenance of Ia expression by murine peritoneal macrophages.[38] PGE$_2$ does not inhibit Ia expression by macrophages but does prevent its induction by interferon.[39] Interestingly, this effect can be counteracted by thromboxane. Although the expression of Ia by peritoneal macrophages is transient following the injection of most antigens,[40] PGE$_2$ does not alter the kinetics of Ia loss. Additionally, PGE$_2$ does not affect continuous Ia expression by macrophages following the injection of BCG or *Corynebacterium parvum* into BCG-resistant mice.[41,42] The LPS-induced inhibition of Ia expression has been reported to be mediated by PGE$_2$ in one study[39] but was not affected by the addition of indomethacin in another.[41]

B. Antitumor Activity

Following the development of antitumor activity, macrophages in culture progressively lose the ability to kill neoplastic cells.[43,44] This loss has been attributed to an increase in PGE$_2$.[44,45] In a series of studies by Russell and co-workers[44,46,47] it was shown that the levels of PGE$_2$ increased rapidly after the addition of LPS to macrophage cultures. Nevertheless, despite the presence of PGE$_2$ in sufficient quantity to inhibit antitumor activity, macrophages initially continued to destroy tumor cells. However, a rapid loss in cytolytic activity occurred after 16 to 20 hr of culture. The addition of indomethacin to these cultures prevented both the PGE$_2$ synthesis and the loss of cytolytic activity. Further studies showed that the inhibitory effect of PGE$_2$ could be prevented and the cytolytic activity maintained despite its presence by the continued addition of gamma-interferon (IFNγ) to the culture medium. Thus, it appears that interferon blocks PGE$_2$-mediated inhibition of macrophage antitumor activity by some effect other than its reported ability to block phospholipase activation.

PGE$_2$ has also been shown to inhibit the response of macrophages to chemotactic stimuli,[48] to colony-stimulating factor-1 (CSF-1),[49,50] to migration inhibitory factor,[51] and to inhibit interleukin-1 (IL-1) production by macrophages.[52]

V. MODULATION OF cAMP

Macrophage activation in response to immunological, as well as nonimmunological stimuli is a complex, dynamic process initiated when the cell comes in contact with an external signal via plasma membrane receptors. Transmission of external signals through the plasma membrane into the cytoplasmic compartment is mediated by a number of regulatory pathways. Ligand-receptor interaction can result in depolarization of the plasma membrane,[53] fluxes in intracellular calcium levels,[54] turnover of plasma membrane phospholipid,[55,56] increased levels of cGMP, and activation of membrane-bound adenylate cyclase.[58] In the macrophage several studies have shown that intracellular levels of cAMP are modulated in response to stimulation with various hormones. Similarly, treatment of macrophages with a number of agents identified as having a role in activation or associated with the acquisition of various effector functions, also results in modulation of cAMP levels in the cell.

A. Stimulation of Adenylate Cyclase

cAMP was first identified as a "second messenger" which transduces signals received following binding of hormones to receptors, across the plasma membrane, and into the cytosol of the cells.[59] Receptors for catecholamines, peptide hormones, and prostaglandins are found in the cell membrane. Ligand binding to these receptors leads to activation of adenylate cyclase resulting in an increase in intracellular cAMP (Figure 2). Stimulation of adenylate cyclase involves an intermediate protein called the guanine nucleotide binding protein (guanine stimulatory Gs).[60,61] The Gs protein binds to guanosine triphosphate (GTP) or its nonhydrolyzable analogs in addition to guanosine diphosphate (GDP). Interaction of Gs with hormone receptors promotes binding of GTP by displacement of GDP which is normally bound in the basal state. The GTP-Gs complex functions to activate adenylate

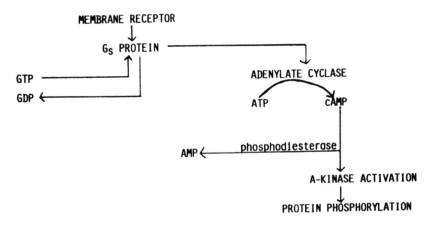

MEMBRANE RECEPTOR

G_S PROTEIN

GTP

GDP

ADENYLATE CYCLASE

ATP   cAMP

AMP ← phosphodiesterase

A-KINASE ACTIVATION

PROTEIN PHOSPHORYLATION

FIGURE 2.   Receptor-mediated activation of adenylate cyclase. Interaction of Gs protein (guanine nucleotide binding protein) with hormone (PGE_2) receptors promotes binding of GTP by displacement of GDP which is normally bound in the basal state. The GTP-Gs complex activates adenylate cyclase which converts ATP to cAMP. The cAMP activates A-kinases by binding to their regulatory subunits and releasing the catalytic subunit.

cyclase resulting in the hydrolysis of bound GTP. The resultant formation of a GDP-Gs complex removes the activation stimulus from adenylate cyclase until GDP is again displaced by GTP. Once adenylate cyclase has been activated by the Gs protein, it stimulates conversion of ATP into cAMP which then serves as a second messenger for the hormone via activation of specific cAMP dependent A-kinases.[53,59]

Using selective β_2-adrenergic stimulants and blocking agents, Ikegami showed that catecholamines bind to β_2 receptors resulting in an increase in cAMP in rat peritoneal macrophages.[62] Stimulation of adenylate cyclase in the macrophage also occurs in response to several hormones which are not classified as β-adrenergic agonists.[63] Elicited macrophages respond to treatment with parathyroid hormone and calcitonin by a twofold increase in intracellular cAMP.

Macrophages respond to PGE_2 stimulation with an increase in cAMP.[64,65] Membrane-associated receptors for prostaglandins on the macrophage have been detected using a ^3H-PGE_2-binding assay.[66] Macrophages express receptors on their surface which bind PGE_2 via a specific saturable mechanism. Unlabeled prostaglandins compete with ^3H-PGE_2 for binding with a potency series of $PGE_2 > PGE_1 > PGI_2$. The ability to compete correlates with the capacity to stimulate adenylate cyclase. Based upon competition kinetics, it is apparent that macrophages express more than one type of prostaglandin receptor on their surface. Gemsa and associates[67] observed that treatment of macrophages with PGE generated a rapid increase in intracellular cAMP. The increase was accompanied by a progressive accumulation of the nucleotide in the extracellular space. Additional experiments demonstrated that the A-type and F-type prostaglandins elicited a much smaller increase in cAMP levels. The same order of potency was observed when prostaglandins were used to stimulate cAMP production in other leukocytes.[68] Further studies revealed that treatment of macrophages with concanavalin A (Con A) or a microtubule inhibitor, colchicine, increased the sensitivity of cells to the effects of PGE_1.[69] Similar results were obtained when agents were tested in the presence of isoproterenol and cholera toxin. This suggests that sensitivity of the macrophage to agents which increase production of cAMP can be modulated by treatment with substances that affect the organization of plasma membrane components, microtubule function, or ion transport. The effect of Con A and colchicine on macrophage sensitivity to PGE_1, resulting in activation of adenylate cyclase. was primarily due to alterations of the plasma membrane. Enhanced stimulation of adenylate cyclase following the use of agents which alter membrane conformation supports the concept that hormone binding to receptors activates adenylate cyclase indirectly via transducing proteins in the membrane. Interaction of the hormone receptors with Gs protein and adenylate cyclase may be facilitated by treatment with Con A or colchicine.

B. Stimulation of cAMP

Treatment of macrophages with calcium ionophore A23187 has been shown to cause an increase in intracellular cAMP.[70-73] The increase required extracellular calcium and was inhibited by the addition of indomethacin. The increase in cAMP occurred within 1 min following the addition of ionophore and was not due to inactivation of phosphodiesterases. Additional studies[73] found that the increase in cAMP following treatment with A23187 could be blocked by the addition of calcium channel blockers, calmodulin blockers, and inhibitors of phospholipase A_2 or cyclooxygenase. Furthermore, A23187-induced prostaglandin production was markedly reduced when cells were preincubated with 8-bromo-cAMP, dibutyryl cAMP, or cholera toxin. The addition of arachidonic acid alleviated the inhibition. These observations suggest the existence of a self-limiting regulatory mechanism in which A23187-treated macrophages respond to an influx of Ca^{2+} into the cell: the Ca^{2+} stimulates turnover of arachidonic acid which is converted to prostaglandin which in turn activates adenylate cyclase. cAMP then modulates subsequent prostaglandin production in a feedback mechanism by affecting steps prior to formation of arachidonic acid.

The response of macrophages to agents which stimulate cAMP production is a short-lived phenomenon. Treatment with isoproterenol and the phosphodiesterase inhibitor aminophylline resulted in a dose-dependent elevation of cAMP within 1 min followed by a gradual return to basal levels after 2 min.[74] Continuous stimulation by the addition of fresh isoproterenol and aminophylline did not maintain or increase levels of cAMP. The presence of aminophylline in these cultures raises the possibility that phosphodiesterases were not involved in the decrease in cAMP. The results of this study suggest that the addition to macrophage cultures of agents that stimulate cAMP results in the rapid development of a refractory state. A similar desensitization was observed following the addition of PGE_2;[75] pretreatment of macrophages with PGE_2 for as few as 5 min resulted in a significant decrease in cAMP production. Analogous results were obtained when epinephrine was used to pretreat cells. These studies indicate that hormone-specific desensitization is involved in the control of intracellular cAMP concentrations in the macrophage. Stimulation and desensitization of macrophage adenylate cyclase by prostaglandins and catecholamines occur via two separate classes of receptors.[76] The catecholamine-induced stimulation is mediated by β-adrenergic receptors, whereas prostaglandin-induced stimulation is not. Desensitization of macrophages to adenylate cyclase agonists was found to be specific in that incubation of intact macrophages with prostaglandins decreased adenylate cyclase responsiveness to PGE_2 alone. Basal epinephrine and NaF-stimulated adenylate cyclase activity was unaffected. Similarly, treatment of macrophages with epinephrine decreased the adenylate cyclase response when cells were incubated with catecholamines but not with PGE_2.

Verghese and Snyderman[77] characterized the molecular mechanisms involved in activation of adenylate cyclase by prostaglandins. Significant stimulation of adenylate cyclase in macrophage membranes was observed following treatment with guanine nucleotide. The addition of GTP resulted in a twofold increase in adenylate cyclase activity which subsided after 15 min. In contrast, the nonhydrolyzable analog Gpp(NH)p caused a persistent hormone-dependent activation of adenylate cyclase. Isoproterenol and PGE_1 did not activate adenylate cyclase in the absence of guanine nucleotide; however, a threefold increase in adenylate cyclase was observed to occur in the presence of guanine nucleotides alone. Based on these findings the authors proposed that the mechanism of adenylate cyclase activation in the macrophage involves a ternary complex composed of the specific hormone receptor, adenylate cyclase, and guanine nucleotide regulatory protein Gs, which transduces the hormone signal from the receptor to adenylate cyclase. Activation of adenylate cyclase and increased levels of cAMP have been shown following treatment of macrophages with agents that have the ability to activate the cell to acquisition of effector function. Snider et al.[19] measured increased intracellular levels of cAMP in macrophage subpopulations elicited with peptone or BCG as compared to resident cells. An increased state of activation, as defined by cytolytic effector function, correlated with high levels of cAMP within the cell.

Products of activated lymphocytes also result in enhancement of macrophage adenylate cyclase.[78] Addition of lymphokines to macrophage cultures increases adenylate cyclase activity after 24 to 48 hr of incubation. Lymphokine does not act by binding to β-adrenergic receptors because the addition of β-adrenergic agonists or blockers to the cultures did not affect adenylate cyclase activation by lymphokine. Macrophages treated with conditioned medium from Con A-stimulated lymphocytes that contained macrophage activating factor produced increased amounts of prostaglandins. The addition of indomethacin to these cultures increased the sensitivity of adenylate cyclase to activation by lymphokine following removal of the cyclooxygenase inhibitor. Confirmation of the role of lymphokine in stimulating intracellular levels of cAMP was provided by Vogel and co-workers who demonstrated that treatment of macrophages with conditioned medium from Con A-stimulated lymphocytes for 48 hr resulted in a 60% increase in the levels of macrophage intracellular cAMP.[79]

β-Interferon and binding of immune complexes to Fc receptors also increase intracellular cAMP.[80] The maximal response to β-interferon occurred 5 hr after the addition of 1000 units. As described earlier, Suzuki and co-workers reported that binding of both IgG_{2a} and IgG_{2b} immune complexes resulted in an increase of cAMP.[10,26-29] The increase mediated by binding to $Fc\gamma_{2a}$ was a result of direct triggering of adenylate cyclase. In contrast, $Fc\gamma_{2b}$ stimulation of adenylate cyclase was not direct and was mediated through Gs protein following the binding of PGE_2 to its receptor. Interestingly, Walker has reported that IgG_{2a} antibodies were active in stimulating phagocytosis by the IC-21 macrophage cell line, whereas IgG_{2b} antibodies were active in promoting extracellular killing of target cells.[81] This observation suggests that the binding of different Fc receptors, both of which result in an increase in cAMP, promotes different functions.

VI. EFFECTS OF cAMP ON MACROPHAGE FUNCTION

cAMP has numerous effects on macrophage function as demonstrated by studies utilizing cAMP analogs or agents which stimulate adenylate cyclase. Preincubation of macrophages with 8-bromo or dibutyryl analogs of cAMP, with phosphodiesterase inhibitors, or with PGE_2, causes a significant inhibition of oxygen radical production following the stimulation with A23187.[73] The production and secretion of proteolytic enzymes by macrophages have also been shown to be inhibited by cAMP.[82,83] In variants of the macrophage-like cell line J774.2 that lack cAMP-dependent A-kinase, plasminogen activator secretion cannot be inhibited by the addition of either 8-bromo-cAMP or cholera toxin. This observation raises the possibility that the inhibitory action of cAMP involves activation of A-kinases. In contrast to the inhibitory effect of cAMP on production and secretion of plasminogen activator, cAMP has been shown to stimulate collagenase production by macrophages.[30,84] The addition of indomethacin to LPS-stimulated guinea pig macrophages was found to inhibit not only prostaglandin production, but also increases in cAMP and the production of collagenase. The addition of dibutyrl cAMP or cholera toxin to cultures pretreated with indomethacin restored macrophage collagenase production but not prostaglandin synthesis. Additionally, dibutyryl cAMP and cholera toxin were shown to potentiate collagenase production by LPS-stimulated macrophages.

Early studies on the mechanism of action of migration inhibitory factor (MIF) indicated that agents which increased cellular cAMP inhibited the activity of MIF.[51] The addition of dibutyryl cAMP to cultures also prevented inhibition of macrophage migration by the MIF. Subsequent studies by Higgins and David,[74] carried out to determine whether the action of MIF on macrophages involved the lowering of cAMP levels, found that the addition of MIF to macrophage cultures did not cause a decrease below basal levels. In contrast, studies by Pick showed that incubation of macrophages with MIF for 1 to 2 hr resulted in a moderate but consistent decrease in intracellular cAMP.[85] Furthermore, MIF was found to decrease the response of macrophages to PGE_1, PGE_2, isoproterenol, and cholera toxin. These results indicate that MIF does not inhibit macrophage migration by increasing cAMP. MIF activity may be due to its ability to decrease cAMP or to inhibit macrophage responses to agents that stimulate cAMP production.

Increased cAMP has been reported to have both stimulatory and inhibitory effects on phagocytosis. In one study, treatment of murine peritoneal macrophages with interferon (IFN) was found to stimulate phagocytic activity and production of cAMP.[80] Incorporation of the adenylate cyclase inhibitor N-ethylmaleimide into cultures treated with IFN prevented the increase in cAMP but did not affect phagocytic activity. It was concluded that cAMP levels in the cell do not affect phagocytosis. In contrast, dibutyryl cAMP has been reported to inhibit phagocytosis of starch particles.[22] The increased oxidation of ^{14}C-glucose to $^{14}CO_2$, which normally accompanies phagocytosis, was also found to be decreased in the presence of theophylline, a phosphodiesterase inhibitor. Phagocytosis of antibody-coated sheep RBC has also been shown to be sensitive to agents which inhibit phosphodiesterase activity such as theophylline, 5'-AMP, 3',5'-AMP, and 2-dichloroadenosine.[86] Increased concentrations of cAMP resulting from phosphodiesterase inhibitors caused a 40 to 80% decrease in phagocytosis of sheep RBCs. As expected, imidazole and phenylimidothiazole, agents which potentiate phosphodiesterase action, were found to increase phagocytic activity above control levels.

Other studies have also reported the down regulation of phagocytosis by cAMP or agents which stimulate its production. Fibronectin-mediated phagocytosis by macrophages is inhibited by PGI_2 and PGE_2.[87] In both instances, the action of the prostaglandins is due to their ability to stimulate cAMP production. Finally, uptake of the parasite *Trypanosoma cruzi* was decreased following treatment of macrophages with isoproterenol, PGE_1, theophylline, and dibutyryl cAMP.[88]

Despite these observations, and as described earlier, receptor-mediated phagocytosis appears to be enhanced by cAMP or cAMP agonists. Razin et al. reported that prostaglandins potentiated phagocytosis of opsonized sheep RBCs by murine macrophages.[23] Vogel and Rosenstreich[89] examined macrophages from LPS-unresponsive C_3H/HeJ mice which characteristically lose the ability to phagocytize opsonized sheep RBC in vitro. Treatment with lymphokine was able to restore macrophage phagocytic function. Because of the known ability of lymphokine to increase intracellular cAMP, studies were conducted to determine if cAMP itself could restore phagocytic activity.[24] The addition of 8-bromo-cAMP, dibutyryl cAMP, isoproterenol, and PGE_1 all restored the ability of macrophages from the nonresponder mice to bind sheep RBC and to ingest them at a rate comparable to that of macrophages from LPS-responsive mice of the strain C_3H/HeN. In a series of studies using variants of the macrophage cell line J774.2 which were unable to ingest opsonized sheep RBCs, although they could rosette IgG-coated sheep RBCs and ingest latex particles, the addition of cAMP analogs and agonists of cAMP restored phagocytic capability in 50% of the variants tested.[90-92] More recently the effects of IFN on Fc-receptor-mediated phagocytosis and on intracellular levels of cAMP in the J774.2 cell line and its variants were examined.[25] Interferon increased phagocytic activity in the parental cell line as well as in the cAMP responsive variants. No potentiation of sheep RBC ingestion was observed in cultures of cAMP-unresponsive variants or adenylate cyclase-deficient or A-kinase-deficient variants.

Under conditions in which interferon augmented phagocytosis, an increase in intracellular cAMP also occurred. These experiments clearly show that receptor-mediated uptake of opsonized sheep RBC is dependent on cAMP and the presence of A-kinases.

Differences in the effects of cAMP on the antitumor activity of macrophages have also been reported. Schultz and co-workers have reported that increases in intracellular cAMP in macrophages result in a loss of macrophage-mediated cytostatic activity.[45,93,94] The inhibitory effect of PGE_2 was also shown to be by a cAMP-dependent process. In contrast, Taffet et al.[95] reported that PGE_2 but not PGI_2 inhibited macrophage cytolytic activity. Both PGE_2 and PGI_2 are potent stimulators of adenylate cyclase. It was expected that both prostaglandins would inhibit antitumor activity by increasing the intracellular levels of cAMP. However, when this was not observed, it was concluded that cAMP was not directly involved in the inhibition of cytolytic function by PGE_2.

VII. cAMP-DEPENDENT A-KINASES

Although it has been demonstrated that hormones and other agents increase intracellular levels of cAMP in the macrophage, little is known regarding the mechanism through which elevated cAMP affects the cell or its functions. Extensive evidence in other cell systems suggests that cAMP modulates cellular processes via a specific type of protein, the cAMP-dependent A-kinases.[53] The presence of A-kinases has been demonstrated in a wide spectrum of mammalian tissues[96] and the enzyme has been identified as the major cAMP binding protein in eukaryotic cells.[97,98] Binding of cAMP to A-kinase regulates the activity of this enzyme which catalyzes the transfer of the γ-phosphoryl group from MgATP to serine or threonine residues at specific sites on substrate proteins. It is the major, if not the only, function carried out by A-kinases following activation by cAMP.[99] Although it is likely that the effects of cAMP on a cell are mediated by A-kinase alone, Krebs[100] suggested five criteria which should be met before an effect mediated by cAMP can be said to occur via phosphorylation of a protein. These criteria are that the cell type involved contains an A-kinase, a protein substrate exists which bears a functional relationship to the process mediated by cAMP, phosphorylation of the substrate alters its function in vitro, the protein substrate is modified in vivo in response to cAMP, and that a phosphoprotein phosphatase exists to reverse the process. Currently, only the first criterion has been fulfilled for the macrophage.[101,102]

A-kinases can be separated by ion exchange chromatography into two major peaks, designated type I or type II.[103,104] These two major forms of A-kinases are similar in size, composition, and mechanism of activation. They differ, however, in their regulatory (R) subunits. Both isozymes occur as inactive tetramers composed of two catalytic (C) and two R subunits. The binding of cAMP results in the formation of an unstable intermediary complex containing cAMP, R dimer, and C subunits.[105] Spontaneous dissociation of the intermediate yields two free C monomers and a R dimer. The R subunits from type I and type II kinase (RI and RII) have molecular weights of 45 kdalton and 54 kdalton, respectively, on SDS-PAGE.[104] C subunits isolated from type I or type II A-kinases have identical molecular weights of 40 kdalton and exhibit similar chemical, physical, and C properties.[98] The type I isozyme exhibits a higher affinity for cAMP than does type II, resulting in preferential activation at lower concentrations of cAMP.[106]

cAMP exerts many effects on cells by virtue of its role as a second messenger for steroid hormones, prostaglandins, and other substances. Changes in cell growth, function, and differentiation caused by cAMP are brought about by phosphorylation of endogenous protein substrates by A-kinases. Mechanisms by which substrate phosphorylation is controlled include: (1) differential activation kinetics for the type I and II isozymes, (2) changes in the ratio of type I to type II isozyme within a cell, and (3) subcellular location of the A-kinases and/or substrates.[107]

In general it is believed that type I A-kinase is involved in cellular growth processes, whereas type II is associated with differentiation. Recent studies have indicated that the activity of A-kinase may be controlled in part by subcellular localization of the type I and type II isozymes.[97,108] The distribution of the A-kinase isozymes is, in turn, controlled by differences in the R subunits which act to direct them to specific locations within a cell. Subcellular localization of kinase activity provides a mechanism by which the cell can control the type and availability of endogenous protein substrates that can be phosphorylated. The existence of two isozymes with different activation kinetics and compartmentalization within a cell creates a finely tuned system for regulating kinase function. Localization of type I and type II A-kinases can occur via association with subcellular components. In addition, several studies have shown that the A-kinase isozymes actually translocate within the cell from one compartment to another in response to various stimuli.[107] Initial studies demonstrated both membrane-associated and soluble forms of A-kinase.[109-110]

The nucleus is also an important target for the action of the A-kinases. Evidence for this includes the following: (1) low endogenous levels of A-kinase exist in the nucleus, (2) certain stimuli appear to cause a translocation of A-kinase subunits into the nucleus from the cytoplasm, (3) cAMP-dependent phosphorylation of histone and nonhistone proteins occurs, and (4) dibutyryl cAMP and other agents which elevate cAMP have been shown to stimulate increases in specific mRNAs in vivo.[107] Alterations in genomic activity by A-kinase may occur via one or more of the following mechanisms: (1) activation of endogenous nuclear A-kinase, (2) translocation of cytosolic protein kinase into the nucleus in holoenzyme or subunit form, or (3) translocation into the nucleus of a phosphoprotein formed by kinase in the cytosol.[107] Participation by A-kinase subunits in the control of genomic activity could take place as a result of phosphorylation of nuclear proteins by C subunits or via binding of the R subunit to DNA or nuclear proteins associated with DNA. The observations that cytosolic levels of A-kinase C subunit decrease while, at the same time, there is an increase in nuclear levels and that no cAMP-stimulatable A-kinase can be detected in nuclei from unstimulated cells, support the hypothesis that translocation of A-kinase from the cytosol to the nucleus can occur.[111]

Translocation of the type II R subunit into the nucleus appears to be dependent upon the intracellular level of cAMP.[112] Decreased levels of cAMP were found to inhibit movement of the R subunit into the nucleus. Following translocation into the nucleus, the RII subunits bind to chromosomal structures and interact specifically with homologous DNA. Translocation of the RII subunit was found to induce the synthesis of specific proteins and may be associated with topoisomerase activity. The C subunit may translocate separately or in association with the R subunit.[113]

A. Changes in Macrophage cAMP-Dependent A-Kinase

Several studies have examined A-kinases in macrophages. Stimulation of the J774.2 macrophage cell line with LPS or 8-bromo-cAMP results in the phosphorylation of nonhistone nuclear proteins.[114] Incubation of nuclei from unstimulated cells with cytoplasmic extracts from LPS-treated cells increased phosphorylation in the nuclei. Incubation of nuclei and cytoplasm from unstimulated cells in the presence of cAMP also induced phosphorylation of nonhistone proteins. This suggests that an LPS-induced increase in cAMP activates a cAMP-dependent, nonhistone-protein-specific, protein kinase in the cytoplasm which translocates into the nucleus. The phosphorylation of nonhistone nuclear proteins occurs prior to elaboration of IL-1, suggesting a possible involvement in IL-1 production.

Another study reported that the activity of A-kinases was significantly higher in thioglycollate-stimulated macrophages than in resident rat peritoneal macrophages and that the calcium ionophore A23187 stimulated increases in kinase activity for both the resident and elicited populations via a prostaglandin-dependent mechanism.[115] Additionally, prostaglandins, 8-bromo-cAMP, and cholera toxin also stimulated A-kinase activity.

More recently Wenger and O'Dorisio[101] reported that differentiation of human peripheral blood monocytes into macrophages is accompanied by the induction of type I R subunit. Monocytes expressed the type II isozyme in their cytoplasm following isolation from whole blood. No type I R subunit could be detected following extraction of particulate fractions with NP-40. This suggests that the presence of the type I subunit in macrophages was due to *de novo* synthesis. The A-kinase type I from macrophages was found to have a higher affinity for binding of cAMP than did type II A-kinases from either monocytes or macrophages. An increase in the level of cAMP was shown to occur in association with differentiation of monocytes into macrophages.

Work in our laboratory further supports the possibility that cAMP may play a role in the differentiation process via alterations in A-kinase isozyme levels.[102] We have shown that the macrophage cell line RAW 264.7 contains both isozymes of the A-kinase enzyme. The RI subunit was no longer detectable in the cytoplasm following activation of the cell line with lymphokine and LPS, and its disappearance was associated with triggering by LPS. Furthermore, the loss of antitumor activity was associated with the reappearance of RI in the cytosol. These experiments suggest that there is a direct correlation between the presence of RI in the cytosol and cytolytic activity of the macrophage.

The disappearance of RI from the cytosol of activated macrophages may represent a mechanism by which the cell regulates effects of cAMP on the state of activation. Two possibilities exist which may explain the disappearance of RI: (1) degradation or decreased synthesis of the type I isozyme so that the predominant form of A-kinase is type II or (2) translocation of either the type I holoenzyme or the RI subunit into the nucleus or other particulate fraction. Differences in the binding affinity of regulatory subunits of type I or type II for cAMP, together with alterations in the ratio of one isozyme to the other, could provide a mechanism by which the macrophage's responsiveness to cAMP is controlled.

VIII. SUMMARY AND CONCLUSIONS

Prostaglandins and agents that stimulate an increase in intracellular cAMP alter the functional capacity of the macrophage. Their effects on the cell can be stimulatory or inhibitory. These differences may be attributed to the effects of different levels of prostaglandin and/or the state of differentiation of the macrophage. Although it is not yet clear what accounts for the different signals received by the cell following binding of prostaglandin to its receptor, part of the differences may be due to compartmentalization of the cAMP-dependent A-kinases which are regulated by the level of intracellular cAMP.

Caution must be exercised in interpreting experiments which implicate a role for prostaglandin or cAMP in cellular processes. The oxygenation pathways of arachidonic acid are complex and the addition of a prostaglandin or cAMP to the culture or inhibition of cyclooxygenase may result in the production of excess lipoxygenation products which could also affect macrophage function.

Most of the effects of prostaglandins on macrophage function have been attributed to the activation of adenylate cyclase, an increase in cAMP, and activation of A-kinases. New phosphorylated proteins have yet to be identified that may account for the alteration in cell function. The ultimate biochemical mechanism of prostaglandin regulation of macrophage function remains to be determined.

REFERENCES

1. **Cook, J. A., Wise, W. C., and Halushka, P. V.,** Thromboxane A_2 and prostacyclin production by lipopolysaccharide-stimulated macrophages, *J. Reticuloendothel. Soc.,* 30, 445, 1981.
2. **Pawlowski, N. A., Kaplan, G., Hamill, A. L., Cohn, Z. A., and Scott, W. A.,** Arachidonic acid metabolism by human monocytes. Studies with platelet-depleted cultures, *J. Exp. Med.,* 158, 393, 1983.
3. **Humes, J. L., Bonney, R. J., Pelus, L., Dahlgren, M. E., Sadowski, S. J., Kuehl, F. A., Jr., and Davis, P.,** Macrophages synthesize and release prostaglandins in response to inflammatory stimuli, *Nature (London),* 269, 149, 1977.
4. **Bonney, R. J., Davies, P., Kuehl, F. A., Jr., and Humes, J. L.,** Arachidonic acid oxygenation products produced by mouse peritoneal macrophages responding to inflammatory stimuli, *J. Reticuloendothel. Soc.,* 28, 113s, 1980.
5. **Hamilton, T. A., Rigsbee, J. E., Scott, W. A., and Adams, D. O.,** γ-interferon enhances the secretion of arachidinoc acid and metabolites from murine peritoneal macrophages stimulated with phorbol diesters, *J. Immunol.,* 134, 2631, 1985.
6. **Hansch, A. M., Seitz, M., Martionotti, G., Betz, M., Rauterberg, E. W., and Gemsa, D.,** Macrophages release arachidonic acid, prostaglandin E_2 and thromboxane in response to late complement components, *J. Immunol.,* 133, 2145, 1984.
7. **Schenkein, H. A.,** Prostaglandin E and thromboxane B_2 release by PMA-induced U93 or cells in response to C3b, *J. Leukocyte Biol.,* 39, 511, 1986.
8. **Bonney, R. J., Naruns, P., Davies, P., and Humes, J. L.,** Antigen-antibody complexes stimulate the synthesis and release of prostaglandins by mouse peritoneal macrophages, *Prostaglandins,* 18, 605, 1979.
9. **Rouzer, C. A., Scott, W. A., Kempe, J., and Cohn, Z. A.,** Prostaglandin synthesis by macrophages requires a specific receptor-ligand interaction, *Proc. Natl. Acad. Sci. U.S.A.,* 77, 1279, 1980.
10. **Suzuki, T., Saito-Taki, T., Sadasiuan, R., and Nitta, T.,** Biochemical signal transmitted by Fcγ receptors: phospholipase A_2 activity of Fcγ2b receptor of murine macrophage cell line P388D$_1$, *Proc. Natl. Acad. Sci. U.S.A.,* 79, 591, 1982.
11. **Darte, C. and Beaufay, H.,** Subcellular localization of the PGE$_2$ synthesis activity in mouse resident peritoneal macrophages, *J. Exp. Med.,* 159, 89, 1984.
12. **Kurland, J. I. and Bockman, R.,** Prostaglandin E production by human blood monocytes and mouse peritoneal macrophages, *J. Exp. Med.,* 147, 952, 1978.
13. **Kennedy, M. S., Stobo, J. D., and Goldyn, M. G.,** In vitro synthesis of prostaglandins and related lipids by populations of human peripheral blood mononuclear cells, *Prostaglandins,* 22, 135, 1980.
14. **Bray, M. A. and Gordon, D.,** Prostaglandin production by macrophages and the effect of anti-inflammatory drugs, *Br. J. Pharmacol.,* 63, 635, 1978.
15. **Scott, W. A., Zrike, J. M., Hamill, A. L., Kempe, J., and Cohn, Z. A.,** Regulation of arachidonic acid metabolites in macrophages, *J. Exp. Med.,* 152, 324, 1980.
16. **Bockman, R. S.,** Prostaglandin production by human blood monocytes and mouse peritoneal macrophages: synthesis dependent on in vitro culture conditions, *Prostaglandins,* 21, 9, 1981.
17. **Scott, W. A., Pawlowski, N. A., Andreach, M., and Cohn, Z. A.,** Resting macrophages produce distinct metabolites from exogenous arachidonic acid, *J. Exp. Med.,* 155, 535, 1982.
18. **Scott, W. A., Pawlowski, N. A., Murray, H. W., Andreach, M., Zrike, J., and Cohn, Z. A.,** Regulation of arachidonic acid metabolism by macrophage activation, *J. Exp. Med.,* 155, 1148, 1982.
19. **Snider, M. E., Fertel, R. A., and Zwilling, B. S.,** Production of arachidonic acid metabolites by operationally defined macrophage subsets, *Prostaglandins,* 25, 491, 1983.
20. **Humes, J. L., Burger, S., Galavage, M., Kuehl, F. A., Wightman, P. D., Dahlgren, M. E., Davies, P., and Bonney, R. J.,** The diminished production of arachidonic acid oxygenation products by elicited mouse peritoneal macrophages: possible mechanisms, *J. Immunol.,* 124, 2110, 1980.
21. **Goldyne, M. E. and Stobo, J. D.,** Synthesis of prostaglandins by subpopulations of human peripheral blood monocytes, *Prostaglandins,* 18, 687, 1979.
22. **Cox, J. P. and Karnovsky, M. L.,** The depression of phagocytosis by exogenous cyclic nucleotides, prostaglandins and theophylline, *J. Cell Biol.,* 59, 480, 1973.
23. **Razin, E., Bauminger, S., and Globerson, A.,** Effect of prostaglandins on phagocytosis of sheep erythrocytes by mouse peritoneal macrophages, *J. Reticuloendothel. Soc.,* 23, 237, 1978.
24. **Vogel, S. N., Weedon, C. L., Oppenheim, J. J., and Rosenstreich, D. L.,** Defective Fc-mediated phagocytosis in C3H/HeJ macrophages. II. Correction by cAMP agonists, *J. Immunol.,* 126, 441, 1981.
25. **Schneck, J., Rosen, O. M., Diamond, B., and Bloom, B. R.,** Modulation of Fc-receptor expression and Fc-mediated phagocytosis in variants of a macrophage-like cell line, *J. Immunol.,* 126, 745, 1981.
26. **Nitta, T. and Suzuki, T.,** Fcγ_{2b} receptor-mediated prostaglandin synthesis by a murine macrophage cell line (P388D$_1$), *J. Immunol.,* 128, 2527, 1982.

27. **Nitta, T. and Suzuki, T.**, Biochemical signals transmitted by Fc receptors: triggering mechanisms of the increased synthesis of adenosine-3',5'-cyclic monophosphate mediated by Fcγ_{2a}- and Fcγ_{2b}-receptors of a murine macrophage-like cell line (P388D$_2$), *J. Immunol.*, 129, 2708, 1982.

28. **Nitta, T., Saito-Taki, T., and Suzuki, T.**, Phospholipase A$_2$ activity of Fcγ_{2b} of thioglycollate-elicited murine peritoneal macrophages, *J. Leukocyte Biol.*, 36, 493, 1984.

29. **Hanaumi, K., Gray, P., and Suzuki, T.**, Fcγ receptor-mediated suppression of γ-interferon-induced Ia antigen expression on a murine macrophage-like cell line (P388D$_1$), *J. Immunol.*, 133, 2852, 1984.

30. **McCarthy, J. B., Wahl, S. M., Rees, J. C., Olsen, C. E., Sandberg, A. L., and Wahl, L. M.**, Mediation of macrophage collagenase production by 3'-5' cyclic adenosine monophosphate, *J. Immunol.*, 124, 2405, 1980.

31. **Passwell, J. H., Dayer, J-M., Gass, K., and Edelson, P. J.**, Regulation by Fc fragments of the secretion of collagenase, PGE2 and lysozyme by mouse peritoneal macrophages, *J. Immunol.*, 125, 910, 1980.

32. **Takemura, R. and Webb, Z.**, Regulation of elastase and plasminogen activator secretion in resident and inflammatory macrophages by receptors for the Fc domain of immunoglobulin G, *J. Exp. Med.*, 159, 152, 1984.

33. **Sitrin, R. G., Kaltreider, H. B., and Goldyne, M. E.**, Prostaglandin E is required for the augmentation of procoagulant activity of LPS-stimulated rabbit alveolar macrophages, *J. Immunol.*, 132, 867, 1984.

34. **Drysdale, B. E. and Shin, H. S.**, Activation of macrophages for tumor cell cytotoxicity: identification of indomethacin sensitive and insensitive pathways, *J. Immunol.*, 127, 760, 1981.

35. **McCarthy, M. E. and Zwilling, B. S.**, Differential effects of prostaglandins on the antitumor activity of normal and BCG-activated macrophages, *Cell. Immunol.*, 60, 91, 1981.

36. **Snider, M. E., Fertal, R. H., and Zwilling, B. S.**, Prostaglandin regulation of macrophage function: effect of endogenous and exogenous prostaglandins, *Cell. Immunol.*, 74, 234, 1982.

37. **Mochizuki, M., Zigler, J. S., Russell, P., and Gery, I.**, Cytostatic and cytolytic activities of macrophages. Regulation by prostaglandins, *Cell. Immunol.*, 83, 34, 1984.

38. **Snyder, D. S., Beller, D. I., and Unanue, E. R.**, Prostaglandins modulate macrophage Ia expression, *Nature (London)*, 299, 163, 1982.

39. **Steeg, P. S., Johnson, H. M., and Oppenheim, J. J.**, Regulation of murine macrophage Ia antigen expression by an immune interferon like lymphokine: inhibitory effect of endotoxin, *J. Immunol.*, 129, 2402, 1982.

40. **Beller, D. I. and Unanue, E. R.**, Regulation of macrophage populations. II. Synthesis and expression of Ia antigens by peritoneal exudate macrophages is a transient event, *J. Immunol.*, 126, 263, 1981.

41. **Vespa, L., Johnson, S. C., Aldrich, W. A., and Zwilling, B. S.**, Modulation of macrophage I-A expression: lack of effect of prostaglandins and glucocorticoids on macrophages that continuously express I-A, *J. Leukocyte Biol.*, 41, 47, 1987.

42. **Johnson, S. C. and Zwilling, B. S.**, Continuous expression of I-A antigen by peritoneal macrophages from mice resistant to *Mycobacterium bovis* (strain BCG), *J. Leukocyte Biol.*, 38, 635, 1985.

43. **Ruco, L. and Meltzer, M. S.**, Macrophage activation for tumor cytotoxicity: development of macrophage cytotoxic activity requires completion of a sequence of short-lived intermediary reactions, *J. Immunol.*, 121, 2035, 1978.

44. **Taffet, S. M. and Russell, S. W.**, Macrophage mediated tumor cell killing: regulation of expression of cytolytic activity by prostaglandin E, *J. Immunol.*, 26, 424, 1981.

45. **Schultz, R. M., Stoychkov, J. N., Pavlidis, N., Chirigos, M. A., and Olkowski, Z. L.**, Role of E-type prostaglandins in the regulation of interferon-treated macrophage cytotoxic activity, *J. Reticuloendothel. Soc.*, 26, 93, 1979.

46. **Taffet, S. M., Pace, J. L., and Russell, S. W.**, Lymphokine maintains macrophage activation for tumor cell killing by interfering with the negative regulatory effect of prostaglandin E$_2$, *J. Immunol.*, 127, 121, 1981.

47. **Russell, S. W. and Pace, J. L.**, Both the kind and magnitude of stimulus are important in overcoming the negative regulation of macrophage activation by PGE$_2$, *J. Leukocyte Biol.*, 35, 291, 1984.

48. **Gallin, J. I., Sandler, J. A., Clyman, R. I., Manganullo, V. C., and Vaughan, M.**, Agents that increase cyclic AMP inhibit accumulation of cGMP and depress human monocyte locomotion, *J. Immunol.*, 120, 492, 1978.

49. **Moore, R. N., Pitruzzello, F. J., Larsen, H. S., and Rouse, B. T.**, Feedback regulation of colony-stimulating factor (CSF-1) induced macrophage proliferation by endogenous E prostaglandins and interferon-α/β, *J. Immunol.*, 133, 541, 1984.

50. **Inouye, L. K. and Wharton, W.**, The relationship between intracellular cyclic AMP concentrations and the in vitro growth of macrophages, *J. Leukocyte Biol.*, 39, 657, 1986.

51. **Koopman, W. J., Gillis, M. H., and David, J. R.**, Prevention of MIF activity by agents known to increase cAMP, *J. Immunol.*, 110, 1609, 1973.

52. **Durum, S. L., Schmidt, J. A., and Oppenheim, J. J.**, Interleukin. I. An immunological perspective, *Annu. Rev. Immunol.*, 3, 263, 1985.

53. **Greengard, P.,** Phosphorylated proteins as physiological effectors, *Science,* 199, 146, 1978.
54. **Tsien, T., Pozzar, T., and Rink, T. J.,** Calcium activities and fluxes inside small intact cells as measured with intracellularly trapped chelators, *Adv. Cyclic Nucleotide Protein Phosphoryl. Res.,* 17, 535, 1984.
55. **Emilsson, A. and Sunder, R.,** Differential activation of phosphatidylinositol deacylation and a pathway via diphosphoinositide in macrophages responding to zymosan and ionophore A23187, *J. Biol. Chem.,* 259, 3114, 1984.
56. **Myers, R. F. and Single, M. I.,** The appearance of phospholipase activity in the human macrophage-like cell line U937 during dimethyl sulfoxide induced differentiation, *Biochem. Biophys. Res. Commun.,* 118, 217, 1984.
57. **Murad, F., Arnold, W. P., Mittal, C. K., and Brougher, J. M.,** Properties and regulation of guanylate cyclase and some proposed functions for cGMP, *Adv. Cyclic Nucleotide Res.,* 11, 175, 1979.
58. **Feder, D., Arad, H., Gay, A., Hekman, M., Helmreich, E. J., and Levitzki, A.,** Resolution, reconstitution and mode of action of the β-adrenergic receptor-dependent adenylate cyclases, *Adv. Cyclic Nucleotide Protein Phosphoryl. Res.,* 17, 61, 1984.
59. **Nimmo, H. G. and Cohen, P.,** Hormonal control of protein phosphorylation, *Adv. Cyclic Nucleotide Res.,* 8, 145, 1977.
60. **Pfeuffer, T.,** Guanine nucleotide-controlled interactions between components of adenylate cyclase, *FEBS Lett.,* 101, 85, 1979.
61. **Smigel, M., Katada, T., Northrup, J. K., Bokoch, G., Ui, M., and Gilman, A. G.,** Mechanisms of guanine nucleotide-mediated regulation of adenylate cyclase activity, *Adv. Cyclic Nucleotide Protein Phosphoryl. Res.,* 17, 1, 1984.
62. **Ikegami, K.,** Modulation of adenosine 3',5'-monophosphate contents of rat peritoneal macrophages mediated by B₂-adrenergic receptors, *Biochem. Pharmacol.,* 26, 1813, 1977.
63. **Minkin, C., Blackman, L., Newbry, J., Pokress, S., Posek, R., and Walling, M.,** Effects of parathyroid hormone and calcitonin on adenylate cyclase in murine mononuclear phagocytes, *Biochem. Biophys. Res. Commun.,* 76, 875, 1977.
64. **Bonney. R. J., Burger, S., Davies, P., Kuehl, F. A., Jr., and Humes, J. L.,** Prostaglandin E₂ and prostacyclin elevate cAMP levels in elicited populations of mouse peritoneal macrophages, *Adv. Prostaglandin Thromb. Res.,* 8, 1691, 1980.
65. **Bonta, I. L., Adolfs, J. P., and Fieren, J. A.,** Cyclic AMP levels and their regulation by prostaglandins in peritoneal macrophages of rats and humans, *Adv. Cyclic Nucleotide Protein Phosphoryl. Res.,* 17, 615, 1984.
66. **Opmeer, F. A., Adolfs, M. J. P., and Bonta, I. L.,** Direct evidence for the presence of selective binding sites for (³H) prostaglandin E₂ on rat peritoneal macrophages, *Biochem. Biophys. Res. Commun.,* 114, 155, 1983.
67. **Gemsa, D., Steggeman, L., Menzel, J., and Till, G.,** Release of cyclic AMP from macrophages by stimulation with prostaglandins, *J. Immunol.,* 114, 1422, 1975.
68. **Henney, C. S., Bourne, H. R., and Lichtenstein, L. M.,** Cyclic AMP affects macrophage migration, *J. Immunol.,* 108, 1526, 1972.
69. **Gemsa, D., Steggeman, L., Till, G., and Resch, K.,** Enhancement of the PGE₁ response of macrophages by concanavalin A and colchicine, *J. Immunol.,* 119, 524, 1977.
70. **Gemsa, D., Seitz, M., Kramer, S. W., Grim, M. W., Till, G., and Resch, K.,** Ionophore A23187 raises cyclic AMP levels in macrophages by stimulating prostaglandin E formation, *J. Immunol.,* 118, 55, 1979.
71. **Lim, L. M., Hunt, N. H., Evans, T., and Weidemann, M. J.,** Rapid changes in the activities of the enzymes of cyclic AMP metabolism after addition of A23187 to macrophages, *Biochem. Biophys. Res. Commun.,* 103, 745, 1981.
72. **Lim, L. M., Hunt, N. H., Eichner, R. D., and Weidemann, M. D.,** Cyclic AMP and the regulation of prostaglandin production by macrophages, *Biochem. Biophys. Res. Commun.,* 114, 248, 1983.
73. **Lim, L. M., Hunt, N. H., and Weidemann, M. J.,** Reactive oxygen production, arachidonate metabolism and cyclic AMP in macrophages, *Biochem. Biophys. Res. Commun.,* 114, 549, 1983.
74. **Higgins, T. J. and David, J. R.,** Effect of isoproterenol and aminophylline on cyclic AMP levels of guinea pig macrophages, *Cell. Immunol.,* 27, 1, 1976.
75. **Remold-O'Donnell, E. and Alpert, H.,** Alteration of hormone-stimulated cyclic AMP synthesis in guinea pig peritoneal macrophages, *Cell. Immunol.,* 45, 221, 1979.
76. **Remold-O'Donnell, E.,** Stimulation and desensitization of macrophage adenylate cyclase by prostaglandins and catecholamines, *J. Biol. Chem.,* 249, 3615, 1974.
77. **Verghese, M. W. and Snyderman, R.,** Hormonal activation of adenylate cyclase in macrophage membranes is regulated by guanine nucleotides, *J. Immunol.,* 130, 869, 1983.
78. **Remold-O'Donnell, E.,** The enhancement of macrophage adenylate cyclase by products of activated lymphocytes, *J. Biol. Chem.,* 249, 3622, 1974.

79. **Vogel, S. N., Weedon, L. L., Oppenheim, J. J., and Rosenstreich, D. L.,** Defective Fc-mediated phagocytosis in C3H/HeJ macrophages. II. Correction by cAMP agonists, *J. Immunol.,* 126, 441, 1981.

80. **Degre, M. and Rollag, H.,** Effect of a murine beta-interferon preparation on phagocytosis and cyclic AMP levels in mouse peritoneal macrophages, *Interferon Res.,* 2, 151, 1982.

81. **Walker, W. S.,** Mediation of macrophage cytolytic and phagocytic activities by antibodies of different classes and class-specific Fc receptors, *J. Immunol.,* 119, 367, 1977.

82. **Rosen, N., Schneck, J., Bloom, B. R., and Rosen, O. M.,** Inhibition of plasminogen activator secretion by cyclic AMP in a macrophage like cell line, *J. Cyclic Nucleotide Res.,* 5, 345, 1978.

83. **Rosen, N., Piscitello, J., Schneck, J., Muschel, R. J., Bloom, B. R., and Rosen, O. M.,** Properties of protein kinase and adenylate cyclase-dependent variants of a macrophage-like cell line, *J. Cell. Physiol.,* 98, 125, 1979.

84. **Wahl, L. M., Olson, C. E., Sandberg, A. L., and Mergenhagen, S. E.,** Prostaglandin regulation of macrophage collagenase production, *Proc. Natl. Acad. Sci. U.S.A.,* 74, 4955, 1977.

85. **Pick, E.,** The mechanism of action of soluble lymphocyte mediators. IV. Effect of migration inhibitory factor (MIF) on macrophage cyclic AMP and on responsiveness to adenylate cyclase stimulators, *Cell. Immunol.,* 32, 329, 1977.

86. **Liria, A. O., Javierre, M. Q., Dias da Silva, W., and Camara, D. S.,** Immunological phagocytosis: effect of drugs on phosphodiesterase activity, *Experientia,* 30, 945, 1974.

87. **Weinberg, D. A., Weston, L. K., and Kaplan, J. E.,** Influence of prostaglandin I_2 on fibronectin-mediated phagocytosis in vivo and in vitro, *J. Leukocyte Biol.,* 37, 151, 1985.

88. **Wirth, J. J. and Kierszenbaum, F.,** Inhibitory action of elevated levels of adenosine 3′,5′-cyclic monophosphate on phagocytosis: effects on macrophage-*Trypanosoma cruzi* interaction, *J. Immunol.,* 129, 2759, 1982.

89. **Vogel, S. N. and Rosenstreich, D. L.,** Defective Fc receptor mediated phagocytosis in C3H/HeJ macrophages. I. Correction by lymphokine induced stimulation, *J. Immunol.,* 123, 2842, 1979.

90. **Bloom, B. R., Diamond, B., Muschel, R., Rosen, N., Schneck, J., Damiani, G., Rosen, O., and Scharff, M.,** Genetic approaches to the mechanism of macrophage function, *Fed. Proc. Fed. Am. Soc. Exp. Biol.,* 37, 2765, 1978.

91. **Muschel, R. J., Rosen, N., and Bloom, B. R.,** Isolation of variants in phagocytosis of a macrophage-like continuous cell line, *J. Exp. Med.,* 145, 175, 1977.

92. **Muschel, R. J., Rosen, O. M., and Bloom, B. R.,** Modulation of Fc-mediated phagocytosis by cyclic AMP and insulin in a macrophage cell line, *J. Immunol.,* 119, 1813, 1977.

93. **Schultz, R. M., Pavlidis, N. A., Stoychkov, J. N., and Chirigos, M. A.,** Prevention of macrophage tumoricidal activity by agents known to increase cellular cyclic AMP, *Cell. Immunol.,* 42, 71, 1979.

94. **Schultz, R. M.,** E-type prostaglandins and interferons: Yin-Yang modulation of macrophage tumoricidal activity, *Med. Hypothesis,* 6, 831, 1980.

95. **Taffet, S. M., Ewell, T. E., and Russell, S. W.,** Regulation of macrophage-mediated tumor cell killing by prostaglandins: comparison of the effects of PGE_2 and PGI_2, *Prostaglandins,* 24, 763, 1982.

96. **Kuo, J. F. and Greengard, P.,** Cyclic nucleotide-dependent protein kinases. IV. Widespread occurrence of adenosine 3′,5′-monophosphate-dependent protein kinase in various tissues, and phyla of the animal kingdom, *Proc. Natl. Acad. Sci. U.S.A.,* 64, 1349, 1969.

97. **Beavo, J. A. and Mumby, M. C.,** Cyclic AMP-dependent protein phosphorylation, in *Handbook of Experimental Pharmacology,* Vol. 58/I, Nathanson, J. A. and Kebabian, J. W., Eds., Springer-Verlag, Berlin, 1982, 363.

98. **Flockhart, D. A. and Corbin, J. D.,** Regulatory mechanisms in the control of protein kinases, *Crit. Rev. Biochem.,* 12, 133, 1982.

99. **Greengard, P.,** Possible role for cyclic nucleotides and phosphorylated membrane proteins in postsynaptic actions of neurotransmitters, *Nature (London),* 260, 101, 1976.

100. **Krebs, E. G.,** The mechanism of hormonal regulation by cyclic AMP, in *Endocrinology Proceedings of the 4th International Congress,* Scow, R. O., Edling, F. J. G., and Henderson, I. W., Eds., Excerpta Medica, Amsterdam, 1973, 17.

101. **Wenger, G. D. and O'Dorisio, M. S.,** Induction of cAMP-dependent protein kinase I during human monocyte differentiation, *J. Immunol.,* 134, 1836, 1985.

102. **Justement, L. B., Aldrich, W. A., Wenger, G. D., O'Dorisio, M. S., and Zwilling, B. S.,** Modulation of cyclic AMP dependent protein kinase isozyme expression with activation of a macrophage cell line, *J. Immunol.,* 136, 270, 1986.

103. **Corbin, J. D., Keely, S. L., and Park, C. K.,** The distribution of cAMP-dependent protein kinase in adipose, cardiac and other tissues, *J. Biol. Chem.,* 250, 218, 1975.

104. **Hofman, F., Beavo, J. A., Bechtel, P. J., and Krebs, E. G.,** Comparison of adenosine 3′,5′-monophosphate-dependent protein kinases from rabbit skeletal and bovine heart muscle, *J. Biol. Chem.,* 250, 7795, 1975.

105. **Armstrong, R. N. and Kaiser, E. T.**, Sulfhydryl group activity of adenosine 3',5'-monophosphate-dependent protein kinase from bovine heart: a probe of holoenzyme structure, *Biochemistry*, 17, 2840, 1978.

106. **Beavo, J. A., Bechtel, P. J., and Krebs, E. G.**, Activation of protein kinase by physiological concentration of cyclic AMP, *Proc. Natl. Acad. Sci. U.S.A.*, 71, 3580, 1974.

107. **Lohman, S. M. and Walter, U.**, Regulation of the cellular and subcellular concentrations and distribution of cyclic nucleotide-dependent protein kinases, *Adv. Cyclic Nucleotide Protein Phosphoryl. Res.*, 18, 63, 1984.

108. **Kapoor, C. L. and Steiner, A. L.**, Immunocytochemistry of cyclic nucleotides and their kinases, in *Handbook of Experimental Pharmacology*, Vol. 58/I, Nathanson, J. A. and Kebabian, J. W., Eds., Springer-Verlag, Berlin, 1982, 333.

109. **Corbin, J. D., Sugden, P. H., Lincoln, T. M., and Keely, S. L.**, Compartmentalization of adenosine 3',5'-monophosphate and adenosine 3',5'-monophosphate-dependent protein kinase in heart tissue, *J. Biol. Chem.*, 252, 3854, 1977.

110. **Hofman, F., Bechtel, P. J., and Krebs, E. G.**, Concentrations of cyclic AMP-dependent protein kinase subunits in various tissues, *J. Biol. Chem.*, 252, 1441, 1977.

111. **Palmer, W. K., Castagna, M., and Walsh, D. A.**, Nuclear protein kinase activity in glucagon-stimulated perfused rat livers, *Biochem. J.*, 143, 469, 1974.

112. **Nesterova, M. V., Ulmasov, K. H. A., Abdukarimov, A., Aridzhanov, A. A., and Severin, E. S.**, Nuclear translocation of cAMP-dependent protein kinase, *Exp. Cell Res.*, 132, 367, 1981.

113. **Nesterova, M. V., Sashchenko, L. P., Vasiliev, V., and Severin, E. S.**, A cyclic adenosine 3',5'-monophosphate dependent histone kinase from pig brain. Purification and some properties of the enzyme, *Biochim. Biophys. Acta*, 377, 271, 1981.

114. **Kikutani, H., Kishimoto, T., Sakaguchi, N., Nishizawa, Y., Ralph, P., and Yamamura, Y.**, Activation of cyclic AMP-dependent protein kinase activity during LPS stimulation of macrophage tumor cell line J774.1, *Int. J. Immunopharmacol.*, 3, 57, 1981.

115. **Hunt, N. H., Lim, L. K., Eichner, R. D., Buffinton, G. D., and Weidemann, M. J.**, Activation of cyclic AMP-dependent protein kinase in macrophages, *Biochem. Biophys. Res. Commun.*, 119, 1082, 1984.

Chapter 5

GENETIC CONTROL OF MACROPHAGE ANTITUMOR RESPONSES

Mary M. Stevenson and Emil Skamene

TABLE OF CONTENTS

I. INTRODUCTION

Macrophage-mediated defense against tumor growth represents a cascade of events involving both differentiation within the mononuclear cell lineage and modulation by numerous host-derived cytokines. One could, therefore, intuitively expect that the whole basis of such a response would be genetically determined. Severe defects in macrophage responses are likely to be incompatible with the survival of the host, mainly due to the role of this cell in antimicrobial defenses. However, more subtle qualitative or quantitative differences in macrophage responses to tumor cells have often been observed among individuals of a given species and have been found to be the result of genetic variation. The recent explosion of knowledge of the genetics of experimental animals, mainly mice, and the increasing availability of new techniques for gene mapping have led to an upsurge of interest and progress in this area.

II. GENETIC ANALYSIS OF MACROPHAGE RESPONSES IN MICE

The general strategy for these studies is the establishment of a genetic linkage of the trait of altered resistance to tumor growth with a certain facet of the macrophage response that normally develops during the course of host-tumor interaction. Alternatively, a genetically determined alteration of a well-defined macrophage trait can be correlated with the overall level of resistance to a tumor target. Such investigations are usually initiated when an intraspecies variation in the expression of a particular macrophage-related trait is observed. When confirmed in inbred mice, each with a unique genetic background, such variation implies a difference in the genetic control of the given trait. Appropriate breeding studies can then be initiated with the aims of establishing the mode of inheritance and of analyzing the phenotypic expression of such regulation. In some cases, the "macrophage genes" have been mapped and their action is well understood, whereas in other situations the only hint of genetic control stems from the description of deviation in the particular macrophage function in one or several inbred strains. The finding of only one variant strain usually suggests that a mutation at a particular locus controlling that response has taken place while variation observed in several inbred strains implies control by polymorphic gene(s). The best example of a single gene profoundly affecting macrophage function is the Lps^d mutation in C3H/HeJ mice. This mutation resulted in macrophage hyporesponsiveness to endotoxin (more specifically to the lipid A moiety of lipopolysaccharide, LPS), and, as a result, all the usual endotoxin-stimulated facets of the macrophage response (increase in macrophage production, chemotaxis, inflammatory response, and activation for tumoricidal kill) are severely depressed. This observation provided an excellent impetus to look for other genetically determined defects in macrophage responses in our attempts to understand fully the role of the macrophage in resistance to malignancy.

The overall host resistance function of the macrophage defense system may be considered as a sequence of processes which must proceed in a stepwise fashion in order that the demands on the host brought about by malignant transformation and by tumor growth can be met.

1.   Production of adequate numbers of macrophage precursors in the bone marrow
2.   Recruitment and delivery of macrophage precursors to the blood
3.   Margination and emigration of macrophages into tissues and immobilization of macrophages within malignant foci
4.   Establishment of contact between macrophages and tumor cells
5.   Tumoricidal activity

These steps represent unique cellular mechanisms which are regulated by distinct gene products. The genetic control of macrophage responses is, therefore, best considered as an interplay of genetically determined events at each of these steps.

III. GENETIC CONTROL OF MONOCYTOPOIESIS

The relationship between genetic variation of the proliferative potential of mononuclear phagocyte precursors and host response to neoplasia is presently undefined. However, variation among inbred strains of mice in macrophage proliferation has been described and genetic regulation is apparent at each of several, distinct developmental stages. Genetic regulation of the kinetics of proliferation of the multipotential stem cell has been well described.[1-3] The earliest step of myelo-monocytopoiesis, namely in vitro granulocyte-macrophage colony-forming cell (CFC-GM) formation, has been found to vary quantitatively among inbred mouse strains, with the C57BL-derived strains exhibiting high bone marrow responsiveness to colony-stimulating factor (CSF).[4,5] Such interstrain differences could be due to an augmented CSF-responsive bone marrow pool, to an intrinsic enhancement of the precursor cell's responsiveness to CSF, to the magnitude of CFC-GM differentiation, or even possibly to the presence of CFC-GM inhibitors in the autologous sera used in the in vitro assay. The observation that the longevity of myelopoiesis in vitro (i.e., duration of generation of CFC-GM formation) varies markedly among strains of mice suggests that genetic regulation of CFC-GM formation is expressed as an intrinsic property of the precursor cell itself.[6]

Alterations in the development of macrophage colonies in vitro by bone marrow cells from tumor-bearing mice have been described. In 1972, Baum and Fisher[7] observed increased production of macrophage colonies by bone marrow cells from C3H mice bearing implants of a syngeneic, spontaneous mammary tumor. The increase was apparent between 4 days and 2 weeks after subcutaneous tumor implantation, after which time colony production returned to normal. It is of interest to note that in later studies, Baum[10] and Fisher et al.[8,9] demonstrated that antitumor agents, such as *Mycobacterium bovis*, strain Bacillus Calmette Guerin (BCG), or *Corynebacterium parvum*, had a marked stimulatory effect on macrophage colony production in vitro.

Otu and his colleagues[11] observed that an early depression in macrophage colony formation in vitro by bone marrow cells from C57BL mice bearing transplants of the syngeneic, spontaneously arisen Lewis lung carcinoma line was followed by a marked enhancement at 1 week. The response was again severely depressed by 2 to 3 weeks after tumor implantation.

In vitro infection of mouse bone marrow cells with murine leukemia viruses resulted in increased production of granulocyte-macrophage colony-forming unit (culture), CFUc-GM.[12] The mechanism of this increase was enhanced production of CSF by macrophages in virus-infected bone marrow cultures or peritoneal exudates. Balducci and Hardy[13] similarly observed an increased rate of CFUc production early in tumor growth in C57BL/6 mice transplanted with Lewis lung carcinoma and an increased CSF activity in the serum of tumor-bearing mice in comparison to that of control animals. Increased serum CSF has likewise been observed, clinically and in other animal models.[14-16] The results of these studies as well as further work by Hardy and Balducci[17] demonstrated that increased serum colony-stimulating activity (CSA) in tumor-bearing hosts is not only a product of the tumor-stimulated immune system but is also elaborated by the tumor cells themselves. A growing tumor may also cause alterations in the microenvironment of the bone marrow as suggested by the studies of DeGowin et al.[18] which demonstrated that the clonal growth of marrow stromal cells is decreased in tumor-bearing animals.

It was more recently observed that the proliferative capacity of bone marrow cells from B16 melanoma-bearing C57BL mice to form macrophage colonies in vitro was similar to cells from normal mice.[19] Moreover, a threshold level of LPS, which was substantially less than that required for optimal macrophage tumoricidal activation, was required for optimal CFUc production in both bone marrow populations.

It is clear from these studies that, in some cases, tumor growth affects monocytopoiesis. What is not clear is the influence of genetically determined differences in monocytopoiesis on this facet of host response to tumor growth. While such differences have not been described in relation to tumor development, they have been described in relation to host responses to infection.

Wilson et al.[20] examined the responses in vitro of colony-forming cells in the bone marrow of *Salmonella typhimurium*-resistant CBA and susceptible C57BL mice. The resistant strain responded within hours after Salmonella infection with increased numbers of CFC-GM. Increased macrophage production was evident for the first 2 to 3 days. In contrast, susceptible mice exhibited a slowly increasing response which never exceeded 1.2 times normal and eventually fell to less than normal by 2 to 3 days after infection.

Infection with another facultative, intracellular bacterium, *Listeria monocytogenes*, also resulted in changes in the number of colony-forming cells and increased levels of serum CSF.[21,22] A transient increase in CSF was apparent in both resistant C57BL mice and susceptible BALB/c mice following Listeria infection so that the ability to produce CSF is apprently not related to resistance to Listeria.[22] In this study, however, resistant C57BL mice were found to have a larger and more responsive population of colony-forming cells, that is CFC-GM, than did either susceptible BALB/c or CBA mice. Thus, superior mono-cytopoiesis in response to infection appears to be related both to the infecting organism and to the level of genetically determined host response to that organism. Study of the in vitro colony-forming potential of macrophage precursors in bone marrow of tumor-bearing mice would probably also reveal that this facet of host response to neoplasia is dependent both on the genetic background of the host as well as on the origin and type of tumor, that is, whether the tumor arose spontaneously or was chemically or virally induced.

IV. GENETIC CONTROL OF PERIPHERAL BLOOD MONOCYTOSIS

Induction of inflammation, for example, in the peritoneal cavity by injection of nonspe-cific, sterile stimuli, is characterized by the accumulation of young, recently blood-derived macrophages. This response is accompanied by monocytosis in the peripheral blood as a result of increased bone marrow production of mononuclear phagocytes in response to a soluble factor, factor increasing monocytopoiesis (FIM), produced by macrophages at the site of inflammation.[23,24]

If the site of tumor growth, either as a result of experimental implantation or spontaneous development, is considered as an inflammatory focus, monocytosis would be a likely con-sequence. Indeed, there are reports that the number of blood monocytes is increased in both lymphoid and nonlymphoreticular malignant states in cancer patients as well as in experi-mental rodent models.[25-27] It is quite likely that monocytosis during tumor growth, just as during inflammation, is due to a bone marrow stimulatory factor which is either FIM or a molecule with very similar abilities produced by the growing tumor.

Genetic variation has been described in the response of monocyte precursors to FIM in a murine model using latex beads and a saline extract of *L. monocytogenes* as inflammatory inducing agents.[28] In contrast, no genetic restriction in the production of FIM was evident.

Another indication of genetic variation of monocytosis in inbred mice is an observation using the model of resistance to Listeria.[29] It was found that the Listeria-resistant C57BL-derived B10.A strain responded to infection or to the injection of a Listeria cell wall extract with a rapid decrease of promonocyte generation time, whereas there was no such shortening of promonocyte generation time in susceptible A/J mice. As a result, the mice of Listeria-resistant strain (C57BL/6) exhibited monocytosis at 24 and 48 hr, which was not detected in susceptible mice (A/J). It remains to be established whether the genes regulating the monocyte response to FIM and to components of Listeria are genetically linked. Likewise, investigations to determine whether the gene(s) described as controlling monocytosis to acute inflammation and infection also regulate the response to tumors, need to be undertaken.

Another facet of the monocyte response which is altered during carcinogenesis and which is possibly under genetic regulation is the ability of these cells to mature into macrophages. Monocytes from a variety of patients with cancer, including malignant melanoma, renal cell carcinoma, and breast cancer, were found to have an intrinsic defect in maturation to macrophages in vitro.[30-32] The results of maturation studies with monocytes from renal cell carcinoma patients pre- and postsurgical removal of their tumors correlated with the patients' prognosis and recovery.[32]

V. GENETIC CONTROL OF MACROPHAGE INFLAMMATORY RESPONSES

The observation of the presence of macrophages at the site of progressing tumors has led to the development of the concept that macrophages play a major role in surveillance against neoplastic cells. Eccles and Alexander observed that there was a direct correlation between the macrophage content of rat fibrosarcomas and their immunogenic and metastatic potential.[33] However, more recent results obtained with 33 methylcholanthrene-induced sarcomas, which were growing in either C57BL/6J or BALB/CByJ mice, suggested that in the mouse system there is not a relationship between macrophage content and tumor immunogenicity.[34]

Further studies revealed that macrophage accumulation at the site of a growing tumor is not dependent on the presence of an intact immune system, that is, it occurred in T cell or B cell deficient mice,[35,36] nor does it require the fifth component of complement, that is, macrophage accumulation in tumors occurred equally well in C5-sufficient B10.D2/nSn and C5-deficient B10.D2/oSn mice.[37] However, it was demonstrated that an intact bone marrow system is required in order for effective accumulation of macrophages at the site of tumor growth.[36,38,39]

The latter observation is of interest because of the finding that the level of macrophage accumulation in inflammatory foci is genetically controlled in inbred mice.[40] The level of this response was initially described through its linkage with the trait of resistance to infection with Listeria. Listeria-resistant mouse strains (C57BL-derived strains, SJL) were found to have effective accumulation of macrophages in the peritoneal cavity as well as in subcutaneous sites in response to nonspecific inflammatory agents as well as to Listeria.[40,41] In contrast, Listeria-susceptible BALB/c, CBA, DBA/2, DBA/1, and A/J mice have a defective

The defective macrophage inflammatory response found in C5 deficient mice, such as the BALB/c and CBA mouse strains, must be due to an alternate and as yet undefined genetic mechanism. Genetic analysis of the BALB/c defect using the CXB series (C = BALB/c, B = C57BL/6) of recombinant inbred strains suggests that an allelic difference at a single locus is responsible for the deficiency.[43]

As is clear from the experimental results discussed above, the question of macrophage accumulation in growing tumors should be addressed using various inbred mouse strain-tumor combinations to determine the influence of the genetic background of the host on the level of the macrophage response.

The level of the in vitro macrophage response to chemoattractants has also been observed to be controlled genetically.[40,44,45] Furthermore, recombinant inbred strain analysis using the response which results in a two- to threefold lower number of accumulated macrophages. In the case of the A/J mice, susceptibility to Listeria and the defective macrophage response have been found to be due to the C5 deficiency of this strain which is controlled by the Hc locus on mouse chromosome 2.[42]

AXB series (A = A/J, low responder in all three parameters measured, B = C57BL/6, high responder) revealed that the level of host macrophage response to chemoattractants in vitro correlates with the level of their accumulation in vivo and with their response in the leukocyte-adherence inhibition assay in vitro (LAI).[46] The LAI has been demonstrated to be an in vitro correlate of host response to tumor and is used clinically to evaluate a cancer patient's progress.[47]

Similarly, the chemotactic responsiveness of peripheral blood monocytes from cancer patients has been found to correlate with prognosis after surgery and immunotherapy.[48] In general, the chemotactic responsiveness of monocytes from cancer patients and of peritoneal macrophages from tumor-bearing animals has been found to be depressed in comparison to that of normal, control individuals.[49-53] The depression of chemotaxis in vitro observed with peritoneal macrophages from tumor-bearing animals correlated with depressed macrophage accumulation in vivo.[51] The underlying mechanism of the depression in chemotactic responsiveness in vitro of mononuclear phagocytes from both cancer patients and tumor-bearing animals appears to be related to the production of inhibitors of macrophage chemotaxis by the tumor cells.[54-56]

In addition to producing inhibitors of macrophage chemotaxis, tumors have also been found to produce macrophage chemoattractants.[57,58] These factor(s) have been described in supernatants of both human and murine tumor cells, as well as in supernatants of human and murine embryo fibroblast lines. The tumor-produced chemotactic activity has a molecular weight of 12,000 to 15,000 and, thus, is different from lymphocyte-derived chemotactic factor. It has recently been demonstrated that the inhibitory factor and the chemoattractant coexist in the same culture supernatants of two human tumor cell lines.[59]

It has also recently been demonstrated that tumor-promoting agents, specifically phorbol esters, can modulate the activity of macrophages, including the induction of chemotaxis.[60-62] This observation, as well as the observations of the production of macrophage chemotaxis inhibitors and macrophage chemoattractants by tumors, raise three points at which the genetic background of the host could regulate the macrophage responsiveness to the development and progression of neoplasia.

VI. GENETIC CONTROL OF MACRPOHAGE MEMBRANE ANTIGENS: Ia ANTIGENS AND ANTIGEN PRESENTATION AND MAC-1 ANTIGEN

As has been so elaborately demonstrated by Unanue and his colleagues,[63,64] the level of immune responsiveness is controlled by regulation of the expression of Ia antigens on the membranes of macrophages. The kinetics of the influx of Ia$^+$ macrophages correlate with the development of immunity as demonstrated using models of acquired resistance to infection. In addition, young, recently blood-derived macrophages can be induced to express Ia antigens in vitro in the presence of gamma-interferon (γ-IFN).[63-65]

Genetic differences in immune responses have been described in inbred mice for the production of antibody to heterologous erythrocytes,[66-68] synthetic protein antigens,[69,70] and naturally occurring proteins, such as staphylococcal nuclease.[71] In general, A/J strain mice are found to be high responders and C57BL-derived mice, low responders. The genetic control of level of antibody production is multigenic and involves both H-2 linked and non-H-2 linked genes.[67,71] In the model of antibody responses to sheep erythrocytes, it was recently demonstrated that high responder A/J mice had twice as many Ia$^+$ macrophages in the peritoneal cavity following intraperitoneal (i.p.) immunization than did low responder C57BL/10 mice.[68] Furthermore, accumulation of L3T4 cells, or the T-helper subset of T cells, occurred in high responder A/J mice in comparison to the accumulation of Ly2$^+$ cells, the T-suppressor subset, in the spleens of low responder B10 mice. It was concluded that insufficient handling and/or processing of antigen (presumably due to the low expression of

Ia antigens by the macrophages of the low responder B10 strains) leads to proliferation and expansion of suppressor cells rather than of antigen-specific helper cells.

The induction of antitumor immune responses likewise requires Ia antigen expression as the initial step. In some instances, including experimental murine models and in clinical situations, macrophage expression of Ia antigens was found to be decreased in tumor-bearing hosts.[72,73] These studies used systemic macrophage populations and the loss of Ia was correlated with decreased T and B cell functions in tumor-bearing animals.[73,74] Decreased Ia antigen expression apparently can be related to the shedding by metastatic but not non-metastatic tumor cell lines of membrane vesicles which inhibited macrophage Ia antigen expression in vitro in the presence of γ-IFN.[75] Membrane vesicles have also been demonstrated to inhibit other macrophage-mediated responses, including tumor cytotoxicity and lymphocyte responses to mitogens. The mechanism of the inhibition of macrophage Ia antigen expression was found to be increased prostaglandin synthesis by macrophages following uptake of the tumor membrane vesicles.

Paradoxically, examination of tumor-associated macrophages revealed that this macrophage population expressed Ia antigens and possessed potent accessory cell function as demonstrated by their ability to reconstitute the primary antiheterologous erythrocyte response of macrophage-depleted spleen cells.[76] The tumor associated macrophage population, however, was found to be deficient in Mac-1 antigen expression. The Mac-1 antigen appears to be identical to the CR3 receptor. This receptor mediates binding and phagocytosis of cells or particles opsonized with C3bi. As well, it acts synergistically with the Fc receptor in phagocytosis and in antibody-dependent cell-mediated cytotoxicity.[76] A deficiency in Mac-1 antigen on the surface of tumor-associated macrophages may result in a defect in the antitumor activity of these cells *in situ* and lead to progressive tumor growth.

Almost no information is available at this time with respect to the genetic control of Ia antigen expression in relation to tumor progression and the accumulation of Ia$^+$ macrophages in tumors. Since the induction of Ia antigen on macrophages represents the initiation of antitumor immunity, this area needs to be evaluated critically.

VII. GENETIC CONTROL OF MONOKINE RELEASE

Genetically determined qualitative and quantitative differences among inbred mouse strains in the ability to produce a wide variety of monokines have been described. Of major importance is the demonstration of variation among inbred mice in the production of interleukin 1 (IL 1), a soluble immunoregulatory peptide produced by macrophages in response to immune or inflammatory stimulation.[77] Differences among inbred strains of mice in the ability to produce IL 1 were initially described by Mortensen and his colleagues.[78] this observation was confirmed and extended by Brandwein et al.[79] in studies using the AXB/BXA series of recombinant inbred strains derived from high responder C57BL/6 and low responder A/J progenitor mice. Their results showed that production of IL 1 in response to LPS was genetically controlled by multiple genes with the major gene controlling the production of IL 1 and with an additional gene or genes controlling the magnitude of the IL 1 response. Comparison of the strain distribution pattern (SDP) of the major gene controlling the IL 1 level with the SDPs of a large number of previously determined traits suggested that the major gene controlling IL 1 production to LPS was genetically linked to several loci on chromosome 1.

The issue of the dependence of the genetic control of IL 1 production on the identity of the stimulus needs to be addressed since other studies demonstrated that peritoneal macrophages from C3HeB/Fe mice released IL 1 in response to LPS but not to muramyl dipeptide (MDP), whereas macrophages from C57BL/6J mice produced IL 1 in response to both LPS and MDP.[80] That production of IL 1, regardless of the stimulus, is a complex process requiring multiple genes, is evident in the results of a recent study showing multigenic control of IL 1 production. Two genes in the mouse genome, IL 1α and IL 1β, were identified using a human IL 1β probe to identify a homologous sequence in a murine cDNA library.[81] The source of macrophages used in this study was the PU5-1.8 macrophage line stimulated to produce IL 1 with phorbol myristic acid (PMA).

Another monokine which has recently been demonstrated to be under genetic control is procoagulant activity (PCA).[82] PCA is a monokine whose production is regulated by T cell products and whose presence is detected by its prothrombin cleaving activity.[83,84] Susceptibility of inbred mice to mouse hepatitis virus strain 3 (MHV-3) was found to correlate with the level of spontaneous expression of PCA activity.[83,84] In a later study, which used recombinant inbred strain analysis, inheritance of the two traits, namely, resistance or susceptibility to MHV-3 and the level of PCA activity was found to be identical and to be determined by two recessive, non-H-2 linked genes.[82]

The release of several other soluble mediators which are related to either the induction of neoplasia or to host antitumor mechanisms has also been demonstrated to vary among inbred mice. These mediators include tumor necrosis factor (TNF), a neutral protease cytolytic factor (CF), reactive oxygen intermediates, and arachidonic acid metabolites.

TNF,[85] which has recently been shown to be identical to cachectin,[86] is produced by macrophages following priming with a stimulus, such as, infection with BCG or *Corynebacterium parvum* followed by exposure to bacterial endotoxin or LPS. When BCG was used as the priming signal, differences in the production of TNF were apparent among inbred strains; C57BL/6, SJL, and AKR produced TNF while A/J mice did not.[85] This strain difference was apparent only when BCG was used; strain differences were not apparent when *C. parvum* was used. In a later study by Mannel and her colleagues,[87] it was demonstrated that C3H/HeJ mice were also unable to produce TNF in response to infection with BCG followed by LPS. A similar finding by Beutler and his colleagues[88,89] demonstrated that although C3H/HeJ mice did not produce cachectin (TNF), macrophages from this strain did so following in vitro incubation with γ-IFN and LPS. As is evident here with production of TNF (cachectin) and in the studies examining differences among inbred strains in IL-1 production, the identity of the stimulating agent appears to be critical in determining genetic regulation.

Lewis and Adams[62] studied the release of reactive oxygen intermediates (H_2O_2 and O_2^-) and metabolites of arachidonic acid by casein-elicited peritoneal macrophages from SENCAR and C57BL/6 mice following exposure to phorbol esters. SENCAR mice are sensitive to the promotion of skin tumors by a tumor promoting agent (TPA) following initiation with a chemical carcinogen while C57BL/6 mice are almost totally resistant to promotion of skin tumors by TPA.[90] Macrophages from SENCAR mice were found to be more sensitive to TPA exposure and to produce significantly more H_2O_2 and metabolites of arachidonic acid than did macrophages from C57BL/6 mice. Release of the two groups of mediators was similar when macrophages from the two mouse strains were stimulated with zymosan. The investigators concluded that the enhanced response to phorbol ester of macrophages from SENCAR mice correlated with their enhanced sensitivity to tumor promotion by phorbol ester. This conclusion can only be confirmed by backcross studies showing linkage of the two traits. It is of interest to point out that leukocytes stimulated with phorbol esters also suffer breakage of their DNA, produce soluble low molecular weight clastogenic factors, and induce increased rates of sister chromatid exchange in co-cultured mammalian cells.[62] Data indicate that these aberrations may be induced by the release of reactive oxygen intermediates and metabolites of arachidonic acid from inflammatory cells (see Chapter 11).[91,92]

In contrast to the results obtained by Lewis and Adams,[62] Boraschi and her colleagues[93] found that saline-induced macrophages from mice with known defects in macrophage-mediated nonspecific tumor cytotoxicity, that is, strain A/J, C3H/HeJ, and P/J mice, produced normal levels of reactive oxygen intermediates and metabolites of arachidonic acid after in vitro exposure to macrophage activating factors. In this study, macrophages were induced to produce mediators with opsonized zymosan. Comparison of the results of the studies by Lewis and Adams[62] and by Boraschi et al.[93] again stresses the importance of the identity of the stimulus used to induce mediator production in macrophage preparations.

Production of another soluble mediator by macrophages, the neutral protease CF which mediates nonspecific macrophage-mediated tumor cytotoxicity,[94] has also been found to vary among inbred mice.[95] This topic will be discussed in the next section on macrophage activation for tumor cell killing.

Of importance to macrophage activity against tumors, as well as to microorganisms, are genetically determined differences in the production of macrophage activating factors by T cells. In analyzing the macrophage defect in tumoricidal ability of macrophages from P/J strain mice, Boraschi and Meltzer[96] observed that spleen cells from these mice were deficient in production of lymphokines, specifically, macrophage activation factor (MAF). Virelizier[97] found that pokeweed-stimulated spleen cells, from BALB/c, A/J, and C3H/He mice, were low producers of γ-IFN which is a potent activator of macrophage tumoricidal and microbicidal activities.[98] C57BL/6, CBA, and AKR mice were high producers. The relationship between genetic control of monokine and lymphokine production and host antitumor defense mechanisms needs to be addressed.

VIII. GENETIC CONTROL OF MACROPHAGE ACTIVATION FOR TUMORICIDAL ACTIVITY

Perhaps the most intensely studied area of genetic control of macrophage response to tumors has been the in vitro destruction of tumor cells by macrophages. Macrophages are able to destroy tumor cells via at least two distinct mechanisms.[98-100] In the presence of antibody specific for target cells, macrophages are able to lyse target cells, either heterologous erythrocytes or tumor targets. This mechanism of tumor cell destruction, the so-called antibody-dependent cell-mediated cytotoxicity or ADCC, occurs within a relatively short period of time (within hours). The second mechanism, the so-called macrophage-mediated tumor cytotoxicity, is a slow process (requires 2 days), is antibody independent, requires contact between macrophages and tumor targets, and is target specific in the sense that neoplastic cells but not normal cells are lysed. In both types of interactions with tumor cells, activated macrophages possess an enhanced ability to lyse tumor targets in comparison to normal macrophages.[101]

Activated macrophages can be recovered from the peritoneal cavity of mice following i.p. injection of a number of agents, including BCG or *C. parvum*. Macrophages can also be activated in vitro by exposure to lymphokines.[102,103] Observations in several experimental systems demonstrate that the development of activated macrophages for contact-dependent tumor cytotoxicity requires the completion of a series of reactions.[102-105] According to Meltzer and his colleagues,[103] the reaction sequence can be divided into three phases: (1) precursor differentiation, (2) priming, and (3) triggering. The first phase involves the recruitment and differentiation of immature, blood-derived mononuclear phagocytes into lymphokine-responsive cells by factors generated at the site of inflammation. Complete expression of nonspecific antitumor activity by activated macrophages occurs after two additional phases; inflammatory macrophages first respond to signals present in lymphokine preparations and enter into a primed state in which they are not yet cytotoxic but can further be triggered by other signals, such as LPS, to express full tumor cytotoxic potential.

The use of mouse strains with genetically determined defects in the development of activated macrophages facilitated the elucidation by Meltzer and his colleagues[103] of the series of reactions required for the full expression of tumoricidal activity. A survey of 26 mouse strains for the ability of peritoneal macrophages to be activated for tumor cytotoxicity by BCG showed that macrophages of 9 strains were not responsive.[106] Nonresponder strains could be grouped into three categories: (1) strains (C3H/HeJ, C57BL/10ScSn) having defective responses to the lipid A region of bacterial endotoxins, a defect which is controlled by the *Lps* gene on chromosome 4;[107,108] (2) strains (A/J, A/HeJ, AL/N) derived from the A strain;[109,110] and (3) P/J strain mice.[96,111] Inflammatory macrophages of all of the defective strains could not develop tumoricidal activity following in vitro incubation with lymphokines.

Although the phenotypic expression of the defect in macrophage activation was found to be almost identical in all three groups of defective strains, the gene(s) controlling the expression of the defect in each strain appears to be unique.[112] In the case of A/J mice, the defect was found to be the inability of activated macrophages to bind to the tumor target cells, whereas activated macrophages from C3H/HeJ mice were found to be unable to produce a neutral, serine protease, described in the preceding section as CF.[95] Both of these events, binding to tumor targets and release of CF, have been demonstrated to be necessary for completion of macrophage-mediated tumor cytotoxicity.[100] Further analysis of these two events would suggest that the induction of binding to target cells is regulated principally by lymphokines while secretion of CF is regulated by LPS.[95,99] This suggests that the defect of C3H/HeJ mice is the inability of its macrophages to respond to LPS which is indeed the case since cells from these animals lack the receptor for LPS.[113] In contrast, the defect of the A/J mouse would appear to be the inability of its macrophages to respond to lymphokines. Recent studies have confirmed the possibility that macrophages from A/J mice have membrane receptors for γ-IFN but these macrophages do not undergo biochemical changes associated with activation by γ-IFN.[114,115] The genetic lesion of P/J mice has been demonstrated to be expressed as not only a defect in the response of macrophages to activating stimuli but also in the production of macrophage-activating lymphokines.[96]

It is now clear that the defects in the activation of macrophages from C3H/HeJ, A/J, and P/J mice are manifested as alterations in host defense against both neoplasia and infectious diseases (numerous examples described in References 116 and 117). For example, both A/J and P/J mice have been described to have a very high incidence of tumors after administration of carcinogens.[118,119] Tumor-bearing C3H/HeJ mice have been found to be unresponsive to intralesional BCG treatment.[102] The response of C3H/HeJ, A/J, and P/J mice for the development of activated macrophages for the in vitro killing of extracellular targets (tumor cells and larvae of *Schistosoma mansoni*) was found to correlate with the development in vivo of concomitant immunity in schistosomiasis.[120] Backcross-linkage analysis of progeny derived from high responder C57BL-derived and low responder A/J mice showed that both macrophage tumoricidal and schistosomulacidal activities are genetically controlled by the same dominant, autosomal, non-H-2 linked gene.[120] This result was confirmed using the AXB/BXA series of recombinant inbred strains and the gene was mapped to the proximal segment of mouse chromosome 7.[121]

In spite of the defect in macrophage-mediated cytotoxicity, BCG-activated macrophages from C3H/HeJ and A/J mice do, however, have an augmented capacity to mediate ADCC against both erythroid and neoplastic targets.[122] It has been demonstrated that H_2O_2 released from activated macrophages is the mediator of ADCC.[99] Additional evidence that activated macrophages from C3H/HeJ, A/J, and P/J mice are not defective in mediating ADCC and that the defect is specific for macrophage-mediated cytotoxicity, is the finding that in vitro activation of these macrophages with lymphokines resulted in enhanced production of oxygen metabolites and metabolites of arachidonic acid similar to that produced by macrophages from strains which exhibit normal development of tumor cytotoxicity.[93] These findings suggest that ADCC and macrophage-mediated tumor cytotoxicity do not share the same genetic regulation. These findings also stress the concept that there are multiple mechanisms of host antitumor defenses, one of which presumably may function in the absence of the other.

IX. USE OF LIPOSOME ENCAPSULATED MACROPHAGE ACTIVATING AGENTS TO OVERCOME DEFECTS IN MACROPHAGE KILLING OF TUMOR CELLS

Recently, liposome-encapsulated macrophage-activating agents (lymphokine preparations containing MAF, γ-IFN and muramyl dipeptide (MDP), and its various lipophilic derivatives) have been demonstrated to activate murine macrophage tumoricidal activity in vitro.[123] The in vitro activation of macrophages by liposome-encapsulated macrophage-activating agents was, furthermore, demonstrated to correlate with the activation in vivo by liposomes containing the immunomodulators of host macrophages, resulting in destruction of metastases.[124] Systemic administration of immunomodulators such as MAF or MDP is ineffective due to the short half-life of these substances in the host. However, encapsulation in liposomes results in this therapy being effective because the immunomodulators are triggered to the target cell, that is, the macrophage. It has been demonstrated that 80 to 90% of liposomes are taken up by the mononuclear phagocytes of the liver, spleen, lung, lymph nodes, bone marrow, and peripheral blood.[125]

It has likewise been demonstrated that peripheral blood monocytes of both normal individuals and patients with colorectal carcinoma are activated in vitro to become tumoricidal by immunomodulators entrapped in liposomes.[126,127] Activation of monocytes from cancer patients is of significance because there have been reports that these cells have impaired spontaneous cytotoxicity.[128,129] It has also been possible to activate certain types of rodent tissue macrophages, which are refractory to activation by free agents, by the use of liposome-encapsulated agents.[130] This strategy led to the successful activation of tumoricidal properties in macrophages of LPS-unresponsive C3H/HeJ mice[131] and it has recently been observed in our laboratory that treatment of macrophages from defective A/J mice with liposome-encapsulated MDP-GDP (glycerol dipalmitate)[132] also overcomes their genetic defect and results in activation of macrophages with the ability to lyse tumor cells in vitro.[133] Thus, an immunopharmacological manipulation resulted in the correction of two genetically distinct macrophage defects. The results of the studies described here on the activation of macrophages suggest that encapsulation of macrophage-activating agents in liposomes may provide a biological approach for therapy in cancer patients by in vivo activation of macrophages, otherwise nonresponsive for either genetic or environmental reasons, for destruction of growing tumors.

X. CONCLUSION

Host genes regulate the macrophage response to tumor cells at various levels. The appreciation of the importance of the genetic control of macrophage-mediated antitumor activity is important for several reasons. First of all, in experimental situations, animals of the appropriate genotype ("responder" vs. "nonresponders") need to be used to assure reproducibility of data and to enable comparison of results obtained in various laboratories. Segregation analysis of genetic variation may lead to a better understanding of the mechanisms underlying the appropriate macrophage trait. In some instances, the discovery that a seemingly identical defective phenotype (e.g., inability of macrophages from several inbred mouse strains to kill tumor cells) is caused by at least three distinct mutations can lead to the precise analysis of the defect on a cellular and molecular level. In other situations, the finding of a pleiotropic effect of a single gene (e.g., the control of macrophage activation for the killing of malignant and parasitic targets) allows us to appreciate and to study a host defense mechanism which developed, in evolution, as a common response to various threats to the integrity of the organism. The identification of macrophage genes in the murine system can, furthermore, lead the way to their analogs in humans. Chromosomal sequences of importance in the survival of the species are usually preserved among mammals and the isolation of the mouse genes will likely result in the availability of probes for the human genome. The finding of a chromosomal location of a particular macrophage gene, furthermore, leads to the identification of closely linked genetic markers. Use of these markers in the human situation can eventually lead to the typing of individuals in the population who may be tumor-prone due to their inherited macrophage defects. Finally, the precise knowledge of the phenotypic expression of genes which regulates macrophage responses will result in targeted manipulation, either pharmacological or biochemical, of the defective traits in favor of the host.

REFERENCES

1. **Russell, E. S. and Bernstein, S. E.**, Blood and blood formation, in *Biology of the Laboratory Mouse*, Green, E. L., Ed., Dover Publ., New York, 1968, 351.
2. **Suzuki, S. and Axelrad, A. A.**, FV-2 locus controls the proportion of erythropoietic progenitor cells (BFU-E) synthesizing DNA in normal mice, *Cell*, 19, 225, 1980.
3. **van Zant, G., Eldridge, P. W., Behringer, R. R., and Dewey, M. J.**, Genetic control of hematopoietic kinetics revealed by analysis of allophenic mice and stem cell suicide, *Cell*, 35, 639, 1983.
4. **McNeill, T. A. and Fleming, W. A.**, Cellular responsiveness to stimulation in vitro: strain differences in hemopoietic colony forming cell responsiveness to stimulation factor and suppression by glucocorticoids, *J. Cell. Physiol.*, 82, 49, 1973.
5. **Metcalf, D. and Russell, S.**, Inhibition by mouse serum of hemopoietic colony formation in vitro, *Exp. Hematol.*, 4, 339, 1976.
6. **Sakakeeny, M. A. and Greenberger, J. S.**, Granulopoiesis longevity in continuous bone marrow cultures and factor dependent cell line generation: significant variation among 28 inbred mouse strains and outbred stocks, *J. Natl. Cancer Inst.*, 68, 305, 1982.
7. **Baum, M. and Fisher, B.**, Macrophage production by the bone marrow of tumor bearing mice, *Cancer Res.*, 32, 2813, 1972.
8. **Fisher, B., Taylor, S., Levine, M., Saffer, E., and Fisher, E. R.**, Effect of *Mycobacterium bovis* (strain Bacillus Calmette-Guerin) on macrophage production by the bone marrow of tumor-bearing mice, *Cancer Res.*, 34, 1668, 1974.
9. **Wolmark, N. and Fisher, B.**, The effect of a single and repeated administration of *Corynebacterium parvum* on bone marrow macrophage colony production in syngeneic tumor-bearing mice, *Cancer Res.*, 34, 2869, 1974.
10. **Baum, M. and Breese, M.**, Antitumor effect of *Corynebacterium parvum*: possible mode of action, *Br. J. Cancer*, 33, 468, 1976.
11. **Otu, A. A., Russell, R. J., Wilkinson, P. C., and White, R. G.**, Alterations of mononuclear phagocyte function induced by Lewis lung carcinoma in C57BL mice, *Br. J. Cancer*, 36, 330, 1970.
12. **Greenberger, J. S., Wroble, L. M., and Sakakeeny, M. A.**, Murine leukemia viruses: induction of macrophage production of granulocyte-macrophage colony-stimulating factor in vitro, *J. Natl. Cancer Inst.*, 65, 841, 1980.
13. **Balducci, L. and Hardy, C.**, High proliferation of granulocyte macrophage progenitors in tumor bearing mice, *Cancer Res.*, 43, 4643, 1983.
14. **Asano, S., Urabe, A., Okabe, T., Sasto, H., Kondo, Y., Ueyama, Y., Chiba, S., Ohsawa, N., and Kosaka, K.**, Demonstration of granulopoietic factor(s) in the plasma of nude mice transplanted with a human lung cancer and in the tumor tissue, *Blood*, 49, 845, 1977.
15. **Burlington, H., Cronkite, E. P., Laissure, J. A., Reincke, U., and Shadduck, R. K.**, Colony stimulating activity in cultures of granulocytosis-inducing tumor, *Proc. Soc. Exp. Biol. Med.*, 154, 86, 1977.
16. **Wu, M. C., Cini, J. K., and Yunis, A. A.**, Purification of a colony-stimulating factor from cultured pancreatic carcinoma cells, *J. Biol. Chem.*, 254, 226, 1979.
17. **Hardy, C. L. and Balducci, L.**, Early hematopoietic events during tumor growth in mice, *J. Natl. Cancer Inst.*, 76, 535, 1986.

18. **DeGowin, R. I., Gibson, D. P., Knapp, S. A., and Wathen, L. M.,** Tumor-induced suppression of marrow stromal colonies, *Exp. Hematol. (Copenhagen),* 9, 811, 1981.
19. **Erickson, K. L. and McNeill, C. J.,** Is there a relationship between macrophage proliferation and tumoricidal activation?, *Proc. Annu. Meet. Am. Assoc. Cancer Res.,* 27, 348, 1986.
20. **Wilson, B. M., Rosendaal, M., and Plant, J. E.,** Early haemopoietic responses to *Salmonella typhimurium* infection in resistant and susceptible mice, *Immunology,* 45, 395, 1982.
21. **Wing, E. J., Waheed, A., and Shadduck, R. K.,** Changes in serum colony stimulating factor and monocytic progenitor cells during *Listeria monocytogenes* infection in mice, *Infect. Immun.,* 45, 180, 1984.
22. **Young, A. M. and Cheers, C.,** Colony-forming cells and colony-stimulating activity during listeriosis in genetically resistant and susceptible mice, *Cell. Immunol.,* 97, 227, 1986.
23. **Sluiter, W., Hulsing-Hesselink, E., and Van Furth, R.,** Synthesis and release of factor increasing monocytopoiesis (FIM) by macrophages, in *Biochemistry and Function of Phagocytes,* Rossi, F. and Patriaca, P., Eds., Plenum Press, New York, 1982, 225.
24. **Van Furth, R. and Sluiter, W.,** Macrophages as autoregulators of mononuclear phagocyte proliferation, in *Progress in Leukocyte Biology,* Vol. 4, Reichard, S. and Kojima, M., Eds., Alan R. Liss, New York, 1985, 111.
25. **Braun, D. P. and Harris, J. E.,** Relationship of leukocyte numbers, immunoregulatory cell function and phytohemagglutinin responsiveness in cancer patients, *J. Natl. Cancer Inst.,* 67, 809, 1981.
26. **Wood, G. W., Neff, J. E., and Stephens, R.,** Relationship between monocytopoiesis and T lymphocyte function in human cancer, *J. Natl. Cancer Inst.,* 63, 587, 1979.
27. **Normann, S. J., Schardt, M., and Sorkin, E.,** Alteration of macrophage function in AKR leukemia, *J. Natl. Cancer Inst.,* 66, 157, 1981.
28. **Sluiter, W., Elzenga-Classen, I., van der Voort, van der Kley van Andel, A., and van Furth, R.,** Differences in the response of inbred mouse strains to the factor increasing monocytopoiesis, *J. Exp. Med.,* 159, 524, 1984.
29. **Punjabi, C., Galsworthy, S. B., and Kongshavn, P. A. L.,** Cytokinetics of mononuclear phagocyte response to listeriosis in genetically determined sensitive and resistant murine hosts, *Clin. Invest. Med.,* 7, 165, 1984.
30. **Krishnan, E. C., Menon, C. D., Krishnan, L., and Jewell, W. R.,** Deficiency in maturation process of macrophages in human cancer, *J. Natl. Cancer Inst.,* 65, 273, 1980.
31. **Sokol, R. J. and Hudson, G.,** Disordered function of mononuclear phagocytes in malignant disease, *J. Clin. Pathol.,* 36, 316, 1983.
32. **Krishnan, E. C., Mebast, W. K., Weigel, J. W., and Jewell, W. R.,** In vitro peripheral monocyte culture: possible use as a prognostic indicator for renal cell carcinoma patients, *J. Natl. Cancer Inst.,* 74, 1185, 1985.
33. **Eccles, S. A. and Alexander, P.,** Macrophage content of tumours in relation to metastatic spread and host immune reaction, *Nature (London),* 250, 667, 1974.
34. **Evans, R. and Lawler, E. M.,** Macrophage content and immunogenicity of C57BL/6J and BALB/cByJ methylcholanthrene-induced sarcomas, *Int. J. Cancer,* 26, 831, 1980.
35. **Szymaneic, S. and James, K.,** Studies on the Fc receptor bearing cells in a transplanted methylcholanthrene induced mouse fibrosarcoma, *Br. J. Cancer,* 33, 36, 1976.
36. **Evans, R. and Eidlen, D. M.,** Macrophage accumulation in transplanted tumors is not dependent on host immune responsiveness or presence of tumor-associated rejection antigens, *J. Reticuloendothel. Soc.,* 30, 425, 1981.
37. **Evans, R.,** Macrophage accumulation in primary and transplanted tumors grown in C5-deficient B10.D2/oSn mice, *Int. J. Cancer,* 26, 227, 1980.
38. **Kaizer, L. and Lala, P. K.,** Post-mitotic age of mononuclear cells migrating into Ta-3(st) solid tumors, *Cell Tissue Kinet.,* 10, 279, 1977.
39. **Acero, R., Polentarutti, N., Bottazzi, B., Alberti, S., Ricci, M. R., Bizzi, A., and Mantovani, A.,** Effect of hydrocortisone on the macrophage content, growth and metastasis of transplanted murine tumors, *Int. J. Cancer,* 33, 95, 1984.
40. **Stevenson, M. M., Kongshavn, P. A. L., and Skamene, E.,** Genetic linkage of resistance to *Listeria monocytogenes* with macrophage inflammatory responses, *J. Immunol.,* 127, 402, 1981.
41. **Kongshavn, P. A. L.,** Genetic control of resistance to Listeria infection, *Curr. Top. Microbiol. Immunol.,* 124, 67, 1986.
42. **Gervais, F., Stevenson, M., and Skamene, E.,** Genetic control of resistance to *Listeria monocytogenes:* regulation of leukocyte inflammatory responses by the *Hc* locus, *J. Immunol.,* 132, 2078, 1984.
43. **Kongshavn, P. A. L. and Anthony, L. S. D.,** Genetic control of the macrophage inflammatory response elicited in a subcutaneous site, *Curr. Top. Microbiol. Immunol.,* 122, 134, 1985.
44. **Stevenson, M. M., Shenouda, G., Thomson, D. M. P., and Skamene, E.,** Genetically-determined defect in chemotactic responsiveness of inflammatory macrophage from A/J mice, in *Genetic Control of Host Resistance to Infection and Malignancy,* Skamene, E., Ed., Alan R. Liss, New York, 1985, 577.

45. **Stevenson, M. M., Skamene, E., and McCall, R. D.,** Macrophage chemotactic response in mice is controlled by two genetic loci, *Immunogenetics,* 23, 11, 1986.

46. **Thomson, D. M. P., Stevenson, M. M., and Skamene, E.,** Correlation between chemoattractant-induced leukocyte adherence inhibition, macrophage chemotaxis and macrophage inflammatory responses in vivo, *Cell. Immunol.,* 94, 547, 1985.

47. **Thomson, D. M. P., Ed.,** *Assessment of the Immune Status by the Leukocyte Adherence Inhibition Test,* Academic Press, New York, 1982.

48. **Snyderman, R., Siegler, H. F., and Meadows, L.,** Abnormalities of monocyte chemotaxis in patients with melanoma: effects of immunotherapy and tumor removal, *J. Natl. Cancer Inst.,* 58, 37, 1977.

49. **Boetcher, D. A. and Leonard, E. J.,** Abnormal monocyte chemotactic response in cancer patients, *J. Natl. Cancer Inst.,* 52, 1091, 1974.

50. **Snyderman, R. and Stahl, C.,** Defective immune effector function in patients with neoplasia and immune deficiency disease, in *The Phagocytic Cell in Host Resistance,* Bellanti, J. A. and Dayton, D., Eds., Raven Press, New York, 1975, 267.

51. **Snyderman, R., Pike, M. C., Blaylock, B., and Weinstein, P.,** Effects of neoplasia on inflammation: depression of macrophage accumulation after tumor implantation, *J. Immunol.,* 116, 585, 1976.

52. **Stevenson, M. M., Rees, J., and Meltzer, M. S.,** Macrophage function in tumor bearing mice: evidence for lactic dehydrogenase elevating virus associated changes, *J. Immunol.,* 124, 2892, 1980.

53. **Normann, S. J., Schardt, M., and Sorkin, E.,** Diphasic depression of macrophage function after tumor implantation, *Int. J. Cancer,* 28, 185, 1981.

54. **Snyderman, R. and Pike, M. C.,** An inhibitor of macrophage chemotaxis produced by neoplasms, *Science,* 192, 370, 1976.

55. **Normann, S. J. and Sorkin, E.,** Inhibition of macrophage chemotaxis by neoplastic and other rapidly proliferating cells in vitro, *Cancer Res.,* 37, 705, 1977.

56. **Snyderman, R., Pike, M. C., and Cianciolo, G. J.,** An inhibitor of macrophage accumulation produced by neoplasms: its role in abrogating host resistance to cancer, in *Mononuclear Phagocytes,* Part 1, van Furth, R., Ed., Martinus Nijhoff, The Hague, 1980, 569.

57. **Meltzer, M. S., Stevenson, M. M., and Leonard, E. J.,** Characterization of macrophage chemotaxins in tumor cell cultures and comparison with lymphocyte-derived chemotactic factors, *Cancer Res.,* 37, 721, 1977.

58. **Bottazzi, B., Polentarutti, N., Balsari, A., Boraschi, D., Ghezzi, P., Salmona, M., and Mantovani, A.,** Chemotactic activity for mononuclear phagocytes of culture supernatants from murine and human tumor cells: evidence for a role in the regulation of the macrophage content of neoplastic tissues, *Int. J. Cancer,* 31, 55, 1983.

59. **Ji-Ming, W., Cianciolo, G. J., Snyderman, R., and Mantovani, A.,** Co-existence of a chemotactic factor and a retroviral P15E-related chemotaxis inhibitor in human tumor cell culture supernatants, *J. Immunol.,* 137, 2726, 1986.

60. **Laskin, D. L., Laskin, J. D., Weinstein, I. B., and Carchman, R. A.,** Induction of chemotaxis in mouse peritoneal macrophages by phorbol ester tumor promoters, *Cancer Res.,* 41, 1923, 1981.

61. **Laskin, D. L., Laskin, J. D., Kessler, F. K., Weinstein, I. B., and Carchman, R. A.,** Enhancement of macrophage-mediated cytotoxicity by phorbol ester tumor promoters, *Cancer Res.,* 41, 4523, 1981.

62. **Lewis, J. G. and Adams, D. O.,** Enhanced release of hydrogen peroxide and metabolites of arachidonic acid by macrophages from SENCAR mice following stimulation with phorbol esters, *Cancer Res.,* 46, 5696, 1986.

63. **Unanue, E. R.,** Antigen presenting function of the macrophage, *Annu. Rev. Immunol.,* 2, 395, 1984.

64. **Unanue, E. R., Beller, D. I., Lu, C. Y., and Allen, P. M.,** Antigen presentation: comments on its regulation and mechanism, *J. Immunol.,* 132, 1, 1984.

65. **Beller, D. I. and Ho, K.,** Regulation of macrophage subpopulations. V. Evaluation of the control of macrophage Ia expression in vitro, *J. Immunol.,* 129, 971, 1982.

66. **Silver, D. M. and Winn, H. J.,** Variations in the responses of C57BL and A mice to sheep red blood cells. II. Analysis of plaque forming cells, *Cell. Immunol.,* 7, 237, 1973.

67. **Rihova, B. and Riha, I.,** Genetic regulation of antibody response to sheep red blood cells: linkage to H-2 complex, *Am. J. Reprod. Immunol.,* 1, 168, 1981.

68. **Rihova, B., Vetvicka, V., Riha, I., and Holan, V.,** Different handling of antigen by macrophages of low responder C57BL/10ScSn strain and high responder A/J strain of mice. I. Presentation of antigen and induction of helper and suppressor cells, *Thymus,* 8, 161, 1986.

69. **Minga, A. M., Segre, A., and Segre, D.,** Numbers and avidity of anti-DNP antibody plaques in different mouse strains, *Immunogenetics,* 2, 369, 1975.

70. **Rihova, B., Riha, I., Rossman, P., and Vetvicka, V.,** Low IgG response of mouse strain C57BL/10ScSn after immunization with protein antigens, *Folia Microbiol.,* 30, 295, 1985.

71. **Pisetsky, D. S., Berzofsky, A., and Sachs, D. H.,** Genetic control of the immune response to staphylococcal nuclease. VII. Role of non-H-2 linked genes in the control of the anti-nuclease antibody response, *J. Exp. Med.,* 147, 396, 1978.

72. **Nagai, H., Fisher, R. I., Cossman, J., and Oppenheim, J. J.,** Decreased expression of Class II major histocompatibility antigens on monocytes from patients with Hodgkin's disease, *J. Leukocyte Biol.,* 39, 313, 1986.

73. **Garner, R. E., Malick, A. P., and Elgert, K. D.,** Variations in macrophage antigen phenotype: a correlation between Ia antigen reduction and immune dysfunction during tumor growth, *J. Leukocyte Biol.,* 40, 561, 1986.

74. **Evans, R.,** Regulation of T and B lymphocyte responses to mitogens by tumor associated macrophages: the dependency on the stage of tumor growth, *J. Leukocyte Biol.,* 35, 549, 1984.

75. **Taylor, D. D. and Black, P. H.,** Inhibition of macrophage Ia antigen expression by shed plasma membrane vesicles from metastatic murine melanoma lines, *J. Natl. Cancer Inst.,* 74, 859, 1985.

76. **Dougherty, G. J. and McBride, W. H.,** Accessory cell activity of murine tumor-associated macrophages, *J. Natl. Cancer Inst.,* 76, 541, 1986.

77. **Dinarello, C. A.,** Interleukin-1, *Rev. Infect. Dis.,* 61, 51, 1984.

78. **Mortensen, R. F., Beisel, K., Zeleznik, N. J., and Le, P. T.,** Acute phase reactants of mice. II. Strain dependence of serum amyloid P-component (SAP) levels and response to inflammation, *J. Immunol.,* 120, 885, 1983.

79. **Brandwein, S. R., Skamene, E., Aubut, J. A., Gervais, F., and Nesbitt, M. N.,** Genetic regulation of lipopolysaccharide-induced interleukin 1 production by murine peritoneal macrophages, *J. Immunol.,* 138, 4263, 1987.

80. **Abehsira, A. O., Demais, C., Parent, M., and Chedid, L.,** Strain dependence of muramyl dipeptide-induced LAF (IL 1) release by murine adherent peritoneal cells, *J. Immunol.,* 134, 365, 1985.

81. **Gray, P. W., Glaister, D., Chen, E., Goeddel, D. V., and Pennica, D.,** Two interleukin 1 genes in the mouse: cloning and expression of the cDNA for murine interleukin 1β, *J. Immunol.,* 137, 3644, 1986.

82. **Dindzans, V. J., Skamene, E., and Levy, G. A.,** Susceptibility/resistance to mouse hepatitis virus strain 3 and macrophage procoagulant activity are genetically linked and controlled by two non-H-2 linked genes, *J. Immunol.,* 137, 2355, 1986.

83. **Levy, G. A., Leibowitz, J. L., and Edington, T. S.,** Induction of monocyte procoagulant activity by murine hepatitis virus type 3 (MHV-3) parallels disease susceptibility in mice, *J. Exp. Med.,* 154, 1150, 1981.

84. **Dindzans, V. P., MacPhee, P., Fung, L. S., Leibowitz, J. L., and Levy, G. A.,** The immune response to mouse hepatitis virus: expression of monocyte procoagulant activity and plasminogen activator during infection in vivo, *J. Immunol.,* 135, 4189, 1985.

85. **Carswell, E. A., Old, O. J., Kassel, R. L., Green, S., Fiore, N., and Williamson, B.,** An endotoxin-induced serum factor that causes necrosis of tumors, *Proc. Natl. Acad. Sci. U.S.A.,* 72, 3666, 1975.

86. **Beutler, B. and Cerami, A.,** Cachectin and tumor necrosis factor as two sides of the same biological coin, *Nature (London),* 320, 584, 1986.

87. **Mannel, D. N., Meltzer, M. S., and Mergenhagen, S. E.,** Generation and characterization of a lipopolysaccharide-induced and serum-derived cytotoxic factor for tumor cells, *Infect. Immun.,* 28, 204, 1980.

88. **Beutler, B., Krochin, N., Milsark, I. W., Luedke, C., and Cerami, A.,** Control of cachectin (tumor necrosis factor) synthesis: mechanisms of endotoxin resistance, *Science,* 232, 977, 1986.

89. **Beutler, B., Tkacenko, V., Milsark, I., Krochin, N., and Cerami, A.,** Effect of gamma interferon on cachectin expression by mononuclear phagocytes: reversal of the *Ips^d* (endotoxin resistant) phenotype, *J. Exp. Med.,* 164, 1791, 1986.

90. **Reiners, J. J., Newnow, S., and Slaga, T. J.,** Murine susceptibility to two-stage skin carcinogenesis is influenced by the agent used for promotion, *Carcinogenesis,* 5, 301, 1984.

91. **Lewis, J. G. and Adams, D. O.,** Induction of 5,6-ring saturated thymidine bases in NIH-3T3 cells by phorbol ester-stimulated macrophages: role of reactive oxygen intermediates, *Cancer Res.,* 45, 1270, 1985.

92. **Lewis, J. G., Hamilton, T. A., and Adams, D. O.,** The effect of macrophage development on the release of reactive oxygen intermediates and lipid oxidations, and their ability to induce oxidative DNA damage in mammalian cells, *Carcinogenesis,* 7, 813, 1986.

93. **Boraschi, D., Pasqualetto, E., Ghezzi, P., Salmon, M., Bartalini, M., Barbarulli, G., Censini, S., Soldateschi, D., and Tagliabue, A.,** Dissociation between macrophage tumoricidal capacity and suppressive activity: analysis with macrophage defective mouse strains, *J. Immunol.,* 131, 1707, 1983.

94. **Adams, D. O., Kao, K. J., Farb, R., and Pizzo, S. V.,** Effector mechanisms of cytolytically activated macrophages. II. Secretion of cytolytic factor by activated macrophages and its relationship to secreted neutral proteases, *J. Immunol.,* 124, 293, 1980.

95. **Adams, D. O., Marino, P. A., and Meltzer, M. S.,** Characterization of genetic defects in macrophage tumoricidal capacity: identification of murine strains with abnormalities in secretion of cytolytic factors and ability to bind neoplastic targets, *J. Immunol.,* 126, 1843, 1981.

96. **Boraschi, D. and Meltzer, M. S.,** Defective tumoricidal capacity of macrophages from P/J mice: tumoricidal defect involves abnormalities in lymphokine-derived activation stimuli and in mononuclear phagocyte responsiveness, *J. Immunol.,* 125, 777, 1980.
97. **Virelizier, J. L.,** Murine genotype influences the in vitro production of Gamma (immune) interferon, *Eur. J. Immunol.,* 12, 988, 1982.
98. **Adams, D. O. and Hamilton, T. A.,** The cell biology of macrophage activation, *Annu. Rev. Immunol.,* 2, 283, 1984.
99. **Adams, D. O., Johnson, W. J., and Marino, P. A.,** Mechanisms of target recognition and destruction in macrophage-mediated tumor cytotoxicity, *Fed. Proc. Fed. Am. Soc. Exp. Biol.,* 41, 2212, 1982.
100. **Adams, D. O. and Nathan, C. F.,** Molecular mechanisms in tumor-cell killing by activated macrophages, *Immunol. Today,* 4, 166, 1983.
101. **Adams, D. O. and Koren, H. S.,** BCG-activated macrophages: comparison as effectors in direct tumor cell cytotoxicity and antibody-dependent cell mediators in cytotoxicity. Part B. macrophages and lymphocytes, *Adv. Exp. Biol. Med.,* 121, 195, 1979.
102. **Meltzer, M. S., Ruco, L. P., Boraschi, D., and Nacy, C. A.,** Macrophage activation for tumor cytotoxicity: analysis of intermediary reactions, *J. Reticuloendothel. Soc.,* 26, 403, 1979.
103. **Meltzer, M. S., Occhionero, M., and Ruco, L. P.,** Macrophage activation for tumor cytotoxicity: regulatory mechanisms for induction and control of cytotoxic activity, *Fed. Proc. Fed. Am. Soc. Exp. Biol.,* 41, 2198, 1982.
104. **Hibbs, J. B., Taintor, R., Chapman, H. A., and Weinberg, J.,** Macrophage tumor killing: influence of the local environment, *Science,* 197, 279, 1977.
105. **Russell, S. W., Doe, W. F., and McIntosh, A. T.,** Functional characterization of a stable, noncytolytic stage of macrophage activation in tumors, *J. Exp. Med.,* 146, 1511, 1977.
106. **Boraschi, D. and Meltzer, M. S.,** Macrophage activation for tumor cytotoxicity: genetic variation in macrophage tumoricidal capacity among mouse strains, *Cell. Immunol.,* 45, 188, 1979.
107. **Ruco, L. P. and Meltzer, M. S.,** Defective tumoricidal capacity of macrophages from C3H/HeJ mice, *J. Immunol.,* 120, 329, 1978.
108. **Ruco, L. P., Meltzer, M. S., and Rosenstreich, D. L.,** Macrophage activation for tumor cytotoxicity: control of macrophage tumoricidal capacity by the Lps gene, *J. Immunol.,* 121, 543, 1978.
109. **Boraschi, D. and Meltzer, M. S.,** Defective tumoricidal capacity of macrophages from A/J mice. I. Characterization of the macrophage cytotoxicity defect after in vivo and in vitro stimuli, *J. Immunol.,* 122, 1587, 1979.
110. **Boraschi, D. and Meltzer, M. S.,** Defective tumoricidal capacity of macrophages from A/J mice. II. Comparison of the macrophage cytotoxic defect of A/J mice with that of lipid A-unresponsive C3H/HeJ mice, *J. Immunol.,* 122, 1592, 1979.
111. **Boraschi, D. and Meltzer, M. S.,** Defective tumoricidal capacity of macrophages from P/J mice: characterization of the macrophage cytotoxic defect after in vivo and in vitro activation stimuli, *J. Immunol.,* 125, 771, 1980.
112. **Boraschi, D. and Meltzer, M. S.,** Defective tumoricidal capacity of macrophages from A/J mice. III. Genetic analysis of the macrophage defect, *J. Immunol.,* 124, 1050, 1980.
113. **Forni, L. and Coutinho, L.,** An antiserum which recognizes lipopolysaccharide-reactive B cells, *Eur. J. Immunol.,* 8, 56, 1978.
114. **Hamilton, T. A., Becton, D. L., Somers, S. D., Gray, P. W., and Adams, D. O.,** IFN-γ modulates protein kinase C activity in murine peritoneal macrophages, *J. Biol. Chem.,* 260, 1378, 1985.
115. **Hamilton, T. A., Somers, S. A., Becton, D. L., Celada, A., Schreiber, R. D., and Adams, D. O.,** Analysis of deficiencies in IFN-γ-mediated priming for tumor cytotoxicity in peritoneal macrophages from A/J mice, *J. Immunol.,* 137, 3367, 1986.
116. **Skamene, E., Kongshavn, P. A. L., and Landy, M., Eds.,** *Genetic Control of Natural Resistance to Infection and Malignancy,* Academic Press, New York, 1980.
117. **Skamene, E., Ed.,** Genetic control of host resistance to infection and malignancy, *Proc. Leukocyte Biol.,* 3, 1985.
118. **Diwan, B. A. and Meier, H.,** Colo-rectal tumors in inbred mice treated with 1:2 dimethylhydrazine, *Proc. Am. Assoc. Cancer Res.,* 17, 106, 1976.
119. **Malkinson, A. M., Nesbitt, M. N., and Skamene, E.,** Susceptibility to urethan-induced pulmonary adenomas between A/J and C57BL/6J mice: use of AXB and BXA recombinant inbred line indicating a three locus genetic model, *J. Natl. Cancer Inst.,* 75, 971, 1985.
120. **James, S. L., Skamene, E., and Meltzer, M. S.,** Macrophages as effector cells of protective immunity in murine schistosomiasis. V. Variation in macrophage schistosomulacidal and tumoricidal activities among mouse strains and correlation with resistance to reinfection, *J. Immunol.,* 131, 948, 1983.
121. **Skamene, E., James, S. L., Meltzer, M. S., and Nesbitt, M. N.,** Genetic control of macrophage activation for killing of extracellular targets, *J. Leukocyte Biol.,* 35, 65, 1984.

122. **Koren, H. S., Meltzer, M. S., and Adams, D. O.**, The ADCC capacity of macrophages from C3H/HeJ and A/J mice can be augmented by BCG, *J. Immunol.*, 126, 1013, 1981.

123. **Fidler, I. J.**, The generation of tumoricidal activity in macrophages for the treatment of established metastases, in *Cancer Invasion and Metastasis: Biologic and Therapeutic Aspects*, Nicolson, G. L. and Milas, L., Eds., Raven Press, New York, 1984, 421.

124. **Fidler, I. J.**, Macrophages and metastasis: a biological approach to cancer therapy, *Cancer Res.*, 45, 4714, 1985.

125. **Schroit, A. J., Hart, I. R., Madsen, J., and Fidler, I. J.**, Selective delivery of drugs encapsulated in liposomes: natural targeting to macrophages involved in various disease states, *J. Biol. Response Modifiers*, 2, 97, 1983.

126. **Kleinerman, E. S., Erickson, K. L., Schroit, A. J., Folger, W. E., and Fidler, I. J.**, Activation of tumoricidal properties in human blood monocytes by liposomes containing lipophilic muramyl tripeptide, *Cancer Res.*, 43, 2010, 1983.

127. **Fidler, I. J., Jessup, J. M., Folger, W. E., Staerkel, R., and Mazumber, A.**, Activation of tumoricidal properties in peripheral blood monocytes of patients with colorectal carcinoma, *Cancer Res.*, 46, 994, 1986.

128. **Kleinerman, E. S., Zwelling, L., Howser, C., Barlock, A., Young, R. D., Deij, J. M., Bull, J., and Muchmore, A. V.**, Defective monocyte killing in patients with malignancies and restoration of function during chemotherapy, *Lancet*, i, 1102, 1980.

129. **Peri, G., Polentarutti, N., Sessa, C., Mangioni, C., and Mantovani, A.**, Tumoricidal activity of macrophages isolated from human ascitic and solid carcinomas: augmentation by interferon, lymphokines and endotoxin, *Int. J. Cancer*, 28, 143, 1982.

130. **Poste, G. and Kirshm, R.**, Rapid decay of tumoricidal activity and loss of responsiveness to lymphokines in inflammatory macrophages, *Cancer Res.*, 39, 2582, 1979.

131. **Fogler, W. E., Talmadge, J. E., and Fidler, I. J.**, The activation of tumoricidal properties in macrophages of endotoxin responder and nonresponder mice by liposome-encapsulated immunomodulators, *J. Reticuloendothel. Soc.*, 33, 165, 1983.

132. **Phillips, N. C., Moras, M. L., Chedid, L., Lefrancier, P., and Bernard, J. M.**, Activation of alveolar macrophage tumoricidal activity and eradication of experimental metastases by freeze-dried liposomes containing a new lipophilic muramyl dipeptide derivative, *Cancer Res.*, 45, 128, 1985.

133. **Phillips, N. C., Skamene, E., and Chedid, L.**, Correction of defective tumoricidal activity of macrophages from A/J mice by liposomal immunomodulators, *Immunopharmocology*, 15, 1, 1988.

Chapter 6

TUMOR-ASSOCIATED MACROPHAGES

Amy M. Fulton

TABLE OF CONTENTS

I. INTRODUCTION

The presence of host inflammatory cells within and at the periphery of neoplasms has been recognized since the 19th century.[1] The significance of this phenomenon has long been questioned. Now, with the recent development of the necessary techniques to isolate and characterize these cells, the first steps towards describing their properties and functions have been taken.

II. CHARACTERISTICS OF TUMOR-ASSOCIATED MACROPHAGES (TAM)(HUMAN TUMORS)

Whereas many early studies focused on lymphocytic infiltrates, until recently, there has been little quantitation of infiltrating macrophages in human cancer due, undoubtedly, to the difficulty in identifying these cells in conventionally prepared tissue. Data from as early as 1959, however, do suggest an important role for macrophages in tumor behavior. The study by Berg[2] of selected cases of human breast cancer with the histologic appearance of anaplastic-infiltrating ductal carcinomas revealed that the cancers of 73% of the patients remaining disease free for longer than 5 years showed round cell infiltration at the junction of normal and cancerous breast tissue. Only 30% of tumors from patients dying within 5 years of diagnosis had such an inflammatory reaction.[2] Histiocytes were the most commonly observed inflammatory cell, second to plasma cells.

Sinus histiocytosis in lymph nodes (a reaction now believed to be due to macrophages) has been considered a favorable prognostic sign.[3] Two studies reported that breast tumor tissue specimens without nodal or skin involvement have higher macrophage content than do metastatic cancers.[4,5] In a recent study of human breast tumors, the majority of specimens had significant mononuclear infiltrates,[6] but few had evidence of monocytic (OKM 1 and acid phosphatase positive) cells. Steele reported that although peripheral blood monocytes from breast cancer patients had high levels of lysozyme relative to normal controls,[7] TAM had virtually none suggesting a defect in activation. Evidence in human colonic tumors for the differential distribution of subpopulations of TAM, identified histochemically by staining for acid phosphatase and α-naphthyl butyrate esterase, was provided by Luebbers et al.[8] Some cells having the morphologic appearance of macrophages stained for one enzyme but not the other. In addition, the concentration and location of these cells (proximal or distal to the tumor) differed in patients with and without metastases. The total number of TAM in human lung carcinomas was reported to be unrelated to clinical stage, although in totally resectable cases, higher cytostatic activity was associated with a lower recurrence rate,[9] again suggesting a differential distribution of macrophage subpopulations in cancers with differing clinical prognoses.

III. CHARACTERISTICS OF TAM (EXPERIMENTAL TUMORS)

Difficulties in studying inflammatory infiltrates in human cancers have been somewhat alleviated in animal tumors. TAM have been isolated from experimental rodent tumors of spontaneous, viral, and chemical origin, and range from 2 to 60% of total isolated cells.[10,11] Haskill et al. described TAM in methylcholanthrene- or benzypyrene-induced rat sarcomas and in murine line T1699 mammary adenocarcinomas.[12,13] In the rat systems, the proportion of macrophages, in relation to tumor cells, was seen to decrease as the tumor grew. Kerbel and Pross described Fc receptor (FcR)-positive cells in both spontaneous murine mammary carcinomas and chemically induced fibrosarcomas.[14] Antigenic analysis of tumors transplanted into F_1 hybrid mice revealed that the infiltrates were of host origin and not part of the tumor inoculum. Analysis of primary and early passaged methylcholanthrene-induced tumors showed that each tumor had a different proportion of TAM that, after an initial reduction following first passage, remained relatively constant for each tumor.[15] Irradiated tumors were rapidly repopulated with macrophages, resulting in a relatively constant ratio of macrophages-to-tumor cells.[16] These studies indicate that the number or nature of TAM is neither random nor a generalized host response to growing tumors. Rather, since each individual tumor contains a reproducible population of TAM, the TAM are, in fact, a tumor-directed characteristic.

With the extensive study of macrophages in both pathologic and nonpathologic conditions, it has become apparent that cells having the morphologic appearance of monocytes or tissue macrophages are not uniform in either physical characteristics or in function.[17] This concept of macrophage heterogeneity is discussed elsewhere in this volume (Chapters 1 and 2). Suffice it to say that TAM are also composed of subpopulations of macrophages that differ in physical, biochemical, and functional properties.

Using the biochemical markers of peroxidase, 5'nucleotidase, and acid phosphatase, two distinct populations of macrophages have been described in immunogenic mouse fibrosarcomas.[18] One population was a small peroxidase-positive cell, the other a larger cell with an enzyme profile resembling protease-peptone-elicited macrophages. When compared to resident peritoneal macrophages (high 5'nucleotidase, low acid phosphatase) and *Corynebacterium parvum*-activated macrophages (low 5'nucleotidase, high acid phosphatase) these TAM had intermediate levels of both enzymes. TAM isolated from human ovarian carcinomas were also heterogeneous by size and cytochemical criteria.[19]

We have, likewise, found that TAM from different transplantable murine mammary adenocarcinomas are heterogeneous in terms of the kinds of macrophage subpopulations and that the TAM profile for any one tumor is relatively constant and reproducible.[20,21] Macrophage subpopulations isolated from single tumors by centrifugal elutriation differed in density and diameter. In addition, these TAM had varying levels of the ectoenzymes leucine aminopeptidase, alkaline phosphodiesterase, and 5'nucleotidase. Noncoordinate expression of ectoenzymes normally associated with activation (leucine aminopeptidase and acid phosphatase) were seen in these TAM.[21] Additionally, macrophages from different elutriation fractions also varied in their ability to synthesize the immunoregulator prostaglandin E_2.

IV. FUNCTION OF TAM

While the function of inflammatory macrophages in host defense against intracellular parasites is established, the role of such cells in destroying or inhibiting tumor cells is less clear. Macrophages isolated from peripheral tissues (spleen, peritoneum) often have demonstrable cytostatic and cytotoxic activity but the significance of this, and more to the point, the function of TAM in this regard, is uncertain.

A. Cytotoxic Activity

Whereas peripheral macrophages, particularly when activated, can usually be shown to be cytostatic and/or cytotoxic to tumor target cells, similar activities of TAM are not always demonstrable. In one of the few functional studies of human tumors, Vose showed that TAM isolated from 17 of 25 tumors were cytotoxic for autologous target cells.[22] In contrast, Mantovani reported poor cytolytic activity in TAM isolated from an ascites form of ovarian tumor.[23] In this system, however, the possible presence of immunosuppressive factors in the ascites fluid may not reflect the situation in solid tumors. Further evidence that TAM play a host-protective role comes from studies showing that transplantable tumor inocula grow faster after transfer, if freed of TAM.[24] Tumor cells are sometimes (but not always) more clonogenic when freed of host cells.[25] Early studies in the Moloney Sarcoma Virus (MSV) system, in which progressing and regressing tumors are available, show that cytotoxic activity of TAM is lost in progressive lesions.[26,27] It is not certain whether this is causal or an effect of progressive growth and, in addition, this model has been criticized due to the infectious nature of the MSV system.

B. Growth Promotion Activity

In contrast to the many reports of TAM cytostatic activity, there is an equal body of evidence that TAM can function to promote tumor growth. TAM isolated from FS6 tumors and held in culture, stimulated tumor growth. TAM isolated from a weakly immunogenic variant of this tumor enhanced tumor cell proliferation regardless of the time in culture.[28] A later study revealed that the dual effects of growth inhibition and stimulation were dependent on the TAM:tumor cell ratio, with low ratios leading to the stimulation of tumor cell proliferation and higher ratios resulting in cytostasis.[29] Whole body irradiation of mice prior to or following implantation of a fibrosarcoma retarded initial growth.[30] This tumor inhibition was accompanied by a relative paucity of infiltrating macrophages. In adoptive Winn assays, thioglycollate-activated peritoneal macrophages in admixture with tumor cells led to larger tumors, as measured by weight.[31] A reduction in TAM populations as a result of hydrocortisone-induced monocytopenia was accompanied by an inhibition of murine tumors.[32] Studies by Mantovani and colleagues also reported that treatment with the anti-macrophage agents, silica and carrageenan, enhanced metastasis, but decreased the weight of primary tumors.[33] It is not clear, however, whether this reflected a real decrease in tumor growth rate, i.e., fewer tumor cells and subsequent increased survival time, or merely a less cellular tumor mass due to the lack of inflammatory cells.

Similar stimulatory effects on tumor cell proliferation in vitro have been observed with resident or elicited peritoneal macrophages.[34,35] Interestingly, *Corynebacterium parvum*-elicited, fully activated macrophages inhibited tumor cell proliferation under certain conditions immediately after isolation. Following culture in vitro, however, these macrophages became growth stimulating. In addition to putative growth factors, macrophages are known to release angiogenesis factors and are stimulated to do so by hypoxic conditions,[36] thus, TAM might support tumor growth in this indirect fashion. Thus, although growth promoting effects can be demonstrated in vitro, it is unclear whether such feeder effects have relevance in vivo; other cells, such as fibroblasts, have similar activities. It is conceivable that stromal macrophages normally serve some growth supportive function but evidence for such a role is scarce. In addition, macrophages rapidly lose cytotoxic activity upon culture probably through the loss of stimulatory signals and by apparent self-regulatory mechanisms such as prostaglandin E_2 synthesis. Such loss of inhibitory activity could unmask opposing effects. Whether such inactivation occurs in vivo is not known.

In many cases, the clonogenicity of human epithelial tumors is reduced by the removal of plastic adherent nonphagocytic cells.[37] This effect can be reversed by the readdition of macrophages below the agar layer containing the tumor cells and thus, implicates a diffusible factor. The cyclooxygenase inhibitor, indomethacin, blocks this feeder effect suggesting that it may be due to macrophage-synthesized prostaglandins.

In an in vitro model of cyclophosphamide-induced tumor cell inhibition, TAM were seen to increase the proliferation of treated methylcholanthrene (MCA) sarcoma or lymphoma cells. Using toxic drug doses, TAM stimulated the proliferation of the few surviving tumor cells.[38] The authors propose that in vivo TAM can support the regrowth of tumors that have been induced to regress with cyclophosphamide.

C. Role in Metastasis

The relationship of TAM phenotypes to other tumor cell properties such as immunogenicity and metastatic potential is also controversial. An early study by Eccles and Alexander reported that the proportion of TAM in 6 different chemically induced rat fibrosarcomas ranged from

8 to 54% of total cells.[39] An inverse relationship was seen between the incidence of spontaneous metastasis and TAM content. A direct relationship was seen between proportion of TAM and immunogenicity (as measured by number of tumor cells required for growth in previously sensitized animals). This study, therefore, suggested that the high percentage of TAM might prevent spontaneous metastasis. Examination of these relationships in other tumor systems has shown that this is not generally the case. In mouse tumors with relatively low levels of TAM (2 to 9%), no relationship was seen with metastatic potential.[40] In chemically induced murine sarcomas, immunogenicity was not related to degree of macrophage infiltration.[41] In a number of rodent tumors, a higher TAM content was associated with longer induction times (time to palpable tumor) but, again, no relationship was apparent between TAM content and subsequent growth rate, metastatic potential, or immunogenicity.[42] Systemic suppression with antimacrophage agents or enhancement with biological response modifiers affects metastatic rate suggesting that macrophages are important, but the function of TAM in this regard is less clear.

Loveless and Heppner evaluated TAM in a series of murine mammary tumor lines varying in tumorigenicity, immunogenicity, metastatic ability, and many other characteristics.[43] The TAM content, as determined by latex bead phagocytosis or presence of Fc receptor, ranged from 20 to 28% for all tumors. Based on morphologic criteria, TAM ranged from 20 to 44%.[20] No relationship was apparent between macrophage content and the biologic behavior of these lines, however, functional and phenotypic differences between TAM from metastatic or nonmetastatic tumors were seen. TAM from two metastatic lines (immunogenic line 410.4 and nonimmunogenic line 66) were always cytotoxic, whereas significant cytotoxicity was detected for TAM from nonmetastatic tumor line 68H in 50% of the experiments, in only 20% of the isolates of tumor line 67, and in none of the isolates of tumor line 168. Both the latter lines are nonmetastatic but line 168 will form lung colonies following intravenous injection. As discussed above, TAM from different tumors were heterogeneous by the criteria of size, density, ectoenzyme, and prostaglandin E levels.[20] Based on centrifugal elutriation fractionation, TAM from metastatic tumors were larger and denser and had higher levels of the ectoenzyme leucine aminopeptidase, indicating a greater proportion of activated TAM in metastatic tumors. Conversely, TAM from nonmetastatic line 67 had the highest amount of acid phosphatase.[21]

Thus, the role of macrophages in controlling metastatic dissemination is still unclear. Although cytotoxic/cytostatic activity can often be demonstrated for TAM, the susceptibility of the tumor cells to such attack must be considered. We and others have shown that metastatic tumor sublines are more resistant to macrophage-mediated growth inhibition than are nonmetastatic counterparts.[44] It is conceivable that this resistance has arisen by selection processes mediated by TAM. In some cases, macrophage tumor cell interactions do lead to more aggressive phenotypes.[45] An interesting recent finding is that normal alveolar macrophages selectively support the growth in vitro of highly metastatic rat fibrosarcoma cells in comparison to low metastatic cells.[46] This raises the possibility that nonmetastatic cells might survive less well in the lungs due to the poorer "soil" provided by local macrophages. Other nonlethal interactions between macrophages and tumor cells, such as the intriguing reports of fusion between host macrophages and tumor cells to induce new phenotypes are also being explored.[47]

D. Other Functions

In addition to their cytostatic/cytotoxic activity, macrophages have potent immunoregulatory functions as well. These are mediated by many factors including interleukin 1 (IL-1) and prostaglandin E (PGE). This latter molecule is well documented as a potent immunoregulator. Under most conditions it serves to down regulate immune responses, although in some suboptimal responses it has the opposite effect. Thus, TAM-PGE could serve to suppress potentially therapeutic infiltrations of host lymphocytes.[48] Less clear is the role of endogenous PGE (either released by tumor cells or from TAM) on macrophage function. Several studies suggest that PGE has opposing effects on macrophage function depending on the initial activation state of the cell;[49-52] that is, resident macrophages appear to express increased tumor cytostatic ability after exposure to PGE, whereas activated macrophage function is depressed by PGE. In addition, peripheral macrophages from tumor-bearing animals or patients more actively synthesize PGE than do normal macrophages,[53-55] and these cells can suppress normal immunologic reactions in vitro. There is also considerable evidence that macrophage PGE serves as a negative feedback inhibitor of macrophage proliferation and differentiation. Thus, it is conceivable that TAM-PGE can suppress immune effector functions and self-regulate its own function.

We have shown that both TAM and tumor cells synthesize PGE.[20] TAM, fractionated by centrifugal elutriation technique, are heterogeneous for PGE production, with different size macrophages having relatively different synthetic activities. Thus, peak PGE production was seen in the larger, more dense macrophages isolated from three nonmetastatic tumor lines, whereas peak PGE activity was seen in smaller (earlier fraction) macrophages from metastatic tumors. As cells expressed more PGE activity, their levels of the activation-associated ectoenzyme, leucine aminopeptidase, declined and vice versa. Unfractionated TAM from these tumors were heterogeneous for cytotoxic activity as well. Thus, metastatic tumors consistently contained the most cytotoxic TAM while nonmetastatic TAM were rarely cytotoxic.[42] While the interactions between PGE, TAM, and activation markers are not yet defined, tumor PGE might be expected to suppress TAM cytotoxicity. On the other hand, if the phenotype of infiltrating TAM is that of a resident macrophage, then PGE would be expected to enhance these activities. The most cytotoxic TAM, however, are present in the metastatic tumors which also have the highest levels of PGE *in situ*.[20] Double labeling studies by Bugelski et al. of infiltrating macrophages at various times indicate that circulating macrophages can be activated for 3 to 5 days after extravasation suggesting that only newly infiltrating macrophages are activated.[56] Thus, the highly active TAM found in our system might be recently arrived cells. If their activity is indeed suppressed by tumor PGE, then tumors with higher cytotoxic activity would be the result of more intensive continuous influx of TAM. To account for the constant number, one would have to postulate that TAM leave these lesions at a greater rate as well. We do not know if functional suppressor macrophages are present in TAM or what their relationship is to cytotoxic cells. Haskill et al.[19] have described suppressor macrophages in human ovarian tumors, however, whether this activity is related to PGE is not known.

TAM may have functions other than cytotoxicity and suppression; Ia-positive murine macrophages isolated from methylcholanthrene-induced fibrosarcomas can serve as accessory cells for antigen presentation in the primary antibody response to sheep red blood cells.[57] While these cells were phagocytic and 20 to 25% were FcR positive, surprisingly, most were Mac-1 antigen negative, a marker previously thought to be present on all macrophages. The tumor's microenvironment may thus, suppress expression of this antigen. PGE is known to suppress Ia antigen expression[58] and it would be interesting to examine a similar effect for Mac antigens.

Other putative functions of TAM may contribute to the invasive and metastatic success of tumor cells. Co-cultured macrophages and Lewis lung carcinoma cells are able to degrade collagen,[59] whereas neither population alone is able to do so. One-way mixing experiments suggest that macrophages release factors that stimulate tumor cells to release collagenase activities. Additionally, inflammatory macrophages or TAM isolated from mammary tumor lines bind the basement membrane component laminin.[60] Laminin may contribute to their locomotory and invasive capacities as well as facilitating interactions with tumor cells by serving as adhesion molecules.

Can TAM support the growth and success of tumor cells by other mechanisms? Tumor progression, a process by which tumor cells acquire more malignant properties with time, is presumably due to the acquisition of new properties via either mutation or through epigenetic mechanisms.[61] Can the constant association of tumor cells with TAM contribute to the acquisition of more aggressive phenotypes? Studies by others using peripheral phagocytic cells,[62] and our own, show that TAM can be mutagenic to bacteria in the Ames assay,[63] and can induce drug resistance in cultured cells.[64,65] In addition, as stated previously, TAM from metastatic tumors are more fully activated and, therefore, would be expected to produce oxidative products that through mutational or epigenetic events might contribute to tumor progression. Thus, through the *selection* of new phenotypes, e.g., tumor cells resistant to macrophage killing and the *induction* of new tumor cell variants, TAM might contribute to tumor progression. These findings are discussed more fully elsewhere in this volume (Heppner and Dorcey, "Macrophages and Development of Cancer").

V. MECHANISMS OF INFILTRATION

A. Chemotaxis

While most investigators would agree that the majority, if not all TAM, arise from the infiltration of circulating blood monocytes, the mechanisms which direct this reaction are not known. That infiltration is not random is shown by the studies discussed earlier in which the character of the TAM infiltrates of different transplantable tumors is a relatively constant feature.[15,16,20,21] Chemotactic factors produced by solid tumors may contribute to the preferential accumulation of macrophages *in situ*. Meltzer et al.[66] described a chemotactic factor, molecular weight about 15,000, released by murine sarcomas. Bacillus Calmette Guerin-activated macrophages were more responsive than were resident macrophages; neutrophils were not responsive. In a series of 11 murine tumors, a positive, although not perfect, correlation was seen for the amount of releasable chemotactic activity and percentage of TAM in vivo.[67] This activity, which was also released by cultured mouse embryo fibroblasts, was not chemotactic for polymorphonuclear leukocytes, distinguishing it from most known chemotactic factors. Production of this factor was decreased by protein synthesis inhibitors, its activity was sensitive to DNase and RNase, and it appeared to have a molecular weight of 12,000.[68] Cultured vascular endothelial cells also release a chemotactic activity for resident peritoneal macrophages,[69] and thus, the tumor-associated vasculature might attract such cells. Chemokinetic activity, or the nondirectional movement of macrophages, can be increased with conditioned medium from a variety of murine tumor lines but not from cultured fibroblasts.[70] Interestingly, this activity could only be demonstrated in fully (*Corynebacterium parvum* or pyran) activated macrophages. Glycogen or thioglycollate-elicited macrophages were unresponsive. This trypsin-sensitive activity had a molecular weight range of 300,000 to 400,000 and lacked chemotactic activity and, therefore, appears to be distinct from the factor described by Bottazzi.[67,68]

On the other hand, many investigators report that peripheral monocytes obtained from cancer patients, most in later stages of disease, have depressed monocyte responses to chemotactic factors.[71] In melanoma patients, either depressed or elevated chemotactic responses were seen in 64% of patients. Snyderman concludes that either of these reactions was associated with a poorer prognosis than was a normal chemotactic response.[72] Others have also reported depressed responses in late stage melanoma.[73] Peripheral blood from both patients with benign breast disease or those apparently free of cancer following surgery demonstrated normal chemotaxis,[74] in contrast to the many patients with active disease in whom this response was often depressed. Several antichemotactic factors isolated from tumors have been reported but the biochemical characterization of these activities differs.[75-81] Other factors, such as prostaglandins, which are present in high levels at tumor sites, can be inhibitory (PGE$_2$) or stimulatory (PGA$_1$, PGF$_{2a}$) to chemotaxis.[82] The chemotactic component of complement C$_{5a}$ may not control TAM, at least in some systems, as a C$_{5a}$-deficient strain of mice accumulated normal levels of TAM.[11] Other exogenous agents, such as the tumor-promoting phorbol esters, characteristically induce inflammatory reactions, are chemotactic for macrophages.[83] This last finding has interesting implications in terms of the contribution of TAM to tumor induction and progression via epigenetic or mutational events.

Most of the anti-inflammatory effects seen in both experimental and human studies appear in later stage disease. Although such compromised host responses are probably important to the ultimate outcome of disease, they are probably less important in determining TAM characteristics and function in early disease.

The finding that some chemotactic and antichemotactic activities have differential effects on macrophages depending on degree of activation may provide an explanation for the diversity of TAM. Ia antigen positive and negative macrophages respond preferentially to different chemotactic agents.[84] In addition, circulating monocytes in patients may fail to respond normally to chemotactic factors that are present.

B. Proliferation *In Situ*

While some studies propose that the entire TAM population can be accounted for by the influx of circulating monocytes,[85] others feel that proliferation of TAM at the tumor site can occur. Haskill et al. reported that radiolabeled TAM were detectable in T1699 mammary tumors as early as 1 hr following injection of ^{3}H-thymidine.[13] Similarly, Stewart has shown that isolation of TAM 30 min after systemic administration of ^{3}H-thymidine led to radiolabeling of 10 to 28% of TAM, depending on the tumor under study.[86] Again, this short labeling period in vivo probably precludes any labeled blood monocytes from entering the tumor in sufficient numbers to account for this high proportion of proliferating cells. Using BrdU (bromodeoxyuridine) to label proliferating cells followed by detection with fluorescent anti-BrdU antibody on a fluorescence-activated cell sorter (FACs), we have also detected proliferating TAM in mammary tumors.[87] In comparing tumor lines with differing metastatic capacity, a similar number of TAM were seen for all tumors as previously reported. However, the number of proliferating TAM, as determined by BrdU uptake, varied. In metastatic tumor 66, 22% of adherent TAM were labeled compared to 13% of TAM from nonmetastatic tumor 67. Tumor 168, which forms lung colonies following intravenous injection but does not metastasize spontaneously, also had high (18%) levels of proliferating TAM. These findings parallel our earlier studies showing that metastatic tumors contain the most activated TAM. This raises the interesting question of how the macrophage-to-tumor ratio is maintained. Given the shorter doubling time of macrophages compared to tumor cells, some mechanism must be active which prevents overpopulation by these macrophages. We are currently investigating this question.

The mechanisms involved in the induction of TAM proliferation and/or differentiation are not known. In addition, the question of whether different macrophage subpopulations migrate to or are induced to become different TAM subpopulations has not been answered. We have proposed that, in addition to the influx of macrophages, local proliferation and differentiation might be induced via growth factors produced locally by tumor cells.[88] These factors would include or resemble known colony-stimulating factors (CSF) that play a role in normal hemopoiesis.

There have been several reports that nonlymphoid human tumors from patients with granulocytosis release colony-stimulating activities.[89,90] Similarly, mouse fibrosarcomas or adrenocortical tumors which cause granulocytosis in vivo also release activities that stimulate the formation of granulocyte and macrophage colonies from normal bone marrow progenitor cells.[91-93] While these studies provide evidence that granulocytosis associated with cancer

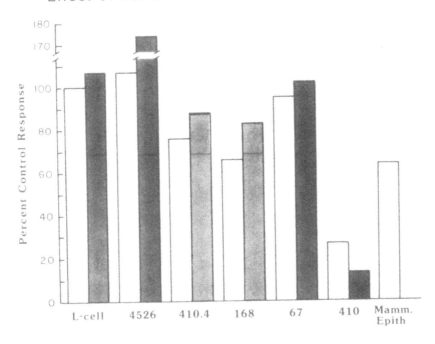

FIGURE 1. Effect of tumor conditioned media on the colony-forming activity of cultured bone marrow cells. Bone marrow cells were plated in soft agar in the presence of conditioned medium from either L-cell fibroblasts, mammary tumor lines, or primary cultures of normal murine lactating mammary epithelium. Colony number is expressed as a percent of the colony number seen in cultures containing L-cell-conditioned medium (open bars). Plates with unconditioned medium have 0 to 1 colonies/dish. Closed bars represent relative colony number for conditioned medium generated in the presence of 1 μM indomethacin.

might be caused by circulating colony-stimulating activities, in some cases a good correlation is not seen for serum levels of activity and numbers of colony forming units detectable in hemopoietic tissues.[94] Indeed, Burlington et al. have, after repeated passages, isolated a tumor variant, which, unlike the parent tumor, did not induce granulocytosis and yet both tumors made colony-stimulating activities in vitro.[95] An interesting recent observation is that highly metastatic clones of a murine mammary carcinoma released more colony-stimulating activity in vitro than did their nonmetastatic counterparts.[96] This association, however, was not seen in vivo again raising questions as to the significance of these observations.

To begin to define the mechanisms that determine the nature of TAM phenotypes, we have focused on the possibility that tumor cells can influence these events. We have tested the effect of conditioned medium prepared from tumor lines with varying properties on the ability of macrophage progenitor cells from the bone marrow to form colonies (CFU-C) in soft agar. We have reported previously[88] and show in Figure 1 that conditioned medium from tumor lines 4526, 410.4, 168, and 67 can support the colony-forming ability of bone marrow cells with quantitatively similar activities to that seen from the L929 fibroblast line (open bars). Conditioned medium from one nonmetastatic tumor line, 410, expressed little CFU activity. Thus, we did not see the relationship reported by Nicoletti et al. for metastatic potential and CFU activity.[96] When bone marrow cells were cultured in unconditioned medium, no colonies were formed. Interestingly, normal mouse mammary epithelium prepared from pregnant mice also expressed CFU activity. These colonies were both macrophage, granulocytic, and mixed macrophage granulocyte colonies. Using these same tumor lines, Thomas et al.[97] have shown that mice bearing tumors of line 410.4 or 168 develop leukocytosis and neutrophilia in vivo.

CSF-1 units vs CFU-C Activity in Tumor Conditioned Media

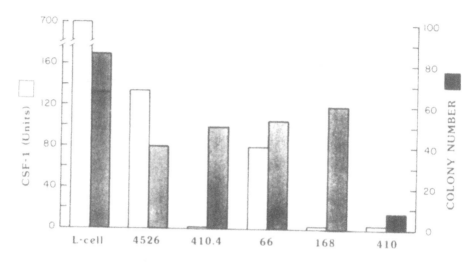

FIGURE 2.   Units of CSF-1, as determined by radioimmunoassay (open bars), and colony number supported by conditioned medium (closed bars) from cultured L-cell fibroblasts or murine mammary tumor lines.

Because of the well documented negative-feedback role of PGE for bone marrow colony formation,[98] and because these tumor lines synthesize PGE,[99] we tested the CFU activity of tumor-conditioned medium generated in the presence of the prostaglandin synthesis inhibitor, indomethacin. As shown in Figure 1 (closed bars), this treatment led to an increase in detection of CFU activity, particularly for line 4526, which produces very high levels of PGE in vitro.[99]

When these conditioned media were assayed for authentic colony-stimulating factor-1 (CSF-1), a good correlation was seen between CSF-1 and colony number for some tumor lines, but not for others (Figure 2). This is not surprising as CSF-1 is specifically stimulatory to macrophages and we saw both macrophage and granulocyte colonies formed. Interestingly, lines 410.4 and 168, in which no relationship was seen for the two activities, were reported to induce granulocytosis by Thomas et al.[97] Thus, the colony-stimulating activities for these tumor lines are more likely to be due to other CSF species such as CSF-GM (granulocyte macrophage), which stimulates both macrophages and granulocytes.[100]

While these experiments describe activities that stimulate very immature cells to proliferate to form colonies, we would suspect that monocytes entering the tumor milieu would be more mature. Thus, while tumor-associated signals might stimulate these cells to proliferate, they might also induce these cells to differentiate, resulting in the heterogeneity of TAM.

VI. SUMMARY AND CONCLUSIONS

Even though TAM have been described in many experimental and human systems, their significance in vivo is still poorly defined. Whether the heterogeneity in function, e.g., suppressor and cytotoxic activities demonstable in vitro, truly reflects multiple and at times conflicting functions in vivo, is still open to question. It is not difficult to imagine that TAM would express such multiple functions just as other macrophages have multiple suppressive, cytotoxic, and growth-promoting cell functions. Although the issue is still debated, (see Chapters 8 and 9) it appears that in some systems, some tumor subpopulations are quite resistant to macrophage effects even when these cells express cytotoxic activity for other targets. Thus, the presence of cytotoxic TAM may only serve to select for more resistant (more metastatic) subpopulations and thus, contribute to tumor progression. The observations that depletion of macrophages sometimes promotes and in some cases inhibits tumor growth, may reflect real differences in the predominant role these cells play in different tumor systems. The seemingly conflicting findings are not readily explained by differences in macrophage-to-tumor cell ratio, tumor immunogenicity, or other obvious differences. Early speculation that high macrophage content was associated with immunogenic lesions and that in these systems macrophages were likely to demonstrate cytotoxicity, have not been supported by later studies by many others including our own, in which the number of TAM was similar for immunogenic and nonimmunogenic tumors, and cytotoxicity for both metastatic TAM was similar regardless of immunogenicity. Studies using many different experimental tumors show that the macrophage response does vary and thus, reflects the heterogeneity of tumors as well as the heterogenous properties of the cells we classify as macrophages. That different tumor populations do contain different but reproducible TAM phenotypes suggests that infiltration is not a random process and therefore, would appear to serve some function.

The role that the tumor microenvironment plays in directing the appearance and function of TAM may be complex. Thus, tumors may contribute both prochemotactic, chemokinetic, and antichemotactic factors. In addition, some of these factors seem to be relatively more or less active for different macrophage populations, e.g., activated vs. resident. CSF activities from tumors have been described in many systems, however, the in vivo role for these activities is, again, in doubt. They may, in fact, be responsible for some systemic effects such as granulocytosis without affecting TAM populations.

The role of TAM in metastatic spread has been studied less extensively than in primary tumor growth. The possibilities that TAM can contribute to invasiveness via collagenase activities to degrade vascular basement membranes, or can facilitate metastatic tumor cell establishment via angiogenesis factors or growth factors are intriguing and are just beginning to be explored. In addition, the potential of TAM to contribute to tumor progression by selecting for macrophage resistant populations, and for inducing other genetic and epigenetic changes resulting in more aggressive tumor cell phenotypes is a new area of research.

ACKNOWLEDGMENTS

Supported by grants CA27437, CA22453 and CA09421 from the National Cancer Institute, by a grant from Concern Foundation, by the E. Walter Albachten Bequest and by the United Foundation of Greater Detroit.

REFERENCES

1. **Underwood, J. C. E.**, Lymphoreticular infiltration in human tumors: prognostic and biological implications: a review, *Br. J. Cancer*, 30, 538, 1974.
2. **Berg, J. W.**, Inflammation and prognosis in breast cancer: a search for host resistance, *Cancer*, 12, 714, 1959.
3. **Cutler, S. J., Black M. M., Mork, T., Harvei, S., and Freeman, C.**, Further observations on prognostic factors in cancer of the female breast, *Cancer*, 24, 653, 1969.
4. **Gauci, C. L. and Alexander, P.**, The macrophage content of some human tumours, *Cancer Lett*, 1, 29, 1975.
5. **Lauder, I., Aherne, W., Stewart, J., and Sainsbury, R.**, Macrophage infiltration of breast tumours: a prospective study, *J. Clin. Pathol.*, 30, 563, 1977.
6. **Hurlimann, J. and Saraga, P.**, Mononuclear cells infiltrating human mammary carcinomas: immuno-histochemical analysis with monoclonal antibodies, *Int. J. Cancer*, 35, 753, 1985.

7. **Steele, R. J. C., Eremin, O., and Brown, M.,** Blood monocytes and tumor-infiltrating macrophages in human breast cancer: differences in activation level as assessed by lysozyme content, *J. Natl. Cancer Inst.,* 71, 941, 1983.

8. **Luebbers, E. L., Pretlow, T. P., Emancipator, S. N., Boohaker, E. A., Pitts, A. M., MacFadyen, A. J., Bradley, E. L., Jr., and Pretlow, T. G.,** Heterogeneity and prognostic significance of macrophages in human colonic carcinomas, *Cancer Res.,* 45, 5196, 1985.

9. **Takeo, S., Yasumoto, K., Nagashima, A., Nakahashi, H., Sugimachi, K., and Nomoto, K.,** Role of tumor-associated macrophages in lung cancer, *Cancer Res.,* 46, 3179, 1986.

10. **Birbeck, M. S. C. and Carter, R. L.,** Observations on the ultrastructure of two hamster lymphomas with particular reference to infiltrating macrophages, *Int. J. Cancer,* 9, 249, 1972.

11. **Evans, R.,** Macrophages and neoplasms: new insights and their implications in tumor immunobiology, *Cancer Metastasis Rev.,* 1, 227, 1982.

12. **Haskill, J. S., Proctor, J. W., and Yamamura, Y.,** Host responses within solid tumors. I. Monocytic effector cells within rat sarcomas, *J. Natl. Cancer Inst.,* 54, 387, 1975.

13. **Haskill, J. S., Key, M., Radov, L. A., Parthenais, E., Korn, J. H., Fett, J. W., Yamamura, Y., DeLustro, F., Vesley, J., and Gant, G.,** The importance of antibody and macrophages in spontaneous and drug-induced regression of the T1699 mammary adenocarcinoma, *J. Reticuloendothel. Soc.,* 26, 417, 1979.

14. **Kerbel, R. S. and Pross, H. F.,** F_c receptor-bearing cells as a reliable marker for quantitation of host lymphoreticular infiltration of progressively growing solid tumors, *Int. J. Cancer,* 18, 432, 1976.

15. **Pross, H. F. and Kerbel, R. S.,** An assessment of intratumor phagocytic and surface marker bearing cells in a series of autochthonous and early passaged chemically induced murine sarcomas, *J. Natl. Cancer Inst.,* 57, 1157, 1976.

16. **Stephens, T. C., Currie, G. A., and Peacock, J. H.,** Repopulation of gamma-irradiated Lewis lung carcinoma by malignant cells and host macrophage progenitors, *Br. J. Cancer,* 38, 573, 1978.

17. **Miller, G. A. and Morahan, P. S.,** Functional and biochemical heterogeneity among subpopulations of rat and mouse peritoneal macrophages, *J. Reticuloendothel. Soc.,* 32, 111, 1982.

18. **Moore, K. and McBride, W. H.,** The activation state of macrophage subpopulations from a murine fibrosarcoma, *Int. J. Cancer,* 26, 609, 1980.

19. **Haskill, S., Koren, H., Becker, S., Fowler, W., and Walton, L.,** Mononuclear cell infiltration in ovarian cancer. III. Suppressor cell and ADCC activity of macrophages from ascitic and solid ovarian tumors, *Br. J. Cancer,* 45, 747, 1982.

20. **Mahoney, K. H., Fulton, A. M., and Heppner, G. H.,** Tumor-associated macrophages of mouse mammary tumors. II. Differential distribution of macrophages from metastatic and non-metastatic tumors, *J. Immunol.,* 131, 2079, 1983.

21. **Mahoney, K. H., Miller, B. E., and Heppner, G. H.,** FACS quantitation of leucine aminopeptidase and acid phosphatase on tumor-associated macrophages from metastatic and nonmetastatic mouse mammary tumors, *J. Leukocyte Biol.,* 38, 573, 1985.

22. **Vose, B. M.,** Cytotoxicity of adherent cells associated with some human tumors and lung tissues, *Cancer Immunol. Immunother.,* 5, 173, 1978.

23. **Mantovani, A., Polentarutti, N., Peri, G., Shavit, Z. B., Vecchi, A., Bolis, G., and Mangioni, C.,** Cytotoxicity on tumor cells of peripheral blood monocytes and tumor-associated macrophages in patients with ascites ovarian tumors, *J. Natl. Cancer Inst.,* 64, 1307, 1980.

24. **Wood, G. W. and Gillespie, G. Y.,** Studies on the role of macrophages in regulation of growth and metastasis of murine chemically induced fibrosarcomas, *Int. J. Cancer,* 16, 1022, 1975.

25. **Siemann, D. W., Lord, E. M., Keng, P. C., and Wheeler, K. T.,** Cell subpopulations dispersed from solid tumors and separated by centrifugal elutriation, *Br. J. Cancer,* 44, 100, 1981.

26. **Taniyama, T. and Holden, H. T.,** Cytolytic activity of macrophages isolated from primary murine sarcoma virus (MSV)-induced tumors, *Int. J. Cancer,* 24, 151, 1979.

27. **Russell, S. W. and McIntosh, T.,** Macrophages isolated from regressing Moloney sarcomas are more cytotoxic than those recovered from progressing sarcomas, *Nature (London),* 268, 69, 1977.

28. **Mantovani, A.,** Effects on *in vitro* tumor growth of murine macrophages isolated from sarcoma lines differing in immunogenicity and metastasizing capacity, *Int. J. Cancer,* 22, 741, 1978.

29. **Mantovani, A.,** *In vitro* effects on tumor cells of macrophages isolated from an early passage chemically induced murine sarcoma and from its spontaneous metastases, *Int. J. Cancer,* 27, 221, 1981.

30. **Evans, R.,** Effect of X-irradiation on host-cell infiltration and growth of a murine fibrosarcoma, *Br. J. Cancer,* 35, 557, 1977.

31. **Evans, R. and Eidlen, L. G.,** The role of the inflammatory response during tumor growth, in *Macrophages and Natural Killer Cells,* Normann, S. J. and Sorkin, E., Eds., Plenum Press, New York, 1982, 379.

32. **Acero, R., Polentarutti, N., Bottazzi, B., Alberti, S., Ricci, M. R., Bizzi, A., and Mantovani, A.,** Effect of hydrocortisone on the macrophage content, growth and metastasis of transplanted murine tumors, *Int. J. Cancer,* 33, 95, 1984.

33. **Mantovani, A., Giavazzi, R., Polentarutti, N., Spreafico, F., and Garattini, S.,** Divergent effects of macrophage toxins on growth of primary tumors and lung metastases in mice, *Int. J. Cancer,* 25, 617, 1980.

34. **Nelson, M. and Nelson, D. S.,** Stimulation of proliferation in mixed cultures of mouse tumor cells and nonimmune peritoneal cells. I. Occurrence of stimulation and cyclical variation in tumor cell activity, *J. Natl. Cancer Inst.,* 74, 627, 1985.

35. **Nelson, M. and Nelson, D. S.,** Stimulation of proliferation in mixed cultures of mouse tumor cells and nonimmune peritoneal cells. II. Stimulation of tumor cells by macrophages and of lymphocytes by a tumor cell product, *J. Natl. Cancer Inst.,* 74, 637, 1985.

36. **Knighton, D. R., Hunt, T. K., Scheuenstuhl, H., Halliday, B. J., Werb, Z., and Banda, M. J.,** Oxygen tension regulates the expression of angiogenesis factor by macrophages, *Science,* 221, 1283, 1983.

37. **Buick, R. N., Fry, S. E., and Salmon, S. E.,** Effect of host cell interactions on clonogenic carcinoma cells in human malignant effusions, *Br. J. Cancer,* 41, 695, 1980.

38. **Evans, R., Duffy, T., and Cullen, R. T.,** Tumor-associated macrophages stimulate the proliferation of murine tumor cells surviving treatment with the oncolytic cyclophosphamide analogue ASTA Z-7557: *in vivo* implications, *Int. J. Cancer,* 34, 883, 1984.

39. **Eccles, S. A. and Alexander, P.,** Macrophage content of tumors in relation to metastatic spread and host immune reaction, *Nature (London),* 250, 667, 1974.

40. **Nash, J. R. G., Price, J. E., and Tarin, D.,** Macrophage content and colony-forming potential in mouse mammary carcinomas, *Br. J. Cancer,* 39, 478, 1979.

41. **Evans, R. and Lawler, E. M.,** Macrophage content and immunogenicity of C57BL/6J and BALB/cByJ methylcholanthrene-induced sarcomas, *Int. J. Cancer,* 26, 831, 1980.

42. **Talmadge, J. E., Key, M., and Fidler, I. J.,** Macrophage content of metastatic and nonmetastatic rodent neoplasms, *J. Immunol.,* 126, 2245, 1981.

43. **Loveless, S. E. and Heppner, G. H.,** Tumor-associated macrophages of mouse mammary tumors. I. Differential cytotoxicity of macrophages from metastatic and non-metastatic tumors, *J. Immunol.,* 131, 2074, 1983.

44. **Yamashina, K., Fulton, A., and Heppner, G.,** Differential sensitivity of metastatic versus nonmetastatic mammary tumor cells to macrophage-mediated cytostasis, *J. Natl. Cancer Inst.,* 75, 765, 1985.

45. **DeBaetselier, P., Kapon, A., Katzav, S., Tzehoval, E., Dekegel, D., Segal, S., and Feldman, M.,** Selecting, accelerating and suppressing interactions between macrophages and tumor cells, *Invas. Metas.,* 5, 106, 1985.

46. **Nagashima, A., Yasumoto, K., Nakahashi, H., Furukawa, T., Inokuchi, K., and Nomoto, K.,** Establishment and characterization of high and low metastatic clones derived from a methylcholanthrene induced rat fibrosarcoma, *Cancer Res.,* 46, 4420, 1986.

47. **Larizza, L., Schirrmacher, V., Graf, L., Pfluger, E., Peres-Martinez, M., and Stohr, M.,** Suggestive evidence that the highly metastatic variant ESb of the T cell lymphoma Eb is derived from spontaneous fusion with a host macrophage, *Int. J. Cancer,* 34, 699, 1984.

48. **Gemsa, D., Leser, H.-G., Deimann, W., and Resch, K.,** Suppression of T lymphocyte proliferation during lymphoma growth in mice: role of PGE_2-producing suppressor macrophages, *Immunobiology,* 161, 385, 1982.

49. **McCarthy, M. E. and Zwilling, B. S.,** Differential effects of prostaglandins on the antitumor activity of normal and BCG-activated macrophages, *Cell. Immunol.,* 60, 91, 1981.

50. **Snider, M. E., Fertel, R. H., and Zwilling, B. S.,** Prostaglandin regulation of macrophage function: effect of endogenous and exogenous prostaglandins, *Cell. Immunol.,* 74, 234, 1982.

51. **Russell, S. W. and Pace, J. L.,** Both the kind and magnitude of stimulus are important in overcoming the negative regulation of macrophage activation by PGE_2, *J. Leukocyte Biol.,* 35, 291, 1984.

52. **Mochizuki, M., Zigler, J. S., Jr., Russell, P., and Gery, I.,** Cytostatic and cytolytic activities of macrophages: regulation by prostaglandins, *Cell. Immunol.,* 83, 34, 1984.

53. **Pelus, L. M. and Bockman, R. S.,** Increased prostaglandin synthesis by macrophages from tumor-bearing mice, *J. Immunol.,* 123, 2118, 1979.

54. **Balch, C. M., Dougherty, P. A., and Tilden, A. B.,** Excessive prostaglandin E_2 production by suppressor monocytes in head and neck cancer patients, *Ann. Surg.,* 196, 645, 1982.

55. **Denbow, C. J., Conroy, J. M., and Elgert, K. D.,** Macrophage derived prostaglandin E modulation of the mixed lymphocyte reaction: an anomaly of increased production and decreased T cell susceptibility during tumor growth, *Cell. Immunol.,* 84, 1, 1984.

56. **Bugelski, P. J., Kirsh, R. L., and Poste, G.,** New histochemical method for measuring intratumoral macrophages and macrophage recruitment into experimental metastases, *Cancer Res.,* 43, 5493, 1983.

57. **Dougherty, G. J. and McBride, W. H.,** Accessory cell activity of murine tumor-associated macrophages, *J. Natl. Cancer Inst.,* 76, 541, 1986.

58. **Snyder, D. S., Beller, D. I., and Unanue, E. R.,** Prostaglandins modulate macrophage Ia expression, *Nature (London),* 299, 163, 1982.

59. **Henry, N., van Lamsweerde, A.-L., and Vaes, G.,** Collagen degradation by metastatic variants of Lewis lung carcinoma: cooperation between tumor cells and macrophages, *Cancer Res.,* 43, 5321, 1983.
60. **Huard, T. K., Malinoff, H. L., and Wicha, M. S.,** Macrophages express a plasma membrane receptor for basement membrane laminin, *Am. J. Pathol.,* 123, 365, 1986.
61. **Nowell, P. C.,** The clonal evolution of tumor cell populations, *Science,* 194, 23, 1976.
62. **Weitzman, S. A. and Stossel, T. P.,** Mutation caused by human phagocytes, *Science,* 212, 546, 1981.
63. **Fulton, A. M., Loveless, S. E., and Heppner, G. H.,** Mutagenic activity of tumor-associated macrophages in *Salmonella typhimurium* strains TA98 and TA100, *Cancer Res.,* 44, 4308, 1984.
64. **Weitzman, A. A. and Stossel, T. P.,** Phagocyte-induced mutation in Chinese hamster ovary cells, *Cancer Lett.,* 22, 337, 1984.
65. **Yamashina, K., Miller, B. E., and Heppner, G. H.,** Macrophage-mediated induction of drug-resistant variants in a mouse mammary tumor cell line, *Cancer Res.,* 46, 2396, 1986.
66. **Meltzer, M. S., Stevenson, M. M., and Leonard, E. J.,** Characterization of macrophage chemotaxins in tumor cell cultures and comparison with lymphocyte-derived chemotactic factors, *Cancer Res.,* 37, 721, 1977.
67. **Bottazzi, B., Polentarutti, N., Acero, R., Balsari, A., Boraschi, D., Ghezzi, P., Salmona, M., and Mantovani, A.,** Regulation of the macrophage content of neoplasms by chemoattractants, *Science,* 220, 208, 1983.
68. **Bottazzi, B., Polentarutti, N., Balsari, A., Boraschi, D., Ghezzi, P., Salmona, M., and Mantovani, A.,** Chemotactic activity for mononuclear phagocytes of culture supernatants from murine and human tumor cells: evidence for a role in the regulation of the macrophage content of neoplastic tissues, *Int. J. Cancer,* 31, 55, 1983.
69. **Quinn, M. T., Parthasarathy, S., and Steinberg, D.,** Endothelial cell-derived chemotactic activity for mouse peritoneal macrophages and the effects of modified forms of low density lipoprotein, *Proc. Natl. Acad. Sci. U.S.A.,* 82, 5949, 1985.
70. **Lane, R. D., Kaplan, A. M., Snodgrass, M. J., and Szakal, A. K.,** Characterization of a macrophage chemokinetic factor in tumor cell culture media, *J. Reticuloendothel. Soc.,* 31, 171, 1982.
71. **Boetcher, D. A. and Leonard, E. J.,** Abnormal monocyte chemotactic response in cancer patients, *J. Natl. Cancer Inst.,* 52, 1091, 1974.
72. **Snyderman, R., Seigler, H. F., and Meadows, L.,** Abnormalities of monocyte chemotaxis in patients with melanoma: effects of immunotherapy and tumor removal, *J. Natl. Cancer Inst.,* 58, 37, 1977.
73. **Rubin, R. H., Cosimi, A. B., and Goetzl, E. J.,** Defective human mononuclear leukocyte chemotaxis as an index of host resistance to malignant melanoma, *Clin. Immunol. Immunopathol.,* 6, 376, 1976.
74. **Snyderman, R., Meadows, L., Holder, W., and Wells, S., Jr.,** Abnormal monocyte chemotaxis in patients with breast cancer: evidence for a tumor-mediated effect, *J. Natl. Cancer Inst.,* 60, 737, 1978.
75. **Cianciolo, G. J., Herberman, R. B., and Snyderman, R.,** Depression of murine macrophage accumulation by low molecular weight factors derived from spontaneous mammary carcinomas, *J. Natl. Cancer Inst.,* 65, 829, 1980.
76. **Snyderman, R. and Pike, M. C.,** An inhibitor of macrophage chemotaxis produced by neoplasms, *Science,* 192, 370, 1976.
77. **Normann, S. J. and Cornelius, J.,** Characterization of anti-inflammatory factors produced by murine tumor cells in culture, *J. Natl. Cancer Inst.,* 69, 1321, 1982.
78. **Fauve, R. M., Hevin, B., Jacob, H., Gaillard, J. A., and Jacob, F.,** Antiinflammatory effects of murine malignant cells, *Proc. Natl. Acad. Sci. U.S.A.,* 71, 4052, 1974.
79. **Cheung, H. T., Cantarow, W. D., and Sundharadas, G.,** Characteristics of a low molecular weight factor extracted from mouse tumors that affects *in vitro* properties of macrophages, *Int. J. Cancer,* 23, 344, 1979.
80. **Cohen, M. C., Brozna, J. P., and Ward, P. A.,** *In vitro* and *in vivo* production of chemotactic inhibitors by tumor cells, *Am. J. Pathol.,* 94, 603, 1979.
81. **Warabi, H., Venkat, K., Geetha, V., Liotta, L. A., Brownstein, M., and Schiffmann, E.,** Identification and partial characterization of a low molecular weight inhibitor of leukotaxis from fibrosarcoma cells, *Cancer Res.,* 44, 915, 1984.
82. **Mokashi, S., Delikatny, S. J., and Orr, F. W.,** Relationships between chemotaxis, chemotactic modulators, and cyclic nucleotide levels in tumor cells, *Cancer Res.,* 43, 1980, 1983.
83. **Honda, M., Yoshimura, T., Watanabe, T., and Hayashi, H.,** Chemotactic macrophage subpopulations defined by macrophage chemotactic factors from delayed hypersensitivity reaction sites, *J. Immunol.,* 131, 2989, 1983.
84. **Sturm, R. J., Smith, B. M., Lane, R. W., Laskin, D. L., Harris, L. S., and Carchman, R. A.,** Antagonist of phorbol ester-mediated chemotaxis in mouse peritoneal macrophages, *Cancer Res.,* 43, 4552, 1983.
85. **Mantovani, A.,** Origin and function of tumor associated macrophages in murine and human neoplasms, *Prog. Immunol.,* 5, 1001, 1983.

86. **Stewart, C. C.**, Local proliferation of mononuclear phagocytes in tumors, *J. Reticuloendothel. Soc.*, 34, 23, 1983.

87. **Mahoney, K. H. and Heppner, G. H.**, FACS analysis of tumor-associated macrophage replication: differences between metastatic and non-metastatic murine mammary tumors, *J. Leukocyte Biol.*, 41, 205, 1987.

88. **Fulton, A., Mahoney, K., and Heppner, G.**, Macrophage differentiation activity in murine mammary tumors, *Proc. Am. Assoc. Cancer Res.*, 26, 306, 1985.

89. **Sato, N., Asano, S., Ueyama, Y., Mori, M., Okabe, T., Kondo, Y., Ohsawa, N., and Kosaka, K.**, Granulocytosis and colony stimulating activity (CSA) produced by a human squamous cell carcinoma, *Cancer (Brussels)*, 43, 605, 1979.

90. **Kondo, Y., Sato, K., Ohkawa, H., Ueyama, Y., Okabe, T., Sato, N., Asano, S., Mori, M., Ohsawa, N., and Kosaka, K.**, Association of hypercalcemia with tumors producing colony stimulating factor(s), *Cancer Res.*, 43, 2368, 1983.

91. **Milas, L. and Basic, I.**, Stimulated granulocytopoiesis in mice bearing fibrosarcoma, *Eur. J. Cancer*, 8, 309, 1972.

92. **Milas, L., Faykus, M. H., Jr., McBride, W. H., Hunter, N., and Peters, L. J.**, Concomitant development of granulocytosis and enhancement of metastases formation in tumor-bearing mice, *Clin. Exp. Metastasis*, 2, 181, 1984.

93. **Pessina, A., Neri, M. G., Muschiato, A., Brambilla, P., Marocchi, A., and Mocarelli, P.**, Colony stimulating factor produced by murine adrenocortical tumor cells, *J. Natl. Cancer Inst.*, 76, 1095, 1986.

94. **Balducci, L. and Hardy, C.**, High proliferation of granulocyte-macrophage progenitors in tumor-bearing mice, *Cancer Res.*, 43, 4643, 1983.

95. **Burlington, H., Cronkite, E. P., Heldman, B., Pappas, N., and Shadduck, R. K.**, Tumor-induced granulopoiesis unrelated to colony-stimulating factor, *Blood*, 62, 693, 1983.

96. **Nicoletti, G., Brambilla, P., DeGiovanni, C., Lollini, P. -L., Del Re, B., Marocchi, A., Mocarelli, P., Prodi, G., and Nanni, P.**, Colony stimulating activity from the new metastatic TS/A cell line and its high and low metastatic clonal derivatives, *Br. J. Cancer*, 52, 215, 1985.

97. **Thomas E., Smith, D. C., Lee, M. Y., and Rosse, C.**, Induction of granulocytic hyperplasia, thymic atrophy, and hypercalcemia by a selected subpopulation of a murine mammary adenocarcinoma, *Cancer Res.*, 45, 5840, 1985.

98. **Kurland, J. I., Broxmeyer, H. E., Pelus, L. M., Bockman, R. S., and Moore, M. A. S.**, Role for monocyte-macrophage derived colony stimulating factor and prostaglandin E in the positive and negative feedback control of myeloid stem cell proliferation, *Blood*, 52, 388, 1978.

99. **Fulton, A. M.**, Effects of indomethacin on the growth of cultured mammary tumors, *Int. J. Cancer*, 33, 375, 1984.

100. **Metcalf, D.**, The granulocyte-macrophage colony stimulating factors, *Science*, 229, 16, 1985.

Chapter 7

MACROPHAGE-LYMPHOCYTE INTERACTIONS IN TUMOR RECOGNITION AND RESPONSE

James L. Urban, Jay L. Rothstein, and Hans Schreiber

TABLE OF CONTENTS

I. INTRODUCTION

Macrophages (Mφ) can show a highly selective cytotoxicity towards cancer cells in vitro and there is evidence that they may also destroy malignant cells in vivo.[1-7] Defining the precise role of activated Mφ in tumor rejection has been difficult. The Mφ is only one of many critical components firmly integrated into the immune network and cooperation between each of these components is required for tumor rejection. Traditionally, interactions between cell populations of the immune system have been dissected in vitro and such interactions may or may not be relevant in vivo. We, therefore, have chosen to use a different approach which is based upon the analysis of tumor variants derived in vivo. In the host, tumors readily develop phenotypic variants which show specific resistance to effector mechanisms that restrain the growth of the parent tumor. These phenotypic changes can, therefore, reflect fingerprints of the action of various types of immunologic effector mechanisms that operate in vivo,[8-14] and these changes provide an insight into the relative importance and hierarchy of the different naturally occurring, interacting immune cells active against neoplastic cells. This type of analysis is analogous to that carried out by the microbiologist who deduces the mechanism of action of a particular antibiotic by studying bacteria which have become resistant to the drug. Using this approach we have dissected the relative contribution of Mφ and T cells as well as their interactions in providing resistance in the normal host to cancer. Ultraviolet (UV)-induced tumors are often so immunogenic that they are rejected by normal syngeneic hosts[15] and, therefore, there is unequivocal evidence for a strong host response in this tumor system. Nevertheless, resistant variants occasionally arise and we have carefully analyzed the selection of variants in this tumor model.[8-14] Our data are consistent with the notion that tumor rejection involves a bidirectional, stimulatory interaction between T cells and Mφ. It is composed of (1) presentation of tumor-specific antigens by Ia+ cells, such as Mφ, to helper T cells and (2) activation of directly tumoricidal Mφ by T cells secreting lymphokines.

II. T CELL REQUIREMENT FOR THE SELECTION OF Mφ-RESISTANT VARIANTS

A. The Role of Host T Cell Competence

Analysis of these progressor variants that arise, rarely, from normal mice injected with the UV-induced regressor tumor 1591 (Figure 1, middle panel) shows that these variants consistently lose expression of a cytolytic T cell-defined rejection antigen; this antigen we have previously designated as "A" antigen.[8,13,16,17] The antigen is not lost in mice that lack intact T cell immunity (Figure 1, left panel). Interestingly, the progressor variants isolated from the normal host also demonstrate a reduced sensitivity to activated Mφ in a 16-hr cytotoxicity assay (Figure 2, middle panel) as well as a 72-hr postlabeling assay,[10] whereas tumors reisolated after injection into T cell-deficient animals show no such reduction of Mφ sensitivity (Figure 2, left panel). In order to determine whether there was an obligatory link between the loss of the 1591 rejection antigen and loss of Mφ sensitivity, we isolated variants by selection in vitro with activated Mφ or with a homogeneous population of cloned T cells that were specific for the rejection antigen.[10,13] The results show that the T cell-selected variants retained Mφ sensitivity (Figure 3) while Mφ-resistant variants retained the cytolytic T cell-recognized antigen (Figure 1, right panel). This indicated that T cell sensitivity could be lost independently of Mφ sensitivity and supported the notion that T cells and Mφ do not recognize the same target structure on 1591 tumor cells. Consistent with this is the fact that loss of Mφ sensitivity appears to precede the loss of sensitivity to cytotoxic T lymphocytes (CTL) as determined by the analysis of sequential reisolates from progressively growing tumors.[14] This, together with the observation that T cell competence is required

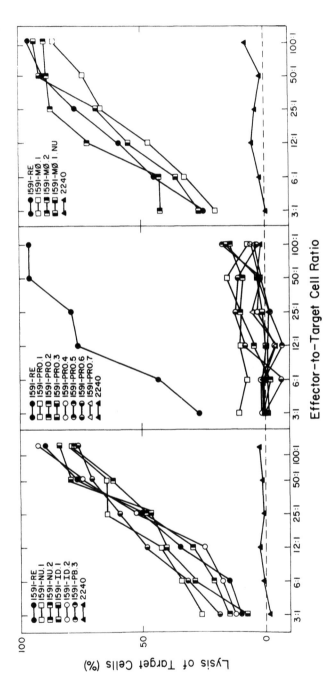

FIGURE 1. Loss of the tumor-specific antigen by progressor variants (1591-PRO) reisolated from T cell-competent mice (middle panel) and retention of the 1591-RE tumor-specific target antigen by the MΦ-resistant tumor cells (1591-MΦ) selected in vitro or by the tumor reisolates from T cell-incompetent mice (left panel). The 1591-RE tumor was implanted subcutaneously into mice (NU, nude; ID, idiotypically suppressed;[35,36] PB, progressor-bearing;[37] PRO, normal mice). One month later, the progressing tumors were adapted to growth in vitro and the resulting cell lines are shown in the three panels. The indicated tumor cell lines were exposed to 1591-RE-specific T cells in a 6-hr ^{51}Cr-release assay. The specific T cells were generated in mixed lymphocyte tumor cell cultures using spleen cells from 1591-RE-immunized mice. Experiments shown in each panel were done independently of those shown in the other panels and were, therefore, individually controlled with 1591-RE and 2240 target cells used in each of the experiments. (From Urban, J. and Schreiber, H., *J. Exp. Med.*, 157, 642, 1983. With permission.)

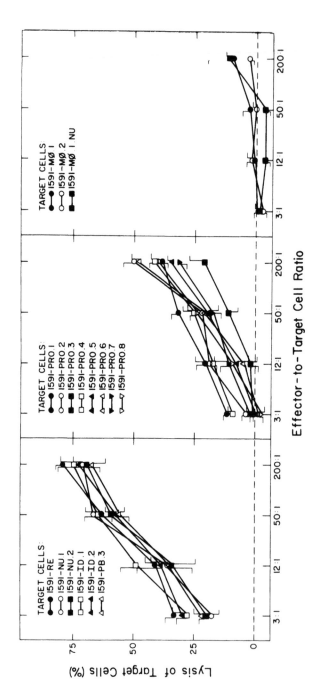

FIGURE 2. Decreased sensitivity to Mφ-mediated lysis in host-selected progressor tumor variants (1591-PRO) isolated after one passage of the parental 1591-RE tumor through normal mice possessing immunocompetent T cells. For tumor subline nomenclature see Figure 1. Adherent peritoneal exudate cells from mice injected intraperitoneally 5 days earlier with Brewer's thioglycollate were cultured for 5 hr with lipopolysaccharide and secondary mixed lymphocyte culture supernatant and used as effectors in a 16-hr ^{51}Cr-release assay against the indicated targets. An E/T of 200:1 corresponds to a Mφ population density of $7.2 \times 10^4/mm^2$. Vertical bars represent the SEM for five separate experiments, each including the parental 1591-RE tumor, at least one 1591-PRO host-selected variant, and at least one 1591-Mφ variant derived in vitro. (From Urban, J. and Schreiber, H., *J. Exp. Med.*, 157, 642, 1983. With permission.)

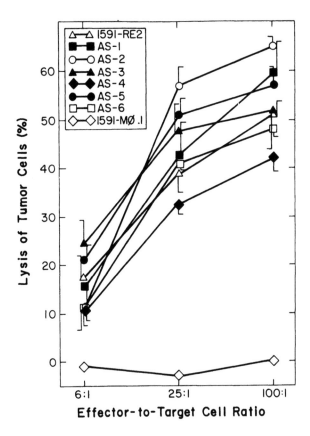

FIGURE 3. Retained sensitivity to activated macrophages of variants selected in vitro with anti-A CTL from 1591-RE for loss of the A antigen (AS variants). The results of four separate experiments with these A antigen-negative variants were similar and, therefore, pooled. Vertical bars indicate the SEM of the results for individual experiments. (From Wortzel, R. et al., *Proc. Natl. Acad. Sci. U.S.A.*, 81, 2186, 1984. With permission.)

for selection of Mφ resistance, suggests that these two cell types interact in the intact host in response to a tumor challenge. Such interaction might occur through lymphokines secreted by T cells, since at least the activation of Mφ in vitro depends upon the addition of lymphokines, and γ-interferon (IFN), in particular,[18,19] and such lymphokines may also be required for the activation of Mφ in vivo. Both helper T cells and cytolytic T cells may secrete Mφ-activating lymphokines, and it might, therefore, be difficult to distinguish the individual contribution of the two subsets in vivo. The fact that the loss of Mφ sensitivity appears to occur in vivo before the cytolytic T cell-recognized antigens are lost (Figure 4) may suggest that helper T cells rather than cytolytic T cells are central.[14] However, cytolytic T cells may still be involved since they may secrete lymphokines before they develop full cytolytic activity.

Several lines of evidence suggest that the observed loss of sensitivity to activated Mφ is biologically significant. First, all of eight independently isolated progressor variants arising in normal animals had lost sensitivity to Mφ (Figure 2). Second, variants that had lost sensitivity to activated Mφ but retained sensitivity to cytolytic T cells showed a significantly increased early growth potential in normal mice (Figure 5) although retention of the cytolytic T cell-recognized antigen seemed to be sufficient to guarantee rejection at a later time (Figure 5). The fact that this growth difference between the Mφ-sensitive and Mφ-insensitive cell

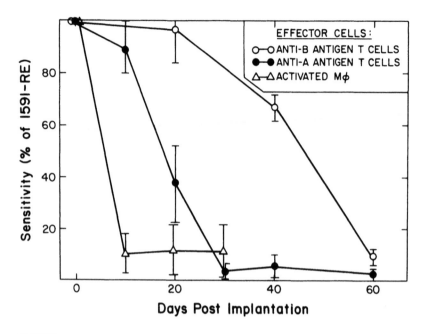

FIGURE 4.   Kinetics of the sequential loss of the macrophage sensitivity, A antigen expression, and B antigen expression during passage of the 1591 regressor tumor through UV-irradiated mice that are partially immunocompetent and, therefore, select for antigen loss variants (g). Injected s.c. were 5×10^7 1591-RE cells into mice 6 weeks after termination of UV irradiation. At the indicated times after challenge, the progressing tumors were excised and adapted to culture. The resultant cell lines were tested for sensitivity to T cells specific for the A or the B antigen in a 6-hr ^{51}Cr-release assay or for sensitivity to activated macrophages in a 16-hr ^{51}Cr-release assay. "Relative sensitivity" was expressed as the percent of the parental 1591-RE sensitivity, i.e., the ratio of the number of T cells or macrophages required to lyse 50% of 1×10^4 parental target cells to the number of T cells or macrophages required to lyse the same number of reisolated tumor cells multiplied by 100. Vertical bars indicate the SEM for the analyses of five tumor cell lines each reisolated independently at each of the five time points. (From Urban, J. L., Kripke, M. L., and Schreiber, H., *J. Immunol.*, 137, 3036, 1986. With permission.)

lines was only observed in normal but not in T cell-incompetent nude mice (Figure 5) further suggests that T cells are required for Mφ-mediated tumor resistance.

B. The Role of Tumor Immunogenicity

Since we have previously shown that a tumor can possess multiple tumor-specific antigens,[20] and since we have shown above that T cells are required for immune selection by Mφ,[10] it was important to determine to what degree tumor immunogenicity played a role in the variant selection by activated Mφ. We first analyzed to what degree variants which had only lost the strong T cell-recognized A antigen were still selected for Mφ resistance in the normal T cell-competent host. Consistent with the notion that a T cell response is required for Mφ selection, Table 1 shows that each of four independently derived variants which had lost the strong rejection antigen A and which, therefore, failed to elicit a strong tumor-specific T cell response, also failed to develop resistance to activated Mφ. In contrast, all of three reisolates from mice injected with the A-positive parental tumor became almost completely resistant to activated Mφ. We know that A⁻ variants still retain other T cell-recognized antigens (such as one designated "B") that can elicit a response after preimmunization. It then follows that selection for Mφ resistance should occur when the A⁻ tumor variant is injected into a preimmune host that demonstrates a tumor-specific immune

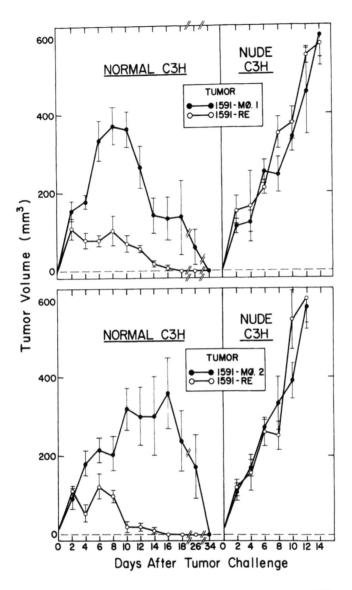

FIGURE 5. Differences in growth kinetics of the A antigen-positive Mφ-sensitive parental 1591-RE tumors and the A antigen-positive Mφ-resistant 1591-Mφ tumors in normal but not in nude mice. The tumors were implanted subcutaneously in the shaved inguinal fossae of groups of ten normal or four nude mice each with two 1-mm³ fragments per mouse. The mean tumor size per mouse was measured every 2 days thereafter with a caliper, and the tumor volume was computed as the average product of three perpendicular tumor diameters. Vertical bars represent the SEM for the individual analysis of the number of mice indicated above. (From Urban, J. and Schreiber, H., *J. Exp. Med.*, 157, 642, 1983. With permission.)

response to this remaining B antigen.[11] Figure 6 shows that two A⁻ variants reisolated from these preimmunized mice (AS-1 immune, AS-2 immune) indeed have developed significant resistance to activated Mφ. In contrast, the same A⁻ tumors passaged through nonimmune mice (AS-1 norm, AS-2 norm) remained completely sensitive to these Mφ. This suggests that the presence of a T cell-recognized antigen on the tumor cell may be a general requirement for Mφ to exert significant tumoricidal effects in vivo.

Table 1
**SELECTION FOR Mφ-RESISTANCE IN VIVO REQUIRES THE
PRESENCE OF A STRONG T CELL-RECOGNIZED Ag ON THE
TUMOR CELLS**

Parental tumor cell line[a]			Subline isolated after passage through normal mice	
Designation	Antigenic phenotype	Mφ sensitivity (% of parental)[b]	Designation	Mφ sensitivity (% of parental)
1591-RE (parental)	A⁺B⁺	100 ± 9[c]	1591-PRO.1	7 ± 4
			1591-PRO.2	9 ± 2
			1591-PRO.3	11 ± 2
AS-1	A⁻B⁺	102 ± 14	AS-1 NORM	90 ± 11
AS-2	A⁻B⁺	98 ± 4	AS-2 NORM	86 ± 4
AS-3	A⁻B⁺	111 ± 7	AS-3 NORM	112 ± 2
AS-6	A⁻B⁺	116 ± 16	AS-6 NORM	98 ± 7

[a] 1591 tumor cell lines either possessed the 1591-A antigen or had lost it during selection in vitro with a 1591-A antigen-specific T cell line. All 1591 tumor cell lines retained the more weakly immunogenic 1591-specific B antigen.

[b] Reciprocal of the no. of Mφ required to lyse 50% of 1×10^4 tumor cells in a 16-hr ^{51}Cr-release assay, normalized to a value of 100% for the parental. Values were determined using linear regression analysis of at least nine different E/T ratios for each tumor cell line. 100% = 4.20×10^{-6}.

[c] Mean ± SEM for 2 separate experiments.

C. The Mechanism of Tumor Resistance to Activated Mφ

Mφ may engage a vast array of diverse mechanisms for their tumoricidal and microbiocidal activity which may differ depending on the particular activating event.[21] It was, therefore, important to determine which mechanism(s) would be used by Mφ when made tumoricidal by the activation with T cell-derived factors, and how variants escaped activated Mφ in the intact host. In lower panels of Figure 7 and 8, we show that the in vivo-selected progressor variants had developed selective resistance to tumor necrosis factor (TNF),[22] a cytotoxic protein known to be released by activated Mφ.[23] These variants still show normal sensitivity to osmotic lysis, natural killer (NK) cells, cytolytic T cells, hydrogen peroxide, and interleukin-1 (IL-1). Selective resistance was also observed by variants derived by exposure of the parental 1591 tumor to activated Mφ in vitro (Figures 7 and 8, upper panels). Since a very large number of tumoricidal substances is simultaneously released by activated Mφ,[21] we next wanted to show that the resistance of Mφ-selected variants to TNF was not coincidental. We determined whether selection with the defined recombinant product would lead to full resistance to the lymphokine-activated Mφ. Panel a of Figure 9 shows that variants resistant to the murine recombinant TNF showed complete resistance to lysis by activated Mφ in a 16-hr ^{51}Cr-release assay. The fact that antibodies raised against recombinant murine TNF fully abrogated the cytotoxic activity of the activated Mφ (Figure 9, panel b) supports the evidence that TNF released by activated Mφ is the crucial substance mediating tumor cell killing.

III. SIMILARITY OF THE BIOLOGIC EFFECTS OF LYMPHOTOXIN AND TNF

Although lymphotoxin and TNF only share about 30% sequence homology,[24,27] they compete for binding to the same cellular receptor suggesting that they may share common cellular effector pathways.[28] In order to determine whether the Mφ-resistant variants had

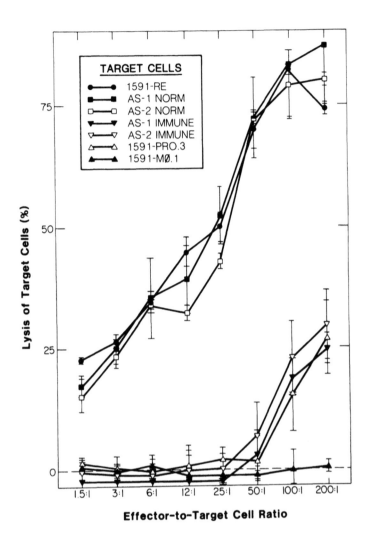

FIGURE 6. Retention of Mφ-sensitivity by A antigen-negative variants injected into and then reisolated from normal (nonimmune) mice showing progressive tumor growth after tumor injection (AS-1 norm, AS-2 norm). In contrast, loss of Mφ-sensitivity was observed in A⁻ variants injected into and then reisolated from preimmune mice (AS-1 immune, AS-2 immune). The tumor cells were isolated 10 days after subcutaneous injection of a nontumorigenic (5×10^7) dose of AS-1 or AS-2 tissue culture-grown tumor cells. A tumor-specific immune response against the B antigen was generated in these mice (data not shown). Mφ-sensitivity was assessed in a 16-hr ^{51}Cr-release assay. The data are pooled from four experiments, each testing AS-1 as a positive control and 1591-PRO.1 as a negative control. Values represent the mean ± SEM.

also become resistant to lymphotoxin, we compared the sensitivity of Mφ-resistant variants and the parental 1591 tumor to the two recombinant cytotoxic proteins. Figure 10 shows that the two proteins had an identical effect on the parental 1591 tumor and both failed to exert a cytotoxic effect on two Mφ-resistant variants. Although the gene from which the recombinant lymphotoxin had been produced was originally isolated from a lymphoblastoid B cell line,[24] it is now clear that only nonmalignant activated T cells express this gene and secrete its product.[38] In unpublished experiments with Drs. Gibb Otten and Frank Fitch from the University of Chicago, we have found that a helper T cell clone,[29] when activated in an

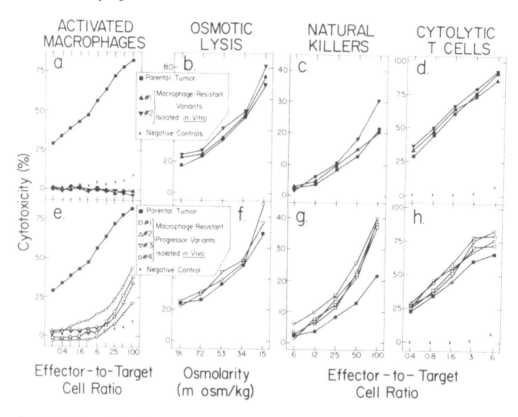

FIGURE 7. Susceptibility of parental and Mφ-resistant UV1591 tumor variants to osmotic lysis, NK cells, and cytolytic T cells. Results utilizing Mφ-resistant tumor variants selected in vitro are shown in a to d and results with variants selected in vivo are shown in e to h. Definitions of the symbols are given in the figures. Mφ were activated 6 hr with lipopolysaccharide and lymphokine and used as effectors in a 16-hr ^{51}Cr-release assay (a and e). 10T1/2 fibroblasts were used as negative controls. Susceptibility to osmotic lysis (b and f) was determined for ^{51}Cr-labeled target cells in a 4.5 hr assay using complete medium diluted with distilled water to the osmolarity indicated. Maximum release (100%) was determined by saponin lysis. NK cells were derived from spleens of poly(I)-poly(C)-injected C3H mice and were used in a 4.5-hr ^{51}Cr-release assay. These NK cells lysed YAC-1 target cells 81, 76, 70, 52, and 33% at the effector:target ratios shown (c and g). NK cells were eliminated in the control with an anti-GM1 antibody and complement. Uninduced spleen cells caused less than 5% lysis of the UV1591-RE tumors. Cytolytic T cells were UV1591-RE tumor-specific cytolytic T cell clones directed against the A antigen which is specific for the parental 1591 regressor tumor (d) or the B antigen (h) (a second independent UV1591-specific antigen retained by host-selected progressor tumor variants) using the independently derived UV-induced C3H tumor 2240-RE as negative control. The SEM for each point indicated was always ≤ 10% of the value of each point shown. The data represent pooled values from three separate experiments. (From Urban, J. et al., *Proc. Natl. Acad. Sci. U.S.A.*, 83, 5233, 1986. With permission.)

I-A^k-restricted antigen-specific way, will secrete lymphotoxin with marked cytotoxic activity toward the TNF-sensitive 1591 parental tumor. In addition, this lymphotoxin had precisely the same reactivity pattern as TNF in that it did not affect the 1591 variants resistant to recombinant murine or human TNF. Therefore, this natural T helper cell-derived lymphotoxin appears to behave similarly to the recombinant lymphotoxin in reactivity towards the parental and the variant tumor cell lines.

IV. Mφ REQUIREMENT FOR ANTIGEN-SPECIFIC T HELPER CELL RESPONSE

Ia-positive immune cells, including Mφ, dendritic cells, or B cells, seem to be required for the recognition of foreign antigens by helper T cells. Likewise, tumor-specific cytotoxic

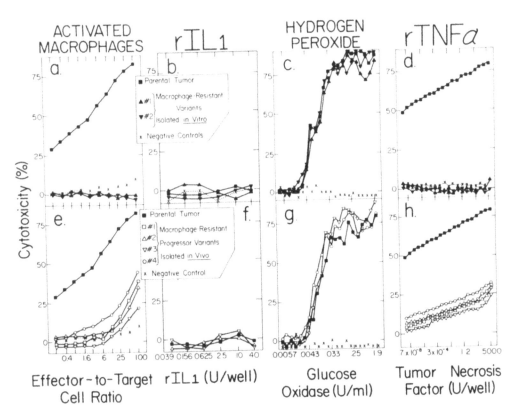

FIGURE 8. Sensitivity of Mφ-resistant UV1591 tumor variants to soluble mediators of cytotoxicity; a and e are repeated from Figure 1. Murine rIL-1 was added to cultures as indicated. Heat-inactivated IL-1 was used as a negative control. The murine rIL-1 was quantified by the standard thymocyte proliferation assay. For measuring sensitivity to enzyme-generated hydrogen peroxide (c and g), target cells were exposed to various concentrations of glucose oxidase for 4 hr as described. The specific activity of glucose oxidase (Sigma Chemical Company, St. Louis, Mo.) was 1200 units per mℓ, where 1 unit is defined as the generation of 1 μmol H_2O_2 per minute. The assay was run for 360 min in a total volume of 0.2 mℓ. The concentration required for 50% lysis in the presence of glucose oxidase was 0.0156 unit per well for the parental 1591 tumor, 0.0156 and 0.0120 unit per well for the progressor variants, and 0.0162 and 0.0136 unit per well for Mφ-resistant variants. The cytotoxic activity of glucose oxidase was due to the generation of H_2O_2, since it was completely eliminated by catalase (40 units per well, negative control). Susceptibility to human rTNF-α was analyzed in a 72 hr ^{51}Cr-postlabeling assay; 0% cytotoxicity represents no difference between test wells (with TNF-α) and control wells (without TNF-α). The negative control shows the neutralization of human rTNF-α activity on the parental 1591 tumor cells after preincubation with monoclonal antiTNF-α antibody at 1.85 μg/mℓ for 16 hr. Similar results were obtained using either a 72-hr [^{3}H]-thymidine release assay or a 16-hr ^{51}Cr-release assay (data not shown). Actinomycin D-treated mycoplasma-free L929 cells, used for standardizing the cytotoxic effects (units) of TNF-α in a 48-hr incubation, are substantially less susceptible to TNF-α and to activated Mφ than the UV1591-RE tumor cells. The data represent pooled values from three separate experiments. (From Urban, J. et al., *Proc. Natl. Acad. Sci. U.S.A.*, 83, 5233, 1986. With permission.)

T cells and other cytolytic T cells are known to usually depend on helper T cells for their maturation.[30-32] Thus, Mφ may be critical as antigen-presenting cells for T cell-mediated tumor rejection. Since many tumors such as the tumor 1591 do not express Ia antigen and since helper T cells can only recognize tumor cells in the context of Ia,[33] helper T cells must recognize the tumor antigen on antigen-presenting cells if an immune response is to occur. Table 2 shows that 1591-immunized mice generated L3T4$^+$ T cells whose restimulation in vitro was selectively inhibited by antibody to Ia. The antigen recognized by the L3T4$^+$ cells was independent of the cytotoxic T lymphocyte (CTL)-defined tumor-specific antigen (Table 2) and appeared to be retained by highly immunoselected variants

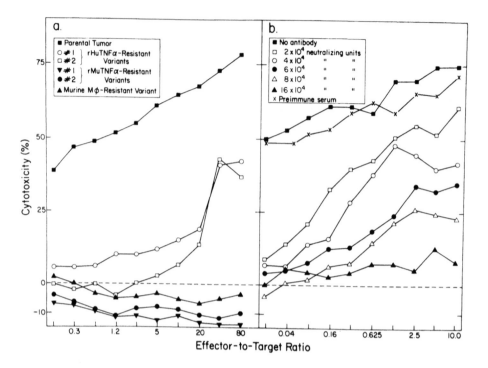

FIGURE 9.   (a) Complete resistance of the variants selected with murine rTNF-α to the cytolytic effects of murine activated macrophages (aMϕ). Variants selected for resistance to human rTNF-α show incomplete resistance to the murine aMϕ, while demonstrating complete resistance to human rTNF-α. The pooled values of two separate 16-hr ^{51}Cr-release assays are shown. (b) Neutralization of tumor cell killing by aMϕ using antibodies raised against murine rTNF-α. The pooled results of two experiments using a modified ^{51}Cr-release assay are shown. aMϕ were preincubated for 16 hr with either media alone, preimmune serum, or the indicated amounts of a rabbit polyclonal antibody that neutralizes the cytotoxic effects of murine rTNF-α. The amount of preimmune serum added was 16 μℓ equal to the largest volume of neutralizing antiserum added. Labeled parental 1591-RE target cells were added without further washing, and the amount of ^{51}Cr released into the supernatant was determined after 16 hr. The data represent pooled values from two separate experiments. (From Urban, J. et al., *Proc. Natl. Acad. Sci. U.S.A.*, 83, 5233, 1986. With permission.)

that had lost all CTL-recognized antigens.[33] This retention demonstrates that T helper cells did not select for antigen-loss variants which may suggest that they did not exert a direct tumoricidal effect. Similarly, lymphotoxin, known to be secreted by T helper cells in vivo, may not necessarily select for tumor variants since the helper T cells only recognize the tumor antigen on the surface of antigen-presenting cells and not on the tumor cell directly. This may be particularly true since close proximity between the lymphotoxin-producing helper cell and the target is required for optimal tumor cell killing.[34]

V. CONCLUSION

This chapter discusses the evidence for a positive-feedback loop between T cells and Mϕ as it may occur in tumor immunity. Ia$^+$ cells, including Mϕ, are required for the presentation of the tumor antigen to L3T4$^+$ helper T cells, which in turn release lymphokines necessary for the maturation of tumor-specific CTL and for the further activation of Mϕ to the tumoricidal state. Although we have used a highly defined tumor model for this dissection, we have analyzed only a single tumor system and, therefore, not all of the important regulatory interactions may be known at the present time. Nevertheless, the data now available clearly show that an activation of T cells is required for selection of variants

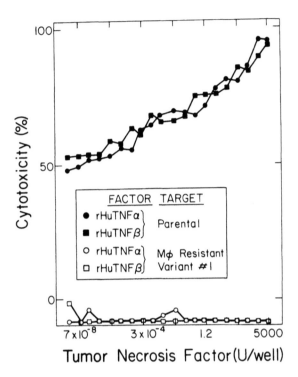

FIGURE 10. Resistance of the Mφ-selected UV1591-RE variant to the cytotoxic effects of recombinant human TNF (rTNF-α) and recombinant human lymphotoxin (rTNF-β). The parental UV1591-RE tumor cells were equally sensitive to both recombinant proteins in a 72-hr ^{51}Cr-postlabeling assay. The sensitivity of the aMφ-resistant variant 1 was not increased by the simultaneous addition of recombinant murine IFN-γ (50 to 5000 units/mℓ) to human rTNF-α or human rTNF-β, each at a concentration of 5000 units/mℓ (not shown). The data represent pooled values from two separate experiments. (From Urban, J. et al., *Proc. Natl. Acad. Sci. U.S.A.*, 83, 5233, 1986. With permission.)

resistant to tumoricidal Mφ and that the nature of this resistance in the model used appears to be resistance to TNF. Although we cannot exclude that lymphotoxin secreted by activated tumor-specific helper T cells may be the actual selecting agent in the normal host, direct interaction between helper T cells and the tumor is unlikely in light of the fact that helper T cells only appear to recognize the tumor antigen on antigen-presenting cells. Thus, the pivotal role of helper T cells in tumor rejection appears more likely to be related to the activation of CTL and the release of lymphokines that can activate Mφ to release TNF. In contrast, CTL and activated Mφ are known to recognize the tumor cells directly and are, therefore, likely to exert direct tumoricidal effects.

Table 2
SENSITIZATION AND ELICITATION OF L3T4 POSITIVE T_h REQUIRE THE PRESENCE OF Ia-POSITIVE CELLS AND SHARING OF A TUMOR LINEAGE-SPECIFIC ANTIGEN WHICH IS INDEPENDENT OF THE CTL-DEFINED TUMOR-SPECIFIC ANTIGENS

Exp.	Tumor antigen[a] Sensitization in vivo	Elicitation in vitro	Blocking mAb specificity[b]	Lysis by helper factor-dependent anti-1591 CTL[c]
1	—	1591-[A$^+$B$^-$]	—	11 ± 3 (control)
	2240-RE[d]	1591-[A$^+$B$^-$]	—	12 ± 4
	1130-RE	1591-[A$^+$B$^-$]	—	15 ± 3
	1591-[A$^+$B$^+$]	1591-[A$^+$B$^-$]	—	37 ± 6[e]
	1591-[A$^+$B$^-$]	1591-[A$^+$B$^-$]	—	40 ± 6[e]
	1591-[A$^-$B$^+$]	1591-[A$^+$B$^-$]	—	30 ± 5[e]
2	1591-[A$^-$B$^+$]	—	—	7 ± 2 (control)
	1591-[A$^-$B$^+$]	1591-[A$^+$B$^-$]	—	40 ± 4[e]
	1591-[A$^-$B$^+$]	1591-[A$^+$B$^-$]	Thy1.2	37 + 4[e]
	1591-[A$^-$B$^+$]	1591-[A$^+$B$^-$]	L3T4	4 ± 1
	1591-[A$^-$B$^+$]	1591-[A$^+$B$^-$]	I-A^k	8 ± 4
	1591-[A$^-$B$^+$]	1591-[A$^+$B$^-$]	D^k	49 ± 4[e]
3	1591-[A$^+$B$^+$]	—	—	12 ± 4 (control)
	1591-[A$^+$B$^+$]	1591-[A$^+$B$^+$]	—	62 ± 4[e]
	1591-[A$^+$B$^+$]	1591-[A$^+$B$^+$]	L3T4	6 ± 1
	1591-[A$^+$B$^+$]	1591-[A$^+$B$^+$]	I-A^k	19 ± 2
	1591-[A$^+$B$^+$]	1591-[A$^+$B$^+$]	D^k	51 ± 5[e]
4	1591-[A$^+$B$^+$]	—	—	6 ± 1 (control)
	1591-[A$^+$B$^+$]	1591-[A$^+$B$^+$]	—	59 ± 2[e]
	1591-[A$^+$B$^+$]	1591-[A$^+$B$^+$]	L3T4	13 ± 3
	1591-[A$^+$B$^+$]	1591-[A$^+$B$^+$]	L3T4 + IL-2	41 ± 3[e]

[a] Nonimmune, 2240-RE, 1130-RE, 1591-RE [A$^+$B$^+$], 1591-BS [A$^+$B$^-$] and 1591-AS [A$^-$B$^+$] tumor-immune spleen cells were cultured with a 1591-specific IL-2-dependent cytolytic T cell line (which is used as a readout for IL-2 production by helper T cells), mitomycin C-treated stimulating tumor cells, and T-depleted filler spleen cells in a limiting dilution assay (for details see Van Waes, C. et al., 1986[33]). The 1591-specific, CTL-defined antigenic phenotypes are shown in brackets.

[b] Anti-Thy1.2, anti-L3T4, anti-IA^k, or anti-D^k mAb or secondary mixed lymphocyte culture supernatant as a source of IL-2 was added at a 1:10 dilution at initiation of culture.

[c] Numbers represent the mean percent lysis ± SEM for 8 replicate cultures in Exps. 1 and 2, and 16 replicates in Exps. 3 and 4 in a 6-hr ^{51}Cr release assay after 7-day culture. Lysis of the unrelated target 2240-RE in duplicate assay was 0% in Exp. 1, 3% or less in Exp. 2, 1% or less in Exp. 3 and 8% or less in Exp. 4 for all culture groups.

[d] The failure to elicit help from spleen cells of mice injected with the tumors unrelated to 1591 in Exp. 1 was apparently not due to less efficient priming by these tumors. This is suggested by the fact that 2240-RE immune spleen cells from the same group of mice provided help when the relevant tumor antigen to which they had been immunized (2240-RE cells) was added (not shown).

[e] Mean response is significantly greater than that of controls as determined by student's test ($p < 0.01$).

From Van Waes, C., et al., *J. Exp. Med.*, 164, 1547, 1986. With permission.

REFERENCES

1. **Hibbs, J. B.,** Control of carcinogenesis: a possible role for the activated macrophage, *Science, 177,* 998, 1972.
2. **Hibbs, J. B., Jr., Lambert, L. H., and Remington, J. S.,** Possible role of macrophage mediated nonspecific cytotoxicity in tumor resistance, *Nature (London) New Biol.,* 235, 48, 1972.
3. **Nathan, C. F., Karnovsky, N. L., and David, J. R.,** Alterations of macrophage functions by mediator from lymphocytes, *J. Exp. Med.,* 133, 1356, 1971.
4. **Evans, R. and Alexander, P.,** Mechanism of immunologically specific killing of tumor cells by macrophages, *Nature (London),* 236, 168, 1972.
5. **Meltzer, M. S.,** Macrophage activation for tumor cytotoxicity: characterization of priming and trigger signals during lymphokine activation, *J. Immunol.,* 127, 179, 1981.
6. **Pace, J. L. and Russell, S. E.,** Activation of mouse macrophages for tumor cell killing. I. Quantitative analysis of interactions between lymphokine and lipopolysaccharide, *J. Immunol.,* 126, 1963, 1981.
7. **Adams, D. O. and Snyderman, S.,** Do macrophages destroy nascent tumors?, *J. Natl. Cancer Inst.,* 62, 1341, 1979.
8. **Urban, J. L., Burton, R. C., Holland, J. M., Kripke, M. L., and Schreiber, H.,** Mechanisms of syngeneic tumor rejection: susceptibility of host-selected progressor variants to various immunological effector cells, *J. Exp. Med.,* 155, 557, 1982.
9. **Urban, J. L., Holland, J. M., Kripke, M. L., and Schreiber, H.,** Immunoselection of tumor cell variants by mice suppressed with ultraviolet radiation, *J. Exp. Med.,* 156, 1025, 1982.
10. **Urban, J. L. and Schreiber, H.,** Selection of macrophage-resistant progressor tumor variants by the normal host: requirement for concomitant T cell-mediated immunity, *J. Exp. Med.,* 157, 642, 1983.
11. **Wortzel, R. D., Urban, J. L., Philipps, C., Fitch, F. W., and Schreiber, H.,** Independent immunodominant and immunorecessive tumor-specific antigens on a malignant tumor: antigenic dissection with cytolytic T cell clones, *J. Immunol.,* 130, 2461, 1984.
12. **Urban, J. L., Van Waes, C., and Schreiber, H.,** Pecking order among tumor-specific antigens, *Eur. J. Immunol.,* 14, 181, 1984.
13. **Wortzel, R. D., Urban, J. L., and Schreiber, H.,** Malignant growth in the normal host after variant selection *in vitro* with cytolytic T cell lines, *Proc. Natl. Acad. Sci. U.S.A.,* 130, 2461, 1984.
14. **Urban, J. L., Kripke, M. L., and Schreiber, H.,** Stepwise immunological selection of antigenic variants during tumor growth, *J. Immunol.,* 137, 3036, 1986.
15. **Kripke, M. L.,** Immunologic mechanisms in UV-radiation carcinogenesis, *Adv. Cancer Res.,* 34, 69, 1981.
16. **Philipps, C., McMillan, M., Flood, P. M., Murphy, D. B., Forman, J., Lancki, D., Womack, J. E., Goodenow, R. S., Schreiber, H.,** Identification of a unique tumor-specific antigen as a novel class I major histocompatibility molecule, *Proc. Natl. Acad. Sci. U.S.A.,* 82, 5140, 1985.
17. **Stauss, H. J., Van Waes, C., Fink, M. A., Starr, B., and Schreiber, H.,** Identification of a unique tumor antigen as a rejection antigen by molecular cloning and gene transfer, *J. Exp. Med.,* 164, 1516, 1986.
18. **Nathan, C. F., Murray, H. W., Wiebe, M. E., and Rubin, B. Y.,** Identification of interferon-γ as the lymphokine that activates human macrophage oxidative metabolism and antimicrobial activity, *J. Exp. Med.,* 158, 670, 1983.
19. **Schreiber, R. D., Altman, A., and Katz, D. H.,** Identification of a T cell hybridoma that produces large quantities of a macrophage-activating factor, *J. Exp. Med.,* 156, 677, 1982.
20. **Wortzel, R. D., Philipps, C., and Schreiber, H.,** Multiple tumour-specific antigens expressed on a single tumour cell, *Nature (London),* 304, 165, 1983.
21. **Nathans, C. F. and Adams, D. O.,** Molecular mechanisms in tumor-cell killing by activated macrophages, *Immunol. Today,* 4, 166, 1983.
22. **Urban, J. L., Shepard, H. M., Rothstein, J. L., Sugarman, B. J., and Schreiber, H.,** Tumor necrosis factor: a potent effector molecule for tumor cell killing by activated macrophages, *Proc. Natl. Acad. Sci. U.S.A.,* 83, 5233, 1986.
23. **Carswell, E. A., Old, L. J., Kassel, R. L., Green, S., Fiore, N., and Williamson, B.,** An endotoxin-induced serum factor that causes necrosis of tumors, *Proc. Natl. Acad. Sci. U.S.A.,* 72, 3666, 1975.
24. **Gray, P. S., Aggarwal, B. B., Benton, C. V., Bringman, T. S., Henzel, W. J., Jarett, J. A., Leung, D. W., Moffat, B., Ng, P., Svedersky, L. P., Palladino, M. A., and Nedwin, G. E.,** Cloning and expression of cDNA for human lymphotoxin, a lymphokine with tumour necrosis activity, *Nature (London),* 312, 721, 1984.
25. **Pennica, D., Nedwin, G. E., Hayflick, J. S., Seeburg, P. H., Derynk, R., Palladino, M. A., Kohr, W. J., Aggarwal, B. B., and Goeddel, D. V.,** Human tumor necrosis factor: precursor structure, expression and homology to lymphotoxin, *Nature (London).,* 312, 724, 1984.

26. **Pennica, D., Hayflick, J. S., Bringman, T. S., Palladino, M. A., and Goeddel, D. V.,** Cloning and expression in *Eschericha coli* of the cDNA for murine tumor necrosis factor, *Proc. Natl. Acad. Sci. U.S.A.,* 82, 6060, 1985.

27. **Aggarwal, B. B., Moffat, B., and Harkins, R. N.,** Human lymphotoxin: production by a lymphoblastoid cell line, purification, and initial characterization, *J. Biol. Chem.,* 259, 686, 1984.

28. **Aggarwal, B. B., Eessalu, T. E., and Hass, P. E.,** Characterization of receptors for human tumor necrosis factor and their regulation by γ-interferon, *Nature (London),* 318, 665, 1985.

29. **Wide, D. B., Marrack, P., Kappler, J., Dialynas, D. P., and Fitch, W. F.,** Evidence implicating L3T4 in class II MHC antigen reactivity; monoclonal antibody GK 1.5 (anti-L3T4a) blocks class II MHC antigen-specific proliferation, release of lymphokines, and binding by cloned murine helper T lymphocyte lines, *J. Immunol.,* 131, 2178, 1983.

30. **Mosier, D.,** A requirement for two cell types for antibody formation *in vivo, Science,* 158, 1573, 1967.

31. **Steinman, R. M. and Nussenweig, M. C.,** Dendritic cells: features and functions, *Immunol. Rev.,* 53, 127, 1980.

32. **Unanue, E. R.,** The regulatory role of macrophages in antigenic stimulation, *Adv. Immunol.,* 15, 95, 1972.

33. **Van Waes, C., Urban, J. L., Rothstein, J. L., Ward, P. L., and Schreiber, H.,** Highly malignant tumor variants retain tumor-specific antigens recognized by T helper cells, *J. Exp. Med.,* 164, 1547, 1986.

34. **Tite, J. P. and Janeway, C. A.,** Cloned helper T cells can kill B lymphoma cells in the presence of specific antigen: Ia restriction and cognate vs. noncognate interactions in cytolysis, *Eur. J. Immunol.,* 14, 878, 1984.

35. **Flood, P. M., Kripke, M. L., Rowley, D. A., and Schreiber, H.,** Suppression of tumor rejection by autologous anti-idiotypic immunity, *Proc. Natl. Acad. Sci. U.S.A.,* 77, 2209, 1980.

36. **Flood, P. M., Urban, J. L., Kripke, M. L., and Schreiber, H.,** Loss of tumor-specific and idiotype-specific immunity with age, *J. Exp. Med.,* 154, 275, 1981.

37. **Mullen, C. A., Urban, J. L., Van Waes, C., Rowley, D. A., and Schreiber, H.,** Multiple cancers: tumor burden permits the outgrowth of other cancers, *J. Exp. Med.,* 162, 1665, 1985.

38. **Ruddle, N.,** personal communication.

Chapter 8

HETEROGENEITY IN TUMOR AND MACROPHAGE POPULATIONS IN THE RECOGNITION, CYTOSTASIS, AND CYTOLYSIS OF NEOPLASTIC CELLS

Susan M. North, Tatsuro Irimura, and Garth L. Nicolson

TABLE OF CONTENTS

I. INTRODUCTION

The relationship between a tumor and its host environment is complex. During the course of this discussion we will address two of the many factors that contribute to this complexity; namely, the functional heterogeneity of macrophages that infiltrate and reside within tumors, and the heterogeneity of tumor cells and their abilities to evade host immunological and nonimmunological defenses.

Macrophages possess a range of effector functions, including the capacity to phagocytose invading organisms, become cytotoxic, and kill aberrant or neoplastic cells.[1-4] They also possess a number of affector functions, such as the processing of antigens for interaction with T-lymphocytes and the binding of opsonins.[5,6] It has become increasingly apparent that not all macrophages are able to perform all the functions attributed to them. The ability to carry out these functions may depend on a macrophage's tissue origin or stage of development. Tissue differences in macrophage effector potentials and morphologies have been demonstrated in a number of studies.[7-9] Thus, macrophages are a heterogeneous group of cells (see Chapter 1).

The functional heterogeneity of peritoneal macrophages was shown by Walker.[10,11] He considered a number of parameters, including antigen-binding activity, Fc-Receptor (Fc-R) content, and antigen-processing ability. Peritoneal macrophages were obtained from rabbits and purified on Ficoll density gradients. The denser macrophages in these gradients possessed higher levels of Fc-R activity than the less-dense macrophages. Using the IC-21 macrophage cell line established by SV40 transformation of mouse peritoneal macrophages, Walker[12] showed that phagocytic and cytolytic activities of macrophages are separate functions, although they can be competitive in vivo during the interactions of macrophages with target cells.[12] Interestingly, macrophages appear to have more than one Fc-R receptor,[13] but whether such Fc-Rs on macrophages isolated from different tissue sites are functionally disparate was not determined.[14] It is known that mice have specific Fc-R receptors for IgG_{2a} and IgG_{2b} antibody isotypes.[15] These studies, in concert with Walker's[12] data, indicate that antibody-dependent phagocytic and cytolytic activities are mediated by different antibody isotypes interacting with distinct Fc-Rs.[12] Cytolytic activity was mediated primarily by IgG_{2b}, whereas phagocytosis required both IgG_{2a} and IgG_{2b} antibodies.[12]

Considering the multiple functions of macrophages, it is reasonable that they are involved in the surveillance and elimination of neoplastic cells as a first line of defense in preventing the development and progression of tumors. However, the situation in vivo is complex, and the role of macrophages in influencing surveillance against neoplasia remains controversial. The review that follows will illustrate that the views of researchers in this field are as heterogeneous as the macrophages and tumors they study.

II. MACROPHAGE HETEROGENEITY AND TUMOR INFILTRATION

A. Early Studies

That macrophages can infiltrate tumors is well established,[16] but whether such infiltrating macrophages carry out specific functions that affect tumor survival and progression is still largely unknown.[17] It should be pointed out that tumors are very complex structures, and in addition to tumor cells, there are a number of normal host cells that form an integral part of tumors. These include stromal cells, the vascular system stimulated by the tumor, and infiltrating macrophages, lymphocytes, polymorphonuclear leukocytes, and other host cells. Before considering the significance of macrophages and their heterogeneity, it is important to note that host-tumor environments are also heterogeneous and will influence both affector and effector macrophage functions.

A number of studies have investigated the relationship between the macrophage content of rodent tumors and tumor growth, immunogenicity, and dissemination. Eccles and Alexander[18] showed a good correlation between the immunogenicity of a number of murine and rat sarcomas and the macrophage contents relative to tumor cells of these sarcomas.[19] These and other in vivo studies indicated that a low intratumoral macrophage content correlated with a high spontaneous metastatic potential.[18-21] The presence of macrophages in these tumors was attributed to a response to tumor antigens, in a manner comparable to macrophage entry into sites of delayed-type hypersensitivity.[21] Confirmation of the immune nature of this recruitment was obtained by injecting the same tumor cells into either congenitally athymic nude rats,[22] or syngeneic rats immunosuppressed with the peptide cyclosporin A.[23] In these experiments immunosuppression reduced the recruitment of macrophages into the growing tumors by up to 50% of that found in tumors growing in immunocompetent rats. A similar relationship between tumor immunogenicity and macrophage recruitment was observed by Wood and Gillespie.[24] They found that tumors of low immunogenicity had lower numbers of infiltrating macrophages. However, other investigators, notably Evans and Lawler,[25] were unable to establish a similar correlation in the murine sarcomas they examined. Therefore, it remains to be established whether tumor antigens specifically elicit the recruitment of tumor-infiltrating macrophages.

B. Functional Status of Intratumoral Macrophages

Once the presence of macrophages in tumors was established, it was necessary to demonstrate the significance of tumor-infiltrating macrophages to tumor growth and progression. A number of approaches have been explored. One attempt to demonstrate the functional importance of intratumoral effector macrophages was to deplete the host of effector macrophages. The consequence of this manipulation was a significant reduction in the number of tumor-infiltrating macrophages with a corresponding increase in tumor growth and pulmonary metastases.[21] Moore and Moore[26] examined a number of rodent tumors, including immunogenic sarcomas, a squamous cell carcinoma, and a spontaneously arising mammary carcinoma, and were able to demonstrate a relationship between tumor growth and macrophage infiltration. Unfortunately, most tumors progress irrespective of their macrophage contents, and it has been argued that intratumoral macrophages are nontumoricidal and irrelevant to the process of tumor progression.[27] Studies were initiated to test this prediction. For example, Russell and McIntosh[28] proposed that the macrophages in progressing tumors were less "activated", and hence less cytotoxic than those in spontaneously regressing tumors. They tested this hypothesis by isolating macrophages from both regressing and progressing Moloney virus-transformed sarcomas. The isolated macrophages were tested in vitro for tumoricidal activity against the sarcoma cells. In the majority of the tumors they examined there was a correlation between in vitro macrophage cytotoxicity and the biological characteristics of the tumor. Macrophages isolated from progressing tumors were less cytotoxic than macrophages from regressing tumors. The former population of tumor cells was able to lyse tumor target cells, but much less efficiently than macrophages from regressing tumors. It was also established that the ability of macrophages to penetrate progressing tumors was reduced compared to the ability of macrophages isolated from regressing tumors. To explain the difference in tumoricidal abilities of these two macrophage isolates, Russell and McIntosh[28] proposed that macrophages in progressively growing Moloney virus-transformed sarcomas were inadequately activated by intratumoral lymphocytes. The reasons for this were not explored.

Considering the diversity of functions that macrophages have, the antitumor characteristics rather than the actual numbers of macrophages infiltrating a tumor must be more important. Mahoney et al.[29] have addressed this question in a series of experiments designed to determine the maturity of macrophages infiltrating mouse mammary tumors of differing metastatic potentials. Using the expression of a number of ectoenzymes to estimate murine macrophage maturity, macrophages of various differentiation states were quantitated. Macrophage maturity correlated with the metastatic potential of the tumors, such that the more metastatic tumors had more mature or more functionally cytotoxic macrophages than did the nonmetastatic mammary tumors. Intratumoral heterogeneity of the macrophages associated with each tumor was shown by the quantitative differences of ectoenzymes and by differential adherence.[30] This showed that not only were different populations of macrophages present in tumors of differing metastatic potential, but also that the macrophages in each tumor consisted of more than one population.

III. TUMOR HETEROGENEITY, METASTASIS, AND MACROPHAGES

The malignant cells composing the overwhelming majority of the cells within a tumor are known to be heterogeneous in a variety of properties.[31-34] One of the most interesting aspects of tumor heterogeneity is the heterogeneous propensity of tumor cells to metastasize. In the previous section we discussed the relationship between tumors growing at their sites of implantation and the heterogeneity of infiltrating macrophages. Although some of these tumors were metastatic, the recruitment of macrophages to metastases was not investigated. To determine whether progressively growing, spontaneous metastases represented subpopulations of tumor cells that had been selected for resistance to macrophage infiltration, the following experiment was carried out by Key et al.[35] Detailed examination of lung and lymph node metastases from the murine tumors — B16-BL6, a metastatic variant of B16 melanoma, and UV-2237 and UV-1422 fibrosarcomas — showed that they were heterogeneous in the degree of macrophage infiltration. The macrophage contents of metastases did not correlate with the numbers of macrophages present in the primary tumor implants, nor did they correlate with metastatic potential.[36] A similar study using iron-dextran to quantify the number of macrophages present in metastatic tumors[37] showed that for the B16 melanoma[38] and a metastatic clone, MTLn3, of the 13762NF rat mammary adenocarcinoma,[39] the size of the spontaneous metastases and degree of macrophage infiltration were related. Individual metastases were examined, and it was found that the numbers of macrophages present in spontaneous metastases decreased with the size of the secondary lesion.

Little is known about the role of macrophages that reside in tumor metastases. For example, are there inherent differences in the macrophages entering a metastatic lesion as opposed to those infiltrating the primary tumor? Are they subjected to immune suppression by factors released in greater quantities by metastatic tumor cells? Although the answers to these questions are unknown, there is some information available. Macrophages isolated from nonmetastatic tumors have been shown to be more cytolytic in vitro than macrophages isolated from metastatic tumors, but macrophages isolated from a lung metastasis were not significantly different in their tumoricidal abilities from either normal macrophages or macrophages isolated from the primary tumor.[40] Therefore, the macrophages infiltrating metastases were not functionally deficient, implying that the tumor itself was responsible for influencing activation of the macrophages after their recruitment.

IV. HETEROGENEITY OF RODENT TUMORS TO MACROPHAGE CYTOLYSIS

A. Introduction

Evans and Alexander[41] were among the first to demonstrate a direct cytotoxic effect of macrophages on tumor cells in vitro. Much of our current knowledge on the abilities of macrophages to recognize and kill tumor cells has been derived from such assays. Tumor cells within a primary neoplasm are heterogeneous for a number of properties, such as expression of cell surface antigens,[42-44] morphology,[45,46] invasiveness,[47,48] and metastatic potential.[31-34,49-51] Considering the extensive literature on tumor heterogeneity[31-34,50] it is reasonable to propose that tumor cells will have different susceptibilities to host-immune effector mechanisms, such as macrophage-mediated cytolysis and cytostasis. Although tumor cell variants resistant to T lymphocyte[52,53] and natural killer cell-mediated killing[54,55] have been selected, variants resistant to macrophage-mediated cytolysis have not been obtained with similar selection procedures (but see Chapter 7). One exception was reported by DeBaetselier et al.,[56] who were able to select a variant of the Lewis lung carcinoma, which after repeated selections in vivo in the presence of thioglycolate-elicited macrophages, grew faster in vitro in their presence. This growth enhancement was not seen in the parental cell line. On the basis of the inability to select macrophage-resistant cell lines and earlier in vitro cytolysis assays performed at high effector:target ratios, it was proposed that all tumor cells are equally sensitive to macrophage-mediated antitumor mechanisms.[57] Evidence for such a conclusion is, at best, circumstantial. In this section we will discuss evidence that suggests that tumor cells are heterogeneous in their susceptibility to macrophage-mediated cytolysis. Three animal tumor models will be discussed in detail: murine B16 melanoma, murine RAW117 lymphosarcoma, and rat 13762NF mammary adenocarcinoma. The conclusion that all tumor cells are not equally susceptible to killing by macrophages was also arrived at by other investigators working with a metastatic murine sarcoma,[58] a murine adenocarcinoma,[59] and a metastatic variant of the liver metastasizing Lewis lung carcinoma.[60] We will also discuss the heterogeneous nature of the macrophages resident within these tumors and how both tumor cell heterogeneity and macrophage heterogeneity are important in determining tumor survival and growth.

B. B16 Melanoma

Miner et al.[61,62] examined the macrophage sensitivities of metastatic B16 sublines selected for their abilities to colonize the brain and lung.[63] They compared B16-B14b, a subline that preferentially colonizes brain meninges and other organs such as lung, and B16-F10, a subline selected for its ability to colonize lung, with the poorly metastatic parental line B16-F1.[64] Using an in vitro cytotoxicity assay with poly I:C-activated peritoneal exudate macrophages (PEM6), they showed that the B16-B14b and B16-F10 cells were more resistant to cytolysis than were the parental B16-F1 cells.[61,62]

Neoplastic monocytic cell lines have been used as effector cells in cytolysis assays with tumor cells of various metastatic properties. The ability of the J774 reticulum cell sarcoma cell line to mediate cytolysis of the B16 melanoma sublines was examined, because this cell line behaves in many respects like PEM.[65] Although both PEM and J774 effector cell populations lysed low and high metastatic B16 cell variants, the J774 cell line was, in general, more efficient in lysing B16 melanoma cells than were the PEMs. In addition to examining direct cell killing by macrophages, the effects of macrophage cytotoxins on tumor cell death were evaluated.[61] Using an indirect killing assay, the ability of effector cell supernatants to induce cytolysis was determined for B16-B14b, B16-F10, and B16-F1. The more metastatic B16-B14b and B16-F10 were consistently more resistant to cytolysis than was the less metastatic B16-F1. Some killing of the tumor cells was always detected; although the more metastatic cell lines showed increased resistance to lysis, they were not totally impervious to the effects of poly I:C-activated macrophages. For example, at an effector:target ratio of 25:1, after incubation with poly I:C for 72 hr, 24% of the B16-F1 cells were lysed, compared with 17% of the B16-B14b and 16% of the B16-F10.

In contrast to the above studies, Fidler[57] was not able to detect differences in macrophage susceptibility between the B16-F10 and B16-F1 cell lines. It is possible that the reasons for this discrepancy reside in the different experimental conditions used by the two groups of investigators. For example, the different methods of activation of the macrophages may be important since macrophage activation can be achieved by more than one route and not all in vitro methods of activation are equivalent.[66] In addition, the densities of macrophages used in the cytolysis assays are important and can influence the ability of the macrophages to interact with their target cells.[67] In general, Miner et al.[61,62] used lower effector:target ratios in their cytolysis assays, more consistent with the known macrophage contents of tumors.

C. RAW117 Large Cell Lymphoma

The RAW117 lymphosarcoma is a large cell lymphoma or lymphosarcoma syngeneic to BALB/c mice. The RAW117 cell line has been sequentially selected for metastatic organ colonization variants in vivo,[68] and for cell surface metastatic variants that show an inability to bind to selected lectins in vitro.[69] These metastatic variants were compared in vitro with the low metastatic potential parental line for their sensitivities to macrophage-mediated cytolysis and cytostasis.[70] The effector cells in these assays were poly I:C-activated PEMs. The low metastatic parental line was the most sensitive to macrophage-mediated cytolysis. At an effector:target ratio of 25:1, 65% of the cells were lysed, whereas only 32% of the metastatic RAW117-H10 were killed after 72 hr. In addition, the highly metastatic RAW117 cells were also much more resistant to macrophage growth inhibition in cytostasis assays than was the low metastatic parental line.[70]

Reading et al.[71] had shown previously that the metastatic potential of the RAW117 sublines was related to the expression of the RNA tumor virus-encoded envelope glycoprotein gp70. They were able to demonstrate by sodium dodecyl sulfate-polyacrylamide gel electrophoresis (SDS-PAGE) and competition radioimmunoassays that the metastatic RAW117-H10 subline had significantly less gp70 than the parental RAW117-P. To test the hypothesis that resistance to macrophage-mediated cytolysis correlated with gp70 expression and metastatic potential, a number of in vivo experiments were carried out in which macrophage function was inhibited by such agents as trypan blue, silica particles, carrageenan, cyclophosphamide, pristane, and chlorinated drinking water. Under these conditions the parental RAW117-P cells became more metastatic, whereas the highly metastatic RAW117-H10 cells were unaffected.[72] If the expression of gp70 were important in macrophage recognition of RAW117 cells, then increasing the concentrations of cell surface gp70 should decrease metastatic potential concomitant with an increased sensitivity to lysis by PEMs. This was accomplished by super-infection of highly metastatic RAW117-H10 cells with endogenous RNA tumor viruses isolated from the parental RAW117 cells.[70] Virus superinfection increased the expression of gp70 on RAW117-H10 cells and increased their sensitivity to macrophage-mediated cytolysis concomitant with loss of liver colonization, confirming that gp70 is related to host macrophage surveillance mechanisms and, therefore, to metastasis, in this system.[73]

D. 13762NF Rat Mammary Adenocarcinoma

The two tumor metastasis models described above, B16 melanoma and RAW117 large cell lymphoma, were derived by repeated in vivo selections. The rat mammary adenocarcinoma model was arrived at in a different manner. A number of cell clones were obtained directly from a primary tumor implant and from its spontaneous metastases. These cell clones have since been characterized biologically,[49,51] biochemically,[42,46] and immunologically.[43,74,75]

Using the 13762NF cell clones MTLn3 (high metastatic potential), MTF7 and MTLn2 (intermediate metastatic potential), and MTC and MTPa (low metastatic potential), we examined the correlation of spontaneous metastatic potential with macrophage infiltration of tumors growing in the mammary fat pads of syngeneic F344 rats.[75] Tumors were established by injection of 10^6 cells subcutaneously, and 23 days later the tumors were removed and enzymatically disaggregated; the number of Fc-R-positive cells infiltrating the tumor were then counted using a rosetting assay. The number of Fc-R-positive cells isolated from such tumors ranged from 8 to 20% (Table 1). Although the most metastatic clone (MTLn3)

Table 1
MACROPHAGE INFILTRATION OF 13762NF
ADENOCARCINOMA

Tumor	Original passage no.	Metastatic potential (ranked by order)[a]	Percent FcR$^+$ cells[b]
MTPa	T13	1	10
MTPa	T11	1	9
MTC	T14	2	12
MTC	T12	2	11
MTF7	T18	3	8
MTF7	T17	3	15
MTLn2	T40	4	10
MTLn3	T18	5	20

[a] Spontaneous metastatic potential assayed as described by Welch et al.[51]
[b] FcR$^+$ cell infiltrate determined on tumors grown s.c. in the mammary fat pad of the syngeneic host for 23 days (10^6 cells/rat).

From North, S. M. and Nicolson, G. L., *Cancer Res.*, 45, 1453, 1985. With permission.

contained the greatest number of macrophages (~20%), there was no correlation between metastatic potential and the ability of macrophages to infiltrate the other 13762NF cell clones.[75]

To determine whether activated PEM or macrophages that infiltrated 13762NF tumors were tumoricidal, we examined their ability to lyse syngeneic tumor cells in vitro. Using PEMs obtained from F344 rats given intraperitoneal (i.p.) thioglycolate 5 days prior to harvest, we first determined the susceptibility of established 13762NF cell lines to cytolysis. The cytolysis assay measured the remaining [^{75}Se]-selenomethionine after the interaction of radiolabeled target cells with effectors for 72 hr.[76] In these assays the PEMs were activated in vitro with lipopolysaccharide (LPS) at a concentration of 50 ng/mℓ. In the absence of LPS, negligible lysis occurred. The 13762NF cell clones were similar in their susceptibility to LPS-activated, PEM-mediated cytolysis (Table 2). At an effector:target ratio of 25:1 clones MTF7 and MTLn2 (intermediate metastatic potential) and MTC (low metastatic potential) showed between 50 and 60% cytolysis after 72 hr, whereas clones MTLn3 (high metastatic potential) and MTPa (low metastatic potential) displayed between 30 and 40% cytolysis. Reduction of the effector:target ratio to 10:1 yielded no significant difference in the susceptibility of the 13762NF cell clones to activated PEM-mediated cytolysis, irrespective of their metastatic potential.

To assay the tumoricidal capabilities of intratumoral macrophages (ITMs), we established tumors in the mammary fat pads of F344 rats. After 21 days these tumors were removed and trypsinized, and tumor cells and macrophages were separated by repeated, differential adherence to plastic. ITMs were then incubated in vitro with the newly isolated, [^{75}Se]-selenomethionine-labeled, in vivo grown tumor cells (Table 3). At the same time PEMs were also incubated with this population of tumor cells so that we could compare the tumoricidal abilities of ITMs and PEMs simultaneously. In such assays the highly metastatic MTLn3 cells were the least susceptible to macrophage killing. At a 10:1 effector:target ratio, with PEMs as the effectors, only 21% of the freshly established MTLn3 cells were lysed, compared with 58% of established, tissue-cultured MTLn3 cells. Newly isolated MTF7, MTLn2, and MTC cells showed lower levels of susceptibility to lysis than did the established cultures of these same cells; for example, 43.5% of uncultured MTLn2 cell targets were

Table 2
IN VITRO CYTOLYSIS OF 13762NF CELL LINES BY
ACTIVATED PERITONEAL MACROPHAGES

Clonal cell line (passage no.)[a]	Effector:target ratio[b]	cpm ± S.D.	Percent cytolysis[c]	Significance[d]
MTLn3	25:1	10327 ± 686	30[e]	0.001
(T18)	10:1	6005 ± 568	58	
	5:1	13738 ± 824	0	
	0	13739 ± 476		
MTLn2	25:1	3056 ± 1007	50[e]	0.001
(T42)	10:1	2144 ± 307	68	
	5:1	4925 ± 833	27	
	0	6771 ± 88		
MTF7	25:1	2910 ± 931	58[e]	0.001
(T18)	10:1	2793 ± 118	60	
	5:1	5033 ± 480	37	
	0	6861 ± 711		
MTC	25:1	1428 ± 114	39	0.010
(T11)	10:1	1648 ± 120	64	
	5:1	3829 ± 341	26	
	0	4535 ± 927		
MPTa	25:1	3297 ± 195	36	0.002
(T12)	10:1	3174 ± 145	38	
	5:1	7216 ± 891	0	
	0	5132 ± 478		

[a]   Clonal cells at passage in vitro indicated by T number.

[b]   Effector cells where thioglycolate-stimulated F344 peritoneal macrophages activated in vitro with 50 ng/mℓ LPS. 0 = no macrophages.

[c]   Percentage of cytolysis was calculated by $(1 - \frac{a_l}{a_t}) \times 100$ where a_l = retained cpm in wells with macrophages, and a_t = retained cpm in wells with no macrophages.

[d]   Significance between control and experimental samples at the indicated level was determined by one-way analysis of variance.

[e]   Significant difference ($p < 0.05$) between metastatic MTLn3, low metastatic MTLn2, and MTF7 sublines was determined by the Kruskal-Wallis test.

From North, S. M. and Nicolson, G. L., *Cancer Res.*, 45, 1453, 1985. With permission.

lysed compared with 68% of the cultured cells. In these experiments the most striking difference in susceptibility to macrophage killing was observed with low metastatic parental MTPa cells. Here cell death was 75% for in vivo passaged tumor cells, but only 36% for in vitro cultured cells. When these same tumor cells were exposed to ITMs isolated from the same tumors, they were less sensitive than when PEMs were used as the effector cells: MTF7 cell death was reduced from 38% with PEMs to 16% with ITMs. Heterogeneity of macrophage killing was apparent in all the 13762NF tumors investigated, but was complex and depended on the tumor cell source in addition to the source of macrophage effectors.

When freshly isolated tumor cells were passaged once in vitro and then reexamined using the cytotoxicity assay, clones MTLn3 and MTC showed susceptibilities similar to that of cells from primary explants, but clones MTLn2, MTF7, and MTPa were markedly reduced in their sensitivities to cytolysis after short-term culture. After isolation from a tumor and one passage in vitro, MTPa cells had a sensitivity to LPS-activated PEMs similar to that of the established cell line (Table 4). In these assays it was necessary to activate the macrophages (PEMs and ITMs) with LPS, in order to detect lysis. In general, the most metastatic line

Table 3
IN VITRO CYTOLYSIS OF 13762NF TUMOR EXPLANTS BY ACTIVATED PERITONEAL AND INTRATUMORAL MACROPHAGES

Tumor (passage no.)[a]	Effector population[b]	Effector: target ratio	cpm ± S.D.	Percent cytolysis[c]	Significance[d]
MTLn3	PEC	10:1	8484 ± 96	21.0[e]	0.001
(T18,P1)	PEC	5:1	9025 ± 403	16.0	
	IT	10:1	9614 ± 468	11.0[e]	
	IT	5:1	9769 ± 560	9.0	
	None	0	10798 ± 560		
MTLn2	PEC	10:1	5235 ± 544	43.5[e]	0.020
(T42,P1)	PEC	5:1	7219 ± 917	23.0	
	IT	10:1	5665 ± 181	39.0[e]	
	IT	5:1	7453 ± 607	19.5	
	None	0	9257 ± 1064		
MTF7	PEC	10:1	2933 ± 148	63.5[e]	0.001
(T18,P1)	PEC	5:1	5643 ± 757	30.0	
	IT	10:1	6764 ± 177	16.0	
	IT	5:1	7116 ± 174	11.5	
	None	0	8033 ± 458		
MTC	PEC	10:1	2428 ± 116	38.0[e]	0.010
(T12,P1)	PEC	5:1	3327 ± 416	20.0	
	IT	10:1	3187 ± 204	16.0	
	IT	5:1	4125 ± 374	5.0	
	None	0	4178 ± 374		
MTPa	PEC	10:1	701 ± 33	75.0[e]	0.002
(T12,P1)	PEC	5:1	1032 ± 83	54.0	
	IT	10:1	1463 ± 550	27.0[e]	
	IT	5:1	2776 ± 72	0	
	None	0	2215 ± 180		

[a] Clonal lines after one passage in vivo at the in vitro passage represented by T number.
[b] PEC-thioglycolate elicited peritoneal macrophages stimulated in vitro with 50 ng/mℓ LPS. IT = intratumoral macrophages isolated from tumors as described in materials and methods, macrophages stimulated in vitro with 50 ng/mℓ LPS.
[c,d] See Table 2.
[e] Significant difference ($p < 0.01$) between metastatic MTLn3, low metastatic MTLn2, MTF7, and nonmetastatic MTC and MTPa sublines determined by the Kruskal-Wallis test.

From North, S. M. and Nicolson, G. L., *Cancer Res.*, 45, 1453, 1985. With permission.

(MTLn3) was the least sensitive to lysis by activated macrophages, whereas the less metastatic lines MTF7, MTLn2, MTC and MTPa were more sensitive to PEM- and ITM-mediated killing. It was apparent from these data that the length of time in culture influenced the susceptibility of the tumor cells to the macrophages. Thus, established cell lines may not be the most suitable system for examining macrophage-mediated cytolysis of syngeneic tumor cells. These data showed that the source of macrophages is also important, and suggested that PEMs are not the most appropriate macrophage population to use in such assays.

Macrophage heterogeneity was clearly discernible in the tumor cell cytolysis assays. Not all the ITMs were equally able to lyse tumor cells, probably for a number of reasons. Tumor cells are known to produce a number of immunologically suppressive factors that may not affect macrophage recruitment but may impair their function.[77-79] It is possible that the highly

Table 4

**IN VITRO CYTOLYSIS OF SHORT-TERM TISSUE CULTURES OF
13762NF CELLS BY ACTIVATED PERITONEAL AND
INTRATUMORAL MACROPHAGES**

Target cells (passage no.)[a]	Effector population[b]	Effector: target ratio	cpm ± S.D.	Percent cytolysis[c]	Significance[d]
MTLn3	PEC	10:1	3665 ± 260	17.0[e]	NS[f]
(T18,P1,T1)	PEC	5:1	4771 ± 322	5.0	
	IT	10:1	4088 ± 470	7.0[e]	
	IT	5:1	5112 ± 570	5.0	
	None	0	4405 ± 229		
MTLn2	PEC	10:1	3136 ± 508	5.0[e]	NS[f]
(T42,P1,T1)	PEC	5:1	4168 ± 227	5.0	
	IT	10:1	3256 ± 899	5.0	
	IT	5:1	2827 ± 500	10.0	
	None	0	3151 ± 477		
MTF7	PEC	10:1	3946 ± 793	22.0	0.01
(T18,P1,T1)	PEC	5:1	3100 ± 242	38.0	
	IT	10:1	3406 ± 212	35.0[e]	
	IT	5:1	5776 ± 507	5.0	
	None	0	5092 ± 325		
MTC	PEC	10:1	2429 ± 116	22.0	NS[f]
(T12,P1,T1)	PEC	5:1	2347 ± 72	20.0	
	IT	10:1	3028 ± 142	10.0	
	IT	5:1	4314 ± 177	5.0	
	None	0	3125 ± 374		
MTPa	PEC	10:1	2363 ± 137	30.0[e]	0.01
(T12,P1,T1)	PEC	5:1	2492 ± 51	26.0	
	IT	10:1	2198 ± 220	10.0	
	IT	5:1	2809 ± 382	17.0	
	None	0	3389 ± 613		

[a]   Clonal lines after one passage in vivo, one passage in vitro from the original tissue culture passage designated by the T number.

[b]   See Table 2,3.

[c,d,e]   See Table 2.

[f]   NS not significant by one-way analysis of variance.

From North, S. M. and Nicolson, G. L., *Cancer Res.*, 45, 1453, 1985. With permission.

metastatic MTLn3 cells produce more of these factors in vivo but lose their ability to generate them after in vitro culture. Urban et al.[80,81] reported that variants of the 15911-RE tumor that were increasingly malignant became more resistant to cytotoxic macrophages after they were passaged in vivo in immunocompetent animals. Experiments such as these indicate that macrophages are important in antitumor surveillance but that host factors and tumor heterogeneity may impair this function. In addition, macrophages also produce and secrete a number of biological mediators, including prostaglandins[82,83] and neutral proteases,[84,85] that can modify the tumor environment.

Activation of macrophages appears to be necessary for effective antitumor responses. Moore and Moore[86] showed that it was necessary to activate ITMs in vitro with LPS before they were tumoricidal. Using Mc40A, an immunogenic rat sarcoma that was subjected to macrophage-mediated lysis by ITMs, they were unable to detect significant lysis even at effector:target ratios up to 50:1, unless the macrophages were first activated with LPS. Tumor cell targets other than the Mc40A were also killed by LPS-activated ITMs, suggesting the nonspecific character of LPS activation. Earlier data from Hibbs[87] showed that the nonspecific activation of macrophages with LPS was important in macrophage cytolytic assays. ITMs isolated from the 13762NF adenocarcinoma also required activation by LPS before they were cytotoxic.[75]

V. HETEROGENEITY OF RODENT TUMORS TO MACROPHAGE CYTOSTASIS

A. Introduction

In the preceding section, we discussed the heterogeneity of tumor cell populations in regard to macrophage-mediated cytolysis. Here we discuss the cytostatic function of macrophages and the differences seen in tumor cell subpopulations in their susceptibility to cytostasis. The cytostatic effects of macrophages on tumor cells is not as well documented as their cytolytic effects, and most of our current knowledge has been obtained from in vitro assays. In vivo the ratio of macrophages to tumor cells is usually less than 1:1; therefore, cytostasis may be more important in vivo than cytolysis in inhibiting tumor cell growth and dissemination. This may be particularly pertinent considering that most tumors progress in vivo even in the presence of tumor-infiltrating macrophages.

B. In Vitro Requirements for Cytostasis

Direct cell contact between the macrophage and tumor cell is considered a prerequisite[88] to initiation of tumor cytostatic or tumoricidal activity, though not by all investigators.[89] Cabilly and Gallily[90] showed that binding of macrophages to syngeneic tumor cells elicited cytostasis but not cytolysis. Raz et al.[91] also concluded that the binding of macrophages to Moloney virus-induced lymphoma (YAC) cells was necessary for cytostasis. Schirrmacher and Appelhaus[92] observed consistently higher binding of PEMs to the low metastatic murine Eb lymphoma than to the high metastatic ESb variant. These results were seen at a number of macrophage-to-tumor-cell ratios. In co-culture experiments a cytostatic effect was observed with Eb but not ESb cells. When macrophages were activated with lymphokines, there was an increase in tumor cell binding with a subsequent increase in tumor cytostatic potential. Schirrmacher and Appelhaus[92] concluded that the growth inhibitory effect they observed in the Eb lymphoma cells was a consequence of direct cell contact. The method of eliciting the peritoneal macrophages for such assays is important. Earlier studies by Gemsa et al.[93] examined the effect of *Corynebacterium parvum* on cytostasis. When Schirrmacher and Appelhaus[92] used *C. parvum*-activated macrophages they detected some growth enhancement of ESb tumor cells in the presence of these macrophages; a growth inhibitory effect was observed on Eb cells only.

Miner et al.[61,70] detected a significant cytostatic effect of poly I:C-activated macrophages on the growth of both B16 melanoma and RAW117 lymphoma subpopulations. In both these tumor models the low metastatic parental lines were more susceptible to growth inhibition than the metastatic lines. However, in this case no difference in binding of macrophages to tumor cell populations was observed. They concluded that products released by activated macrophages acted differently on cell populations of differing metastatic potential.[70]

VI. HETEROGENEITY REVEALED BY BIOCHEMICAL ANALYSIS OF TUMOR-REACTIVE MACROPHAGES

A. Introduction

The biochemical nature of recognition between cell surface molecules on neoplastic cells and macrophages is currently unknown but is under intensive investigation in a number of laboratories.[94-96] Several proteins/glycoproteins have been found to increase in their expression after activation of macrophage populations. Analysis of such cell surface components has been used in attempts to correlate cell surface changes and macrophage function. The approaches used in determining macrophage cell surface changes include analyses of radio-labeled proteins,[97] glycolipids,[98] and lectin-binding sites.[99] For example, Maddox et al.[99] have shown that the *Griffonia simpliciforia*-lectin I-B$_4$ selectively binds to activated murine macrophages. Using the same lectin, Wicha and Huard[100] suggested that the carbohydrate chains recognized by I-B$_4$ interact with cell surface laminin.

B. Heterogeneity in Lectin-Binding Sites of Tumoricidal Macrophages

Using a labeling technique developed in our laboratory,[101,102] the cell surface glycoproteins of macrophages at various stages of activation were examined by a combination of SDS-PAGE and lectin binding.[103] This technique was then applied to the macrophages infiltrating 13762NF tumors established in vivo. Initially, macrophages were isolated from the peritoneal cavities of Fischer F344 rats. Three populations of macrophages were compared, unelicited resident macrophages, thioglycolate-elicited macrophages, and BCG-activated macrophages. The effects of LPS activation on these PEM populations were examined to determine if LPS activation and changes in PEM glycoprotein expression were related. The macrophage populations were lysed in buffered NP-40 and subjected to SDS-PAGE. The binding of lectins to the separated glycoproteins from the macrophage populations was visualized after electrophoretic transfer of the glycoproteins to nitrocellulose paper, incubation with the ^{125}I-labeled lectins, and autoradiography.[101,102]

A number of differences were seen in the amounts and distributions of glycoproteins in unactivated and activated macrophages.[103] One lectin, *Ricinus Communis* agglutinin I (RCA$_1$), showed the presence of several glycoproteins, including two of M$_r$ ~160,000 and ~65,000 that were prominent on resident macrophages (Plate 1).* Of particular interest was the increased expression of a class of glycoproteins that bound a pokeweed mitogen (PWM) isolectin, Pa-4 (Plate 2). This lectin recognizes branched poly-(*N*-acetyl-lactosamine)-type carbohydrate chains.[104] The family of Pa-4-binding glycoproteins ranged from M$_r$ ~70,000 to ~150,000, and the quantitative expression of these glycoproteins increased with the stage of activation of the macrophages as assessed by tumoricidal ability. Histochemical analysis of formaldehyde-fixed macrophages in vitro using biotinyl-Pa-4 also showed an increase in PA-4 reactivity with activation. In addition, resident macrophages did not bind significant amounts of PWM, whereas on the thioglycolate-elicited macrophages the presence of PWM-reactive glycoproteins on the cell surface and perinuclear region was easily demonstrated. Next the presence of the lectin-binding glycoproteins on alveolar and tumor-associated macrophages was examined. In these assays alveolar macrophages showed more reactivity than either resident or thioglycolate-elicited PEMs. Using biotinyl-Pa-4, heterogeneity in the expression of PWM-reactive glycoproteins was shown immunohistochemically. Some macrophages were densely stained at both the cell surface and in the perinuclear region, whereas other macrophages were only lightly stained (Plate 3).

The cytolytic activity of macrophage populations expressing PWM-binding glycoproteins was assessed. The macrophage populations (thioglycollate-elicited, BCG-activated, alveolar, and intratumoral) expressing PWM-reactive glycoproteins were responsive to LPS, but resident peritoneal macrophages unresponsive to LPS did not express detectable amounts of PWM-binding glycoproteins. LPS-activation of the lectin-reactive macrophage populations resulted in increased expression of PWM-binding glycoproteins concomitant with increased cytolytic activity. Only alveolar and BCG-activated macrophages were cytolytic in the absence of LPS, and these two macrophage populations had the highest amounts of PWM-binding sites.

* Plates 1 to 3 appear following page 152.

It is interesting that LPS and PWM probably share the same receptor on B-lympho-cytes.[105,106] PWM is a known B-lymphocyte mitogen, and our data suggest that PWM-binding sites on macrophages are also receptors for LPS. The cell-surface glycoproteins with poly-(N-acetyllactosamine)-type carbohydrate chains appeared at an early stage of activation and were increased in expression during LPS activation of macrophages to the tumoricidal state.

VII. CONCLUSION

The heterogeneity of tumor cells in sensitivity to macrophage-mediated cytolysis has been demonstrated in a number of experimental tumor models of different origin, including murine B16 melanoma and RAW117 large cell lymphoma and rat 13762NF mammary adenocar-cinoma. In such tumor models, the more metastatic tumor cells were more resistant to the effects of macrophages than the less metastatic cells. The heterogeneity of the target tumor cells was demonstrated in these experiments, in addition to the heterogeneity of the effector macrophages. Intratumoral macrophages isolated from metastatic MTLn3 tumors were the least efficient in lysing autologous tumor cells. These highly metastatic tumor cells were also able to inhibit macrophage activation, but the tumor cells lost this ability after in vitro culture. The experiments presented reinforce the hypothesis that the high metastatic potential of some tumors may reside, at least in part, in their ability to circumvent the host's immune system. In general, recruitment of macrophages to highly metastatic tumors was not different from recruitment to less metastatic tumors of the same origin, implying that tumor envi-ronment is also an important factor in determining the tumoricidal abilities of macrophages in vivo.

The observations on tumor cell and macrophage heterogeneity, documented by a number of different laboratories over a period of years, have serious ramifications for the immu-notherapy of tumors. For such therapeutic approaches to be successful, it will be necessary to isolate and characterize not only metastatic subpopulations of tumor cells, but also the subpopulations of macrophages resident within these tumors. Only then will we be able to understand the mechanisms by which tumors progress and disseminate while interacting with and evading the host's immunological defenses.

REFERENCES

1. **Fidler, I. J.,** Activation in vitro of mouse macrophages by syngeneic, allogeneic, or xenogeneic lymphocyte supernatants, *J. Natl. Cancer Inst.*, 55, 1159, 1975.
2. **Nelson, D. S.,** Macrophages as effectors of cell-mediated immunity, in *Phagocytes and Cellular Immunity*, Gradebusch, H., Ed., CRC Press, Boca Raton, Fla., 1978, 57.
3. **Evans, R.,** Macrophage-mediated cytotoxicity: its possible role in rheumatoid arthritis, *Ann. N.Y. Acad. Sci.*, 256, 275, 1975.
4. **Haskill, J. S., Proctor, J. W., and Yamamura, Y.,** Host responses within solid tumors. I. Monocytic effector cells within rat sarcomas, *J. Natl. Cancer Inst.*, 54, 387, 1975.
5. **Haskill, J. S., Key, M. E., Rador, L. A., Parthenais, E., Kara, J. H., Fett, J. W., Yamamura, Y., Delustro, F., Vesley, J., and Gant, G.,** The importance of antibody and macrophages in spontaneous and drug-mediated regression of T1699 mammary adenocarcinoma, *J. Reticuloendothel. Soc.*, 26, 417, 1979.
6. **Haskill, J. S. and Fett, J. W.,** Possible evidence for antibody-dependent macrophage-mediated cytotoxicity directed against murine adenocarcinoma cells in vivo, *J. Immunol.*, 117, 1992, 1976.
7. **Walker, W. S.,** Functional heterogeneity of macrophages, in *Immunobiology of the Macrophage*, Nelson, D. S., Ed., Academic Press, New York, 1976, 91.
8. **Rice, S. G. and Fishman, M.,** Functional and morphological heterogeneity among rabbit peritoneal macrophages, *Cell. Immunol.*, 11, 130, 1974.

9. **Walker, W. S.,** Macrophage functional heterogeneity in the in vitro induced immune response, *Nature, (London), New Biol.*, 229, 211, 1971.

10. **Walker, W. S.,** Functional heterogeneity of macrophages: subclasses of peritoneal macrophages with different antigen-binding activities and immune complex receptors, *Immunology*, 26, 1025, 1974.

11. **Walker, W. S.,** Functional heterogeneity of macrophages in the induction and expression of acquired immunity, *J. Reticuloendothel. Soc.*, 20, 57, 1976.

12. **Walker, W. S.,** Macrophage heterogeneity: membrane markers and properties of macrophage subpopulations, in *Macrophage Regulation of Immunity*, Unanue, E. R. and Rosenthal, A. S., Eds., Academic Press, New York, 1980, 307.

13. **Unkeless, J. C.,** The presence of two Fc receptors on mouse macrophages: evidence from a variant cell line and differential trypsin sensitivity, *J. Exp. Med.*, 145, 931, 1977.

14. **Unkeless, J. C., Fleit, H., and Mellman, I. S.,** Structural aspects and heterogeneity of immunoglobulin Fc receptors, *Adv. Immunol.*, 31, 247, 1981.

15. **Diamond, B. and Scharff, M. D.,** IgG_1 and IgG_{2b} share the Fc receptor on mouse macrophages, *J. Immunol.*, 125, 631, 1980.

16. **Evans, R.,** Macrophages in syngeneic animal tumors, *Transplantation*, 14, 468, 1972.

17. **Alexander, P.,** Surveillance against neoplastic cells. Is it mediated by macrophages?, *Br. J. Cancer*, 33, 344, 1976.

18. **Eccles, S. A. and Alexander, P.,** Macrophage content of tumors in relation to metastatic spread and host immune reaction, *Nature (London)*, 250, 667, 1974.

19. **Eccles, S. A. and Alexander, P.,** Sequestration of macrophages in growing tumors and its effect on the immunological capacity of the host, *Br. J. Cancer*, 30, 22, 1974.

20. **Alexander, P., Eccles, S., and Gauci, C. L. L.,** The significance of macrophages in human and experimental tumors, *Ann. N.Y. Acad. Sci.*, 276, 124, 1976.

21. **Eccles, S. A., Bandlow, G., and Alexander, P.,** Monocytosis associated with the growth of transplanted syngeneic rat sarcomata differing in immunogenicity, *Br. J. Cancer*, 34, 20, 1976.

22. **Eccles, S. A., Styles, J. M., Hobbs, S. M., and Dean, C. J.,** Metastasis in the nude rat associated with lack of immune response, *Br. J. Cancer*, 40, 802, 1979.

23. **Eccles, S. A., Heckford, S. E., and Alexander, P.,** Effect of cyclosporin on the growth and spontaneous metastasis of syngeneic animal tumours, *Br. J. Cancer*, 42, 252, 1980.

24. **Wood, G. W. and Gillespie, G. Y.,** Studies on the role of macrophages in regulation of growth and metastasis of murine chemically induced fibrosarcoma, *Int. J. Cancer*, 16, 1022, 1975.

25. **Evans, R. and Lawler, E. M.,** Macrophage content and immunogenicity of C57BL/6J and Balb/cByJ methylcholanthrene induced sarcomas, *Int. J. Cancer*, 26, 831, 1980.

26. **Moore, K. and Moore, M.,** Intra-tumor host cells of transplanted rat neoplasms of different immunogenicity, *Int. J. Cancer*, 19, 803, 1977.

27. **Evans, R. and Edilen, D. M.,** Macrophage accumulation in transplanted tumors is not dependent on host immune responsiveness or presence of tumor associated rejection antigens, *J. Reticuloendothel. Soc.*, 30, 425, 1981.

28. **Russell, S. W. and McIntosh, A. T.,** Macrophages isolated from regressing Molony sarcomas are more cytotoxic than those recovered from progressing sarcomas, *Nature (London)*, 268, 69, 1977.

29. **Mahoney, K. H., Fulton, A. M., and Heppner, G. H.,** Tumor associated macrophages of mouse mammary tumors. II. Differential distribution of macrophages from metastatic tumors, *J. Immunol.*, 131, 2079, 1983.

30. **Mahoney, K. H., Miller, B. E., and Heppner, G. H.,** FACS quantitation of leucine aminopeptidase and acid phosphatase in tumor-associated macrophages from metastatic and non-metastatic mouse mammary tumors, *J. Leukocyte Biol.*, 38, 573, 1985.

31. **Fidler, I. J.,** Tumor heterogeneity and the biology of cancer invasion and metastasis, *Cancer Res.*, 38, 2651, 1978.

32. **Heppner, G. H.,** Tumor heterogeneity, *Cancer Res.*, 44, 2259, 1984.

33. **Nicolson, G. L. and Poste, G.,** Tumor cell diversity and host responses in cancer metastasis. I. Properties of metastatic cells, *Curr. Probl. Cancer*, 7(6), 1, 1982.

34. **Hart, I. R. and Fidler, I. J.,** The implications of tumor heterogeneity for studies of the biology and therapy of cancer metastasis, *Biochim. Biophys. Acta*, 651, 37, 1981.

35. **Key, M., Talmadge, J. E., and Fidler, I. J.,** Lack of correlation between the progressive growth of spontaneous metastases and their content of infiltrating macrophages, *J. Reticuloendothel. Soc.*, 32, 387, 1982.

36. **Talmadge, J. E., Key, M., and Fidler, I. J.,** Macrophage content of metastatic and non-metastatic rodent neoplasms, *J. Immunol.*, 126, 2245, 1981.

37. **Bugelski, P. J., Kirsh, R., and Poste, G.,** New histochemical method for measuring intratumoral macrophages and macrophage recruitment into experimental metastases, *Cancer Res.*, 43, 5493, 1983.

38. **Bugelski, P. J., Kirsh, R. L., Sowinski, J. M., and Poste, G.,** Changes in the macrophage content of lung metastases at different stages of tumor growth, *Am. J. Pathol.*, 118, 419, 1985.

39. **Bugelski, P. J., Corwin, S. P., North, S. M., Loveitt, S. C., Kirsh, R. L., Nicolson, G. L., and Poste, G.,** The macrophage content of spontaneous metastases at different stages of their growth, *Cancer Res.,* 47, 4141, 1987.

40. **Mantovani, A.,** In vitro effects on tumor cells of macrophages isolated from an early-passage chemically induced murine sarcoma and from its spontaneous metastases, *Int. J. Cancer,* 27, 221, 1981.

41. **Evans, R. and Alexander, P.,** Role of macrophages in tumor immunity. II. Involvement of a macrophage cytophilic factor during syngeneic tumour growth inhibition, *Immunology,* 23, 627, 1972.

42. **Steck, P. A. and Nicolson, G. L.,** Cell surface glycoproteins of 13762NF mammary adenocarcinoma clones of differing metastatic potentials, *Exp. Cell Res.,* 147, 265, 1983.

43. **North, S. M., Steck, P. A., and Nicolson, G. L.,** Monoclonal antibodies against cell surface antigens of the metastatic rat 13762NF mammary adenocarcinoma and their cross-reactivity with human breast carcinomas, *Cancer Res.,* 46, 6393, 1986.

44. **Schirrmacher, V., Fogel, M., Russman, E., Bosslet, K., Altervogt, P., and Beck, L.,** Antigenic variation in cancer metastasis: immune escape versus immune control, *Cancer Metastasis Rev.,* 1, 241, 1982.

45. **Raz, A., McLellan, W. L., Hart, I. R., Bucana, C. D., Hoyer, L. C., Sela, B.-A., Dragsten, P., and Fidler, I. J.,** Cell surface properties of B16 melanoma variants with differing metastatic potential, *Cancer Res.,* 40, 1645, 1980.

46. **Neri, A., Rouslahti, E., and Nicolson, G. L.,** The distribution of fibronectin on clonal cell lines of a rat mammary adenocarcinoma growing in vitro and in vivo at primary and metastatic sites, *Cancer Res.,* 41, 5082, 1982.

47. **Nicolson, G. L., Dulski, K., Basson, C., and Welch, D. R.,** Preferential organ attachment and invasion in vitro by B16 melanoma cells selected for differing metastatic colonization and invasive properties, *Invasion Metastasis,* 5, 144, 1985.

48. **Hujanen, E. S. and Terranova, V. P.,** Migration of tumor cells to organ-derived chemoattractants, *Cancer Res.,* 45, 3517, 1985.

49. **Neri, A., Welch, D. R., Kawaguchi, T., and Nicolson, G. L.,** The development and biologic properties of malignant cell sublines and clones of a spontaneously metastasizing rat mammary adenocarcinoma, *J. Natl. Cancer Inst.,* 68, 507, 1982.

50. **Nicolson, G. L.,** Cancer metastasis: organ colonization and the cell surface properties of malignant cells, *Biochim. Biophys. Acta,* 495, 113, 1982.

51. **Welch, D. R., Neri, A., and Nicolson, G. L.,** Comparison of "spontaneous" and "experimental" metastasis using rat 13762NF mammary adenocarcinoma cell clones, *Invasion Metastasis,* 3, 65, 1985.

52. **Schirrmacher, V. and Bosslet, K.,** Tumor metastasis and cell mediated immunity in a model system in DBA/2 mice. Immunoselection of tumor variants differing in tumor antigen expression and metastatic capacity, *Int. J. Cancer,* 25, 781, 1980.

53. **Schirrmacher, V., Shortz, G., Clauer, K., Komitowski, D., Zimmerman, H. P., and Lohmann-Malthes, M. L.,** Tumor metastasis and cell-mediated immunity in a model system in DBA/2 mice. I. Tumor invasiveness in vitro and metastasis formation in vivo, *Int. J. Cancer,* 23, 233, 1979.

54. **Hanna, N. and Fidler, I. J.,** Relationship between metastatic potential and resistance to natural killer cell-mediated cytotoxicity in three murine tumor systems, *J. Natl. Cancer Inst.,* 66, 1183, 1981.

55. **Talmadge, J. E., Meyers, K. M., Prieur, D. J., and Starkey, J. F.,** Role of natural killer cells in tumor growth and metastasis in C57BL/6 normal and beige mice, *J. Natl. Cancer Inst.,* 65, 929, 1980.

56. **DeBaetselier, P., Kapon A., Katzar, S., Tzehoval, E., Dekegel, D., Segal, S., and Feldman, M.,** Selecting, accelerating and suppressing interactions between macrophages and tumor cells, *Invasion Metastasis,* 5, 106, 1985.

57. **Fidler, I. J.,** Recognition and destruction of target cells by tumoricidal macrophages, *Isr. J. Med. Sci.,* 14, 177, 1978.

58. **Mantovani, A.,** In vitro effects on tumor cells of macrophages isolated from an early passage chemically induced murine sarcoma and from its spontaneous metastases, *Int. J. Cancer,* 27, 221, 1981.

59. **Yamamura, Y., Fischer, B. C., Harnaha, J. B., and Proctor, J. W.,** Heterogeneity of murine mammary adenocarcinoma cell subpopulations. In vitro and in vivo resistance to macrophage cytotoxicity and its association with metastatic capacity, *Int. J. Cancer,* 33, 67, 1984.

60. **Pal, K., Kopper, T., Timar, J., Rajnai, J., and Lapis, K.,** Comparative study on Lewis lung tumor lines with 'low' and 'high' metastatic capacity. I. Growth rate, morphology and resistance to host defence, *Invasion Metastasis,* 5, 159, 1985.

61. **Miner, K. M., Klostergaard, J., Granger, G. A., and Nicolson, G. L.,** Differences in cytotoxic effects of activated murine peritoneal macrophages and J774 monocytic cells on metastatic variants of B16 melanoma, *J. Natl. Cancer Inst.,* 70, 717, 1983.

62. **Klostergaard, J., Miner, K. M., Granger, G. A., and Nicolson, G. L.,** The cancer cell and its environment: macrophage-mediated killing of metastatic tumor cells, in *Cellular Oncology: New Approaches in Biology, Diagnosis, and Treatment,* Moloy, P. J. and Nicolson, G. L., Eds., Praeger Press, New York, 1983, 63.

63. **Miner, K. M., Kawaguchi, T., Uba, G. W., and Nicolson, G. L.**, Clonal drift of cell surface, melanogenic and experimental metastatic properties of in vivo selected brain meninges colonizing murine B16 melanoma, *Cancer Res.*, 42, 4631, 1982.

64. **Nicolson, G. L., Miner, K. M., and Reading, C. L.**, Tumor cell heterogeneity and blood-borne metastasis, in *Fundamental Mechanisms in Cancer Immunology*, Saunders, J. P., Daniels, J. S., Cerou, B., Rosenfeld, C., and Denny, C. B., Eds., Elsevier, Amsterdam, 1981, 31.

65. **Synderman, R., Pike M. C., Fisher, D. G., and Koren, H. S.**, Biologic and biochemical activities of continuous macrophage cell lines P388D1 and J774.1, *J. Immunol.*, 119, 2060, 1977.

66. **Adams, D. O. and Hamilton, T. A.**, The cell biology of macrophage activation, *Annu. Rev. Immunol.*, 2, 283, 1984.

67. **Marino, P. A. and Adams, D. O.**, Interaction of BCG-activated macrophages and neoplastic cells in vitro. I. Conditions of binding and its selectivity, *Cell. Immunol.*, 54, 11, 1980.

68. **Brunson, K. W. and Nicolson, G. L.**, Selection and biologic properties of malignant variants of a murine lymphosarcoma, *J. Natl. Cancer Inst.*, 61, 1499, 1978.

69. **Reading, C. L., Belloni, P. N., and Nicolson, G. L.**, Selection and in vivo properties and lectin-attachment of various malignant murine lymphosarcoma cell lines, *J. Natl. Cancer Inst.*, 64, 1241, 1980.

70. **Miner, K. M. and Nicolson, G. L.**, Differences in the sensitivities of murine metastatic lymphoma/lymphosarcoma variants to macrophage-mediated cytolysis and/or cytostasis, *Cancer Res.*, 43, 2063, 1983.

71. **Reading, C. L., Brunson, K. W., Torriani, M., and Nicolson, G. L.**, Malignancies of metastatic murine lymphosarcoma cell lines and clones correlate with decreased cell surface display of RNA tumor virus envelope glycoprotein gp70, *Proc. Natl. Acad. Sci. U.S.A.*, 77, 5943, 1980.

72. **Reading, C. L., Kraemer, P. M., Miner, K. M., and Nicolson, G. L.**, In vivo and in vitro properties of malignant variants of RAW117 metastatic murine lymphoma/lymphosarcoma, *Clin. Exp. Metastasis*, 1, 135, 1983.

73. **Yoshida, M., Gallick, G., Irimura, T., and Nicolson, G. L.**, Modification of cell surface glycoproteins, macrophage cytostasis and blood-borne metastatic properties of murine RAW117 large cell lymphoma by virus superinfection, *Cancer Res.*, 47, 2558, 1987.

74. **North, S. M. and Nicolson, G. L.**, Effect of host immune status on the spontaneous metastasis of cloned cell lines of the 13762 NF rat mammary adenocarcinoma, *Br. J. Cancer*, 52, 747, 1985.

75. **North, S. M. and Nicolson, G. L.**, Heterogeneity in the sensitivities of the 13762NF mammary adenocarcinoma cell clones to cytolysis mediated by extra- and intra-tumoral macrophages, *Cancer Res.*, 45, 1453, 1985.

76. **Brooks, C. G.**, Studies on the microcytotoxicity test. III. Comparison of (^{75}Se) selenomethionine with (^{3}H)proline, Na_2 $^{51}CrO_4$, and (^{125}I)iododeoxy-uridine for prelabelling target cells in long term cytotoxicity tests, *J. Immunol. Methods*, 22, 23, 1978.

77. **Pike, M. C. and Synderman, R.**, Depression of macrophage function by a factor produced by neoplasms: a mechanism for abrogation of immune surveillance, *J. Immunol.*, 117, 1243, 1976.

78. **Puccetti, P. and Holden, H. T.**, Cytolytic and cytostatic anti-tumor activities of macrophages from mice injected with murine sarcoma virus, *Int. J. Cancer*, 23, 123, 1979.

79. **Synderman, R., Pike, M. C., Blaylock B. L., and Weinstein, P.**, Effects of neoplasms on inflammation: depression of macrophage accumulation after tumor implantation, *J. Immunol.*, 116, 585, 1976.

80. **Urban, J. L., Burton, R. C., Holland, J. M., Kripke, M. L., and Schreiber, H.**, Mechanisms of syngeneic tumor rejection, *J. Exp. Med.*, 155, 557, 1982.

81. **Urban, J. L. and Schreiber, H.**, Selection of macrophage-resistant progressor tumor variants by the normal host, *J. Exp. Med.*, 157, 642, 1983.

82. **Taffet, S. M. and Russell, S. W.**, Macrophage-mediated tumor cell killing: regulation of expression of cytolytic activity by prostaglandin E, *J. Immunol.*, 126, 424, 1981.

83. **Friedman, S. A., Remold-O'Donnell, E., and Piessens, W. F.**, Enhanced PGE_2 production by MAF treated peritoneal exudate macrophages, *Cell. Immunol.*, 42, 213, 1979.

84. **Adams, D. O., Koa, K., Farb, R., and Pizzo, S.**, Effector mechanisms of cytolytically activated macrophages. II. Secretion of a cytolytic factor by activated macrophages and its relationship to secreted proteases, *J. Immunol.*, 124, 293, 1980.

85. **Reidarson, T. H., Levy, W. E., Klostergaard, J., and Granger, G. A.**, Inducible macrophage cytotoxins. I. Biokinetics of activation and release in vitro, *J. Natl. Cancer Inst.*, 69, 879, 1982.

86. **Moore, M. and Moore, K.**, Kinetics and macrophage infiltration of experimental rat neoplasia, in *The Macrophage and Cancer*, James, K., McBride, B., and Stuart, A., Eds., University of Edinburgh Press, Edinburgh, Scotland, 1977, 330.

87. **Hibbs, J. B.**, The macrophage as a tumoricidal effector cell: a review of in vivo and in vitro studies on the mechanisms of the activated macrophage non-specific cytotoxic reaction, in *The Macrophage and Neoplasia*, Fink, M. Ed., Academic Press, New York, 1976, 83.

88. **Johnson, W. J., Somers, S. D., and Adams, D. O.,** Activation of macrophages for tumor cytotoxicity, *Contemp. Top. Immunobiol.,* 14, 127, 1983.
89. **Reidarson, T. H., Granger, G. A., and Klostergaard, J.,** Inducible macrophage cytotoxins. II. Tumor lysis mechanism involving target cell-binding proteases, *J. Natl. Cancer Inst.,* 69, 889, 1982.
90. **Cabilly, S. and Gallily, R.,** Artifical binding of macrophages to syngeneic cells elicits cytostasis but not cytolysis, *Immunology,* 42, 149, 1981.
91. **Raz, A., Inbar, M., and Goldman, R.,** A differential interaction in vitro of mouse macrophages with normal lymphocytes and malignant lymphoma cells, *Eur. J. Cancer,* 13, 605, 1977.
92. **Schirrmacher, V. and Appelhaus, B.,** Interaction of high or low metastatic related tumor lines with normal or lymphokine-activated syngeneic peritoneal macrophages: in vitro analysis of tumor cell binding and cytostasis, *Clin. Exp. Metastasis,* 3, 29, 1985.
93. **Gemsa, D., Kramer, W., Napierski, I., Barlin, E., Tiu, G., and Resch, K.,** Potentiation of macrophage tumor cytostasis by tumor-induced ascites, *J. Immunol.,* 126, 2143, 1981.
94. **Remold-O'Donnell, E. and Lewandrowski, K.,** Decrease of the major surface glycoprotein GP160 in activated macrophages, *Cell. Immunol.,* 70, 85, 1982.
95. **Imber, M., Pizzo, S. V., Johnson, W. J., and Adams, D. O.,** Selective diminution of the binding of mannose by murine macrophages in the latter stages of activation, *J. Biol. Chem.,* 257, 5129, 1982.
96. **Springer, T. A. and Unkeless, J. C.,** Analysis of macrophage differentiation and function and monoclonal antibodies, *Contemp. Top. Immunobiol.,* 14, 1, 1984.
97. **Yin, H. L., Aley, S., and Cohn, S. A.,** Plasma membrane polypeptides of resident and activated mouse peritoneal macrophages, *Proc. Natl. Acad. Sci. U.S.A.,* 77, 2188, 1980.
98. **Mercurio, A. M., Schwarting, G. A., and Robbins, P. W.,** Glycolipids of the mouse peritoneal macrophage, *J. Exp. Med.,* 160, 1114, 1984.
99. **Maddox, D. E., Shibata, S., and Goldstein, I. J.,** Stimulated macrophages express a glycoprotein receptor reactive with *Griffonia simplicifolia* I-B$_4$ isolectin, *Proc. Natl. Acad. Sci. U.S.A.,* 79, 166, 1982.
100. **Wicha, M. S. and Huard, T. K.,** Macrophages express cell surface laminin, *Exp. Cell. Res.,* 143, 475, 1983.
101. **Irimura, T. and Nicolson, G. L.,** Carbohydrate chain analysis by lectin binding to mixtures of glycoproteins, separated by polyacrylamide slab-gel electrophoresis with in situ chemical modification, *Carbohydr. Res.,* 115, 209, 1983.
102. **Irimura, T. and Nicolson, G. L.,** Carbohydrate chain analysis by lectin binding to electrophoretically separated glycoproteins from murine B16 melanoma sublines of various metastatic properties, *Cancer Res.,* 44, 791, 1984.
103. **Irimura, T., North S. M., and Nicolson, G. L.,** Glycoprotein profiles of macrophages at different stages of activation as revealed by lectin binding after electrophoretic separation, *Eur. J. Immunol.,* 17, 73, 1987.
104. **Irimura, T. and Nicolson, G. L.,** The interaction of pokeweed mitogen with poly-N-acetyllactosamine type carbohydrate chains, *Carbohydr. Res.,* 120, 187, 1983.
105. **Yokoyama, K., Terao, T., and Osawa, T.,** Isolation and characterization of membrane receptors for pokeweed mitogen from mouse lymphocytes, *Biochem. J.,* 165, 431, 1977.
106. **Yokoyama, K., Mashimo, J., Kasai, N., Terao, T., and Osawa, T.,** Binding of bacterial lipopolysaccharide to histocompatibility-2-complex proteins of mouse lymphocytes, *Z. Physiol. Chem.,* 360, 587, 1978.

Chapter 9

THERAPEUTIC CIRCUMVENTION OF THE BIOLOGIC HETEROGENEITY IN MALIGNANT NEOPLASMS BY TUMORICIDAL MACROPHAGES

William E. Fogler and Isaiah J. Fidler

TABLE OF CONTENTS

I. INTRODUCTION

The emergence of metastases in organs distant from the primary malignant neoplasm is the most devastating aspect of cancer. There exist several reasons for the current frustration in treating these metastatic lesions. First, by the time many cancers are diagnosed, metastasis has already taken place, and therefore, despite significant advances in surgical technique and general patient care, most deaths from cancer are still due to the uncontrolled growth of metastases resistant to therapy. Second, metastases are typically located in different organs and may also be in different locations within the same organ. This limits the delivery of chemotherapeutic agents and effective radiation therapy to the lesions without damaging normal tissues. The biggest obstacle to the effective treatment of metastases is due, however, to the nonuniformity of the cells populating both primary and secondary neoplasms. By the time of diagnosis, and certainly in clinically advanced lesions, malignant neoplasms contain multiple cell populations exhibiting a wide range of biologic heterogeneity. Cells obtained from individual tumors exhibit differences with respect to cell surface properties, antigenicity, immunogenicity, growth rate, karyotype, sensitivity to various cytotoxic drugs, and the ability to invade and metastasize.[1-3]

Biological heterogeneity is not confined to cells in primary tumors since it is equally prominent among the cells populating metastases. Indeed, many clinical observations suggest that multiple metastases in different organs or even within the same organ of a cancer patient can exhibit diversity in many biological characteristics such as hormone receptors, antigenic determinants, and sensitivity to chemotherapeutic drugs.[1-3] The development of this heterogeneity is multifactorial. Data indicate that metastases can arise from the nonrandom spread of specialized malignant cells that pre-exist within a primary neoplasm,[4] that some metastases can be clonal in their origin,[5] that different metastases can originate from different progenitor cells,[5] and that, in general, metastatic cells can exhibit a higher rate of spontaneous mutation than nonmetastatic but tumorigenic cells.[6,7]

Collectively, such data suggest that successful therapy of disseminated cancer metastases will have to circumvent the problems of neoplastic heterogeneity, development of resistance to therapy by tumor cells, and nonspecific toxicity of therapeutic regimens. There is now an increasing body of data showing that macrophages activated to the tumoricidal state can fulfill these demanding criteria. In this chapter, we review some of this evidence as well as summarize work from our laboratory and many others that deal with methods to achieve the *in situ* activation of macrophages toward the destruction of established metastases.

II. IN VITRO STUDIES

The term ''macrophage activation'' is an operational one and is used by different investigators to denote different, and even unrelated, changes in the phenotype of the same or different macrophage(s). As defined in the context of this chapter, ''macrophage activation'' is the functional acquisition of tumoricidal properties which allows the macrophage to become directly cytotoxic towards neoplastic cells. Much of our knowledge regarding the mechanisms by which mononuclear phagocytes become activated and destroy target cells has been obtained from a variety of in vitro assays, including light microscopy,[8] inhibition of tumor growth (cytostasis),[9,10] cleared zones of tumor cell monolayers,[11,12] decrease in colony formation,[13] release of radioactive labels from target cells,[14,17] cinemicrographic analysis,[18] and sequential scanning and transmission electron microscopy.[19,20] These assays are substantially diverse in many experimental parameters which include population of mononuclear phagocyte, agent(s) used to induce macrophage activation, tumor target cells, and culture conditions. Moreover, even within the same assay subtle changes lead to apparent contradictory results.[21-25] These points are raised here so the reader is aware of the complexities involved in in vitro studies concerning the activation of tumoricidal properties in macrophages and their interaction with tumor cell populations.

A. Mechanisms for the Activation of Tumoricidal Properties in Mononuclear Phagocytes

Mononuclear phagocytes can be rendered tumor cytotoxic following their interaction with various natural and synthetic agents. These include: (1) chronic infection of the host with bacteria, protozoa, or nematodes;[26-28] (2) bacterial cell wall components (endotoxin, lipopolysaccharide (LPS), lipid A,[29-33] and muramyl dipeptide);[34-36] (3) dsRNA;[29] (4) lymphokines (specific macrophage-arming factor,[37-39] macrophage-activation factor,[30-33,40-43] and interferon-gamma, IFN-γ);[33-40,44] (5) aggregated IgG and immune complexes;[45] (6) C-reactive protein;[46] and (7) lysolecithin analogs.[47,48] The cellular and molecular processes by which a nontumoricidal macrophage can become activated to the tumoricidal state are now receiving wide attention.[49,50] Current concepts of this activation process suggest that a series of phenotypic alterations are acquired in a sequential fashion, culminating in the development of tumoricidal properties.[51,52] The rate of appearance or loss of a specific phenotypic alteration depends on the nature and duration of activating factors.

The activation of macrophages by lymphokines such as IFN-γ or macrophage-activating factor (MAF) requires that the agents bind to the macrophage surface.[53,54] Treatment of macrophages with reagents that alter their surface properties influences the extent to which they respond to lymphokines.[53,55,56] Augmentation of macrophage responses to lymphokines was observed subsequent to alteration of amino, sulfhydryl, hydroxyl, or carbonyl groups on the cell surface.[56] In contrast, treatment of macrophages with various proteases or with α-L-fucose decreased their response to MAF, suggesting that fucose-containing moieties could be the receptor for MAF.[53,55] Moreover, the incubation of macrophages with liposomes containing fucoglycolipids enhanced their responses to MAF, suggesting that cell surface fucoglycolipids may be the natural receptor for MAF.[53] More recently, direct evidence has been presented for the existence of cell surface IFN-γ receptors that bind this lymphokine and thus participate in the activation of macrophage tumoricidal properties.[54]

Whether the cellular alterations in lymphokine-treated macrophages result directly from the binding of MAF or IFN-γ to surface receptors or whether the receptor-bound material is internalized to act at an intracellular locus is not clear. In the latter case the surface receptor would merely bind sufficient lymphokine molecules to initiate biological activity. Experimentally, these questions can be studied by assessing the ability to activate macrophages under conditions in which MAF or IFN-γ is allowed to bind to its surface receptor but not be internalized or under conditions in which the agents are introduced directly into the cell without their initial binding to surface receptors. The latter possibility had been investigated by using synthetic phospholipid vesicles (liposomes) as carrier vehicles to deliver MAF or IFN-γ directly into the intracellular matrix of the macrophages.

In studies from our laboratory, lymphokines with MAF activity were obtained from cultures of mitogen-stimulated rat lymphocytes. These lymphokines were encapsulated within liposomes of different size and lipid composition.[55,57,58] The ability of free and liposome-encapsulated MAF to render normal murine or rat macrophages cytotoxic for tumor cells in vitro was compared. Our studies revealed that normal rodent macrophages were rendered tumoricidal after incubation with liposome-encapsulated MAF and that the level of cytotoxicity exceeded that induced by free MAF. Control cultures of macrophages incubated with liposomes alone or liposomes containing supernatants from normal unstimulated lymphocytes did not acquire tumor cytotoxic properties.

In comparing the extent of macrophage activation induced by free MAF and by liposome-encapsulated MAF, it is important to realize that the total amount of free MAF added to macrophages greatly exceeds the total amount of MAF encapsulated within liposomes. By using serial dilution experiments, we found that the total amount of liposome-encapsulated

MAF inducing activation in macrophages was at least 4 logs lower than the volume of free MAF that was used to induce similar activation.[55,57] The activation by liposome-encapsulated lymphokine was not due to liposome-mediated alterations in the macrophage surface that enhanced their responsiveness to MAF. We conclude this from control experiments in which macrophages incubated with liposomes containing saline and suspended in medium supplemented with MAF diluted 10,000-fold did not acquire tumoricidal properties. Further evidence that liposome-entrapped MAF activates macrophages via an intracellular mechanism came from activation experiments in which normal macrophages were incubated with either free MAF or liposome-encapsulated MAF in the presence of several compounds known to inhibit MAF binding to the macrophage surface.[55] Liposome-encapsulated MAF but not free MAF activated tumoricidal properties in macrophages concomitantly treated with γ-L-fucosidase, which removes surface receptors for MAF, or with fucose-binding plant lectins (*Ulex europaeus* I and *Lotus tetragonolobus*), which compete for binding to the MAF receptor on macrophages. Moreover, populations of nontumoricidal inflammatory tissue macrophages, which were inherently unresponsive to free MAF, could be rendered tumoricidal in vitro by incubation with liposome-encapsulated MAF.[55] Finally, liposome-encapsulated MAF activated tumoricidal properties of macrophages obtained from endotoxin-nonresponsive C3H/HeJ mice, whereas free MAF did not.[59] Collectively, our studies indicate that the activation of macrophages by MAF does not require binding of the lymphokine to the macrophage surface receptors. These initial investigations on the activation of tumoricidal properties in rodent liposome-encapsulated MAF have now been expanded to a human system with equivalent results; the activation of normal, noncytotoxic human blood monocytes by human MAF does not require binding of the lymphokine to putative monocyte surface receptors.[60]

Mononuclear phagocytes can also be rendered tumoricidal by a variety of microorganisms and their structural components. One such component of the bacterial cell wall, *N*-acetyl-muramyl-L-alanyl-D-isoglutamine (muramyl dipeptide, MDP) has been shown to be the minimal active unit with immune-potentiating activity that can replace *Mycobacterium* in complete Freund's adjuvant.[61,62] The mechanism by which MDP interacts with monocytes/macrophages has been investigated in both rodent[63-65] and human[66] systems with radiolabeled glycopeptides. The results are in apparent contradiction. Evidence has been presented demonstrating specific MDP-binding sites on the macrophage membrane.[65,65] In contrast, other studies indicate the absence of cell surface MDP receptors and suggest that the activation of tumoricidal properties in mononuclear phagocytes by muramyl peptides occurs as the result of an intracytoplasmic event following pinocytosis of the glycopeptide.[63,66] The absence of cell surface receptors for MDP on mononuclear phagocytes would not be surprising. In contrast to the activation of macrophages by lymphokines, naturally occurring MDP is liberated following the phagocytosis of bacteria and the breakdown of bacterial cell walls within the macrophage cytoplasm.[59,67] In nature, therefore, MDPs are presented to the macrophage through an intracellular pathway. In this regard, several laboratories have documented this ability of liposome-encapsulated MDP (and various analogs) to activate tumoricidal properties in both rodent[36,59,68-71] and human[72-75] macrophages following phagocytosis of the phospholipid vesicle.

The activation of tumor cytotoxic properties in macrophages by lymphokines or bacterial components need not occur independently of each other. A lymphokine such as IFN-γ[76-78] or MAF[79-81] can prime macrophages to respond to a second signal such as endotoxins[79,80,82] or MDP.[80,81] Recent studies from our laboratory have concentrated on the synergistic activation of tumoricidal properties in macrophages by recombinant IFN-γ and MDP.[83-85] We found that human blood monocytes and murine peritoneal exudate macrophages were activated by the combination of subthreshold amounts of MDP and recombinant IFN-γ to become tumoricidal against their human or murine tumorigenic target cells. The activation of human monocytes or murine macrophages by free IFN-γ and MDP was species specific; human IFN-γ did not activate murine macrophages; murine IFN-γ did not activate cytotoxic properties in human monocytes. In both species, the activation of tumoricidal properties in macrophages by IFN-γ occurred as a consequence of intracellular interaction. We based this conclusion on data showing that, whereas free IFN-γ and MDP did not activate macrophages pretreated with pronase, liposome-encapsulated IFN-γ and MDP did.[85] Moreover, the encapsulation of either murine or human IFN-γ with MDP within the same liposome preparation produced synergistic activation of cytotoxic properties in both mouse macrophages and human monocytes without apparent species specificity.[85] These data suggest that, at least functionally, IFN-γ could consist of two separate moieties. One part may be responsible for binding to the macrophage surface to facilitate the internalization of part of or the whole molecule. This moiety of the IFN-γ molecule may be responsible for the intracellular activation of macrophages to the tumoricidal state, which is not species specific. However, this concept is not supported by another investigator.[86] In this report the macrophage-activating ability of both free and liposome-encapsulated IFN-γ could be neutralized completely by a specific antibody to IFN-γ. The authors conclude that IFN-γ must ultimately leak out of the liposome in order to mediate its biological effects and that these effects are triggered after the IFN-γ binds to its cell surface receptor.[86]

B. Cellular Interactions Involved in the Destruction of Tumor Cells by Activated Mononuclear Phagocytes

Although tumor cell populations are heterogeneous with regard to many phenotypes, their apparent sensitivity to destruction by appropriately activated (tumor cytotoxic) macrophages appears to be a common neoplastic characteristic. Once activated, at least in vitro, macrophages acquire the discriminative ability to recognize and destroy neoplastic cells while leaving nonneoplastic cells unharmed.[87-92] The basis of this specific cytocidal response of the activated macrophage is poorly understood. Early reports with peritoneal macrophages from mice chronically infected with *Toxoplasma* or Bacillus Calmette-Guerin (BCG) and syngeneic or allogeneic tumor target cells characterized the effector phase of the cytotoxic process as being immunologically nonspecific requiring direct cell-to-cell contact.[27] Normal macrophages (obtained from the peritoneum of uninfected mice) were not cytotoxic. Subsequent to these reports cinemicrographic analysis demonstrated that BCG-activated murine macrophages interact extensively with the surface of neoplastic, but not nonneoplastic, target cell lines.[18] Evidence that these areas of intercellular contact represented an actual physical binding between neoplastic target cells and activated macrophages was obtained independently in a murine[93,94] and guinea pig[95] system. The binding, which has the same selectivity as cytolysis in regard to both types of macrophage (control or activated) and type of target (tumor or normal), was subsequently shown to be an initial and necessary event in macrophage-mediated cytolysis.[96] These observations are not restricted to rodent systems. Recently, the interaction of control and tumoricidal human blood monocytes (activated in vitro with liposome-entrapped MDP) with allogeneic melanoma cells and normal skin fibroblasts was studied by means of light microscopy and scanning and transmission electron microscopy.[20,97] Activated monocytes clustered around the melanoma cells, but not the fibroblasts, at a higher density than did control monocytes. This initial clustering of activated monocytes around the melanoma cells was followed by the establishment of numerous focal points of binding. It was concluded that the lysis of the susceptible tumor cells by human blood monocytes occurs as the final step in a process that begins with direct cell-to-cell contact.

In conjunction with tumor cell specificity in macrophage-mediated cytolysis, the requirement for cell-to-cell contact implies a common neoplastic "recognition structure" responsible for their interaction with and subsequent destruction by activated mononuclear phagocytes. These sites are present on the tumor cell surface and are shared by tumors of disparate origins.[98] However, the biochemical identities of the "recognition structures" have not been identified. The role of tumor cell surface carbohydrates in the binding and lysis of these cells by activated macrophages is under investigation.[99] In this regard the monosaccharides, *N*-acetyl-D-galactosamine,[100,101] D-galactose,[101] L-fucose,[101,102] and D-mannose,[100] as well as removal of sialic acid residues[103] have been reported to inhibit target cell recognition and destruction by macrophages. The spatial arrangement of simple membrane phospholipids has also been proposed as an important determinant in the binding and lysis of tumor cells by activated mononuclear phagocytes.[97] Target cell characteristics important in macrophage-mediated cytotoxicity have also been investigated. The susceptibility of targets to destruction by tumoricidal rat and mouse macrophages was studied with virus-transformed cell lines in which various elements of the transformed phenotype are only expressed at specific temperatures.[104] These studies demonstrated that the tumor cells were lysed by macrophages regardless of whether they expressed cell surface fibronectin protein or Forssman antigen, displayed surface changes which permit agglutination by low doses of plant lectins, expressed SV40 T antigen, had a low saturation density, or exhibited density-dependent inhibition of DNA synthesis. The susceptibility of tumor cells to destruction by tumoricidal macrophages appears to be independent of the in vitro biological behavior of the tumor cell. Melanoma-variant cell lines that have a low or high metastatic potential,[89] that have invasive or non-invasive characteristics,[89] that are either susceptible or resistant to lysis mediated by syngeneic T cells or natural killer (NK) cells,[89] and that differ in differentiation markers[105] (pigmentation and tryosinase activity) are all lysed in vitro by activated macrophages. Similarly, several cloned cell lines that were isolated from a murine fibrosarcoma induced by ultraviolet (UV) radiation and that vary in their degree of immunogenicity,[106] sensitivity to the anthracycline antibiotic Adriamycin,[107] or invasive and metastatic potential in vivo[106,108] are all susceptible to destruction in vitro by lymphokine-activated macrophages. Not all investigators agree that macrophage-mediated destruction of tumor cells is independent of the metastatic potential of the cancer cell.[109-112] These reports suggest an inverse relationship between the ability of a tumor cell to form metastases and its susceptibility to destruction by activated macrophages. Accordingly, it is only possible to conclude that the cytocidal activity of the activated mononuclear phagocyte is specific for the neoplastic phenotype.

The events responsible for target cell death occurring subsequent to activated macrophage-tumor cell interaction are under investigation. One proposed mechanism of target injury suggests that activated macrophages induce neoplastic cells to undergo a reductive cell division in the absence of DNA synthesis which leads to lysis.[113] Another mechanism of macrophage-mediated tumor cell cytotoxicity may involve inhibition of mitochondrial oxidative phosphorylation.[114] Morphologic studies of the interaction of BCG-activated murine macrophages with susceptible target cells suggest that following macrophage-tumor cell contact, the direct transfer of lysosomes is responsible for target lysis.[115] Evidence to support this concept was provided by ultrastructural studies.[19] Both reports emphasized that macrophage binding to tumor cells followed by destabilization of the target cell membrane constitute integral steps of the cytolytic process. In direct contradiction, examination of murine peritoneal macrophages treated with perfluorochemicals failed to demonstrate transfer of lysosomes from the activated macrophage into the target cell or alterations in the structure of adjacent macrophage-tumor membranes.[116] The release of soluble macrophage secretory products at contact sites with tumor cells has been proposed as another mechanism of target cell lysis.[96]

Persistent binding between activated macrophages and tumor cells may not be a prerequisite for mediation of cytolysis.[117] Macrophages are indirectly able to destroy tumor cells via secretory molecules toxic for neoplastic cells.[118] These include tumor necrosis factor,[119] third component of complement (C3a),[120] hydrogen peroxide,[121,122] arginase,[123] tumor growth inhibitory products such as excess thymidine,[124] and uncharacterized cytotoxins.[125-132] It is

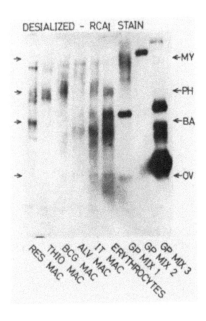

DESIALIZED - RCA₁ STAIN

←MY
←PH
←BA
←OV

RES MAC, THIO MAC, BCG MAC, ALV MAC, IT MAC, ERYTHROCYTES, GP MIX 1, GP MIX 2, GP MIX 3

PLATE 1.   RCA₁ reactive glycoproteins of rat macrophages. Macrophage glycoproteins were electrophoretically transferred to nitrocellulose membranes prior to reacting with ^{125}I-labeled RCA₁. The transblot membrane was first treated with 50 mM sulfuric acid at 80°C for 1 hr to remove sialic acid from the glycoproteins, and washed with 25 mM Tris-HCl buffer pH 7.2 containing 0.14 M NaCl and 0.05% Tween-20, then reacted with ^{125}I-labeled RCA₁ (10^7 M diluted in the same buffer) for 2 hr at room temperature. The macrophage populations were lane 1, resident macrophages incubated in vitro for 18 hr in the absence of LPS; lane 2, thioglycolate-elicited macrophages incubated in vitro for 18 hr in the absence of LPS; lane 3, BCG-activated macrophages incubated for 18 hr in the absence of LPS.; lane 4, alveolar macrophages incubated in vitro in the absence of LPS for 18 hr; lane 5, intratumoral macrophages incubated in vitro for 18 hr in the absence of LPS; lane 6, lysate of rat erythrocyte membranes prepared by hypotonic lysis at 4°C; lane 7, glycoprotein mixture of 1 μg each of porcine thyroglobulin (apparent M_r ~45,000); lane 8, glycoprotein mixture of 1 μg each of bovine serum fibronectin (apparent M_r ~220,000), human serum transferrin (apparent M_r ~75,000), concanavalin-A-unbound hen ovalbumin (apparent M_r ~230,000), and weakly concanavalin-A-bound hen ovalbumin (apparent M_r ~45,000); lane 9, a glycoprotein mixture 1 μg each human lactoferrin (apparent M_r ~80,000), bovine fetuin (apparent M_r ~65,000), human α-acid glycoprotein (apparent M_r ~48,000), and strongly concanavalin A-bound hen ovalbumin (apparent M_r ~45,000). The cellular glycoproteins were separated by NaDodSO₄ polyacrylamide gel electrophoresis, and transferred to a nitrocellulose membrane, where they were labeled with ^{125}I-Pa-4. Molecular weight markers: MY (myosin, M_r ~200,000), PH (phosphorylase b, M_r ~92,000), BA (bovine serum albumin, M_r ~66,000), and OV (hen ovalbumin, M_r ~45,000). (From Irimura, T., North, S. M., and Nicolson, G. L., *Eur. J. Immunol.*, 17, 73, 1987. With permission.)

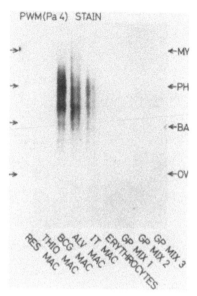

PLATE 2. PWM-reactive glycoproteins of rat macrophages. The caption is the same as Plate 1, except that the transblot was reacted with ^{125}I-Pa-4. (From Irimura, T., North, S. M., and Nicolson, G. L., *Eur. J. Immunol.*, 17, 73, 1987. With permission.)

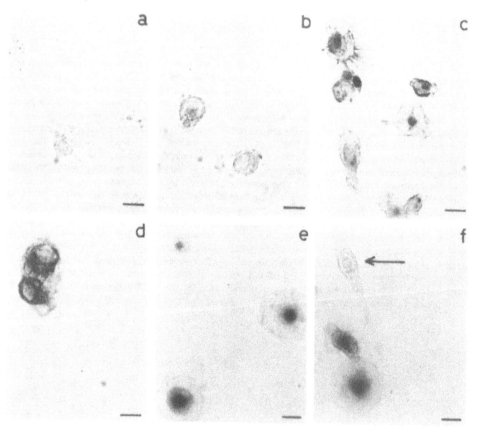

PLATE 3. Histochemical localization of biotinyl-Pa-4 visualized by avidin-peroxidase complex and diaminobenzidine. (a) Resident macrophages; (b) thioglycolate-elicited macrophages; (c) BCG-activated macrophages; (d) alveolar macrophages; (e) and (f) intratumoral macrophages. In (f), a mammary adenocarcinoma cell is seen (arrow) at the top of the plate. Bars indicate 10 μm. (From Irimura, T., North, S. M., and Nicolson, G. L., *Eur. J. Immunol.*, 17, 73, 1987. With permission.)

apparent that the results of an in vitro assay that measures macrophage-mediated cytotoxicity could differ vastly according to the conditions of the experiment. The lack of standardization of many experimental conditions could indeed be responsible for many conflicting reports regarding activation of tumoricidal properties in macrophages and their interaction with tumor cell populations. However, regardless of whether macrophages lyse tumors by direct binding or by release of secretory products, most investigators agree that, at least in vitro, activated macrophages discriminate tumorigenic from nontumorigenic cells. These in vitro studies suggest that macrophage-mediated destruction of malignant tumor cells could provide a new strategy for the therapy of metastatic disease.

III. IN VIVO STUDIES

The macrophage participates in a number of homeostatic mechanisms that include the clearance and catabolism of red blood cells and debris,[133] the controlled recycling of iron stores,[134] and the metabolism of lipids.[135] When host homeostatic mechanisms are stressed, the mononuclear phagocyte system can participate in complex interactions that involve cellular and humoral aspects of the inflammatory and immunologic responses.[136-139] In this regard, the macrophage is an important component of the host defense system against viral, bacterial, fungal and parasitic infections.[136-137] Mononuclear phagocytes also affect the pathogenesis and development of neoplasms.[140-142]

A. Involvement of the Mononuclear Phagocyte System in the Initiation and Progression of Malignant Neoplasms

Macrophages may play a prominent role in the detection and destruction of neoplastic cells by the host immune surveillance system.[11] An early investigation using tumor systems in rabbits produced evidence that the incidence of uterine cancer, dependent on age and strain, was parallel to the natural resistance to infection by tuberculosis (the most resistant strain having the lowest incidence of cancer).[143] In addition, the resistance of the rabbits to tuberculosis was directly related to the bactericidal capacity of their mononuclear phagocytic system.[143] These studies suggested a correlation between the activity of the phagocytes and the observed resistance to neoplasia. Subsequent studies supported this concept. Mice infected with the intracellular protozoa, *Toxoplasma gondii*, were more resistant to viral induction of neoplasms and to tumors resulting from the transplantation of syngeneic tumor cells.[144] The macrophages harvested from the protozoa-infected mice were cytotoxic in vitro to the transplanted tumor cells.[144] The importance of macrophages in carcinogenesis was revealed by studies designed to determine whether treatment of mice with either a macrophage stimulant (pyran copolymer) or macrophage toxins (trypan blue or silica) would influence the latency or incidence of skin carcinogenesis induced by UV radiation.[145] Treatment of mice with pyran copolymer lengthened the latent period of tumor development and reduced the incidence and number of the skin tumors that resulted from suboptimal exposures to UV radiation.[145] Conversely, treatment of mice with macrophage toxins shortened the latent period for induction of skin cancer by UV radiation.[145] Similarly, in transplantable tumor systems, the impairment of macrophage function by agents such as carrageenan or silica was found to be associated with an increase in the incidence of spontaneous[146,147] and experimental[148] metastases. There are also several reports regarding the efficacy of macrophages in the inhibition of metastasis. In an adoptive transfer study, intravenous (i.v.) injections of syngeneic murine macrophages that had been rendered tumoricidal by in vivo or in vitro manipulation reduced the incidence of experimental metastases of the B16 melanoma.[149] Injection of control, nonactivated macrophages either had no effect on metastases[149] or has been reported to augment metastatic formation.[150] Activated macrophages have been shown to eradicate metastases in two other murine tumor systems,[151,152] and to inhibit the growth of tumors at primary sites.[153]

Progressively growing tumors can induce several alterations in macrophage function, such as enhanced carbon clearance in vivo,[154,155] increased expression of monocyte Fc receptors,[156,157] suppressed migration of macrophages into the peritoneal cavity or the site of subcutaneously growing tumors, and suppressed chemotactic response of macrophages in these sites.[158-163] It has been suggested that the elaboration by neoplasms of factors suppressing macrophage function, represents a means of tumor resistance.[157] In this context, studies investigating whether the presence of progressively growing metastases in lung parenchyma of rats influenced the number and function of lung macrophages have been reported.[164] The presence of pulmonary metastases (produced by a syngeneic mammary adenocarcinoma) did not result in a decrease in the number of lung macrophages and the macrophages harvested from rats with metastases were functionally intact.[164] Furthermore, the macrophages harvested from rats with metastases could be rendered cytotoxic to syngeneic tumor cells in response to activation stimuli administered in vitro or in vivo.[164] Such findings suggest that the presence of a large number of tumor cells in organ parenchyma need not interfere with the function of macrophages in that organ. However, tumor cell variants that exhibit increased resistance to activated macrophages have been described.[165,166] Recently, we attempted to select in vitro, tumor cells that were resistant to lysis by activated macrophages,[167] by employing a technique previously used with success to select tumor cells resistant to T lymphocytes[168] or NK cells.[169] Seven different heterogeneous murine neoplasms and one cloned line of a fibrosarcoma were cultured in vitro with syngeneic tumoricidal macrophages. Surviving tumor cells were recovered and expanded to be subsequently exposed once more to tumor cytotoxic macrophages. After six such sequential interactions, all cell lines were examined for their susceptibility to lysis mediated by activated macrophages. In all eight systems, no significant differences were detected between the parent tumor cells and cells that survived the six sequential interactions.[167] Neither macrophage infiltration into tumors growing subcutaneously, nor the experimental or spontaneous metastatic potentials of the parental tumor lines differed from the lines established by the cells surviving six cycles of macrophage-mediated lysis.[167] Collectively, these data suggest that tumor cell destruction by activated macrophages is nonselective and does not lead to the development of resistant tumor cells or to cells with altered metastatic properties.

Several factors influence the extent of macrophage infiltration into tumors. Preliminary studies found that the macrophage content of six carcinogen-induced rat fibrosarcomas correlated directly with their immunogenicity and inversely with their metastic potential, suggesting that some tumors are nonmetastatic because they contain many macrophages.[170,171] However, such observations could not be extended to other tumor systems. Examination of the macrophage content of 16 different rodent tumors did not find a correlation between the extent of macrophage infiltration into neoplasms and the immunogenic or metastic behavior of the tumors.[172] This observation is in agreement with studies by others, who examined the macrophage content and the immunogenicity of the tumors.[173,174] It is also in agreement with reports demonstrating no correlation between the extent of macrophage infiltration into neoplasms and the metastic potential of the tumor.[175] The factors influencing macrophage infiltration into tumors are poorly understood, but both immune and nonimmune factors are clearly involved. In fact, many tumors appear to be nonimmunogenic under conditions of progressive growth, and in these tumors, macrophage infiltration may depend more on nonimmunologic factors such as inflammation and necrosis.[176]

Although the presence of macrophages at the periphery of and within neoplasms is well recognized, their functional activity is unclear. Differences in the cytotoxic activity of tumor-associated macrophages (TAM) isolated from nonmetastasizing and metastasizing tumors have been reported.[177] Mononuclear phagocytes isolated from a nonmetastatic sarcoma demonstrated cytotoxicity in vitro.[177] In contrast, TAM of a weakly immunogenic, metastasizing tumor were not demonstrably cytotoxic. Similar data have been reported for progressing and regressing murine sarcomas.[178] These data are not of a universal nature. Other investigators have observed the converse to be true; i.e., TAM of metastasizing murine mammary tumors and to a lesser extent nonmetastasizing tumors are indeed cytotoxic.[179] However, differences between metastatic and nonmetastatic tumors were seen in the density and size of macrophages, macrophage ectoenzyme concentrations, and macrophage-associated prostaglandin E levels.[180] In a recent report the percentage and antitumor activity of TAM were examined in 77 patients with resectable primary lung cancer.[181] The percentage of recovered TAM increased from Stage I to Stage II and decreased in Stage III (International Union Against Cancer, Geneva, Switzerland, 1978). It also increased in N_1 (node involvement), as compared with N_0 and N_2 but was unrelated to tumor size. However, the cytostatic activity of TAM declined with advance in stage of the disease and an increase of tumor size, but it was relatively unaffected by the presence of metastasis to regional lymph nodes. There was no correlation between the percentage of recovered TAM and the recurrence rate; however, cytostatic activity of TAM was correlated significantly with the prognosis of totally resected cases. The percentage of recovered TAM and cytostatic activity of TAM tended to be lower in palliatively resected cases.[181]

Whether tumors regress or progress can be determined by the degree to which tumoricidal activity of macrophages is generated *in situ*, rather than by the number of macrophages within the tumor.[178] This finding could explain why progressively growing spontaneous metastases often contain as many or more macrophages than the parent tumor.[175] Two recent independent studies reported that the macrophage content of pooled metastases were similar to that of primary tumors[189] and that the metastases did not consist of cells resistant to macrophage-mediated lysis.[183] Clearly, the role of the mononuclear phagocyte system in metastasis varies among different tumors and need not correlate with tumor cell immunogenicity or metastatic properties. In some tumors, numerous infiltrating macrophages can inhibit metastasis, but the absence of macrophage infiltration of a benign neoplasm will not lead to metastasis. Thus, neoplasms with low macrophage content may or may not be metastatic, as demonstrated in studies in which nonmetastatic clones isolated from a highly metastatic neoplasm also exhibited low macrophage content when growing subcutaneously.[175]

B. *In Situ* Activation of the Mononuclear Phagocyte System for Treatment of Disseminated Metastases

The i.v. injection of syngeneic macrophages that were nonspecifically activated in vitro into mice with metastatic lesions has been shown to inhibit tumor growth both at the primary site[153] and in metastatic growths.[149,151,152] These findings suggest that the i.v. administration of tumor cytotoxic macrophages might augment host resistance to disseminated cancer. The clinical feasibility of this approach, however, suffers from two shortcomings; it requires a large number of autologous or histocompatible macrophages for transfusion, and most intravenously injected macrophages arrest in the pulmonary microvasculature and do not reach other visceral organs. A more promising approach, therefore, has been the development of a method to activate host mononuclear phagocytes *in situ*.

One of the major pathways for the activation of macrophages in vitro involves their direct interaction with microorganisms and their structural components. Because such materials are often associated with undesirable side effects, such as delayed type hypersensitivity and granuloma formation,[184] it is preferable to use synthetic compounds that are less toxic yet capable of inducing the in vivo activation of macrophages. One such synthetic agent, MDP (and various analogs), profoundly influences many macrophage functions including cytotoxic activity in vitro.[185,186] Following parenteral administration, however, this compound is rapidly cleared (1 to 2 hr) from the body by the kidneys.[187,188] This short half-life limits the therapeutic potential of MDP.

A second major pathway for macrophage activation in vivo results from the action of lymphokines (MAF and IFN-γ) released from sensitized lymphocytes. Therapeutic use of soluble MAF or soluble IFN-γ has been hindered in the past by the lack of purified preparations of these mediators. Efforts to activate the tumoricidal properties of macrophages in vivo by systemic injection of crude lymphokine preparations have proved unsuccessful. Injection of soluble lymphokines into skin[189] or skin tumors[190,191] provoked local inflammatory reactions and histologic changes suggestive of macrophage activation that resulted in the regression of small cutaneous tumors. Systemic activation of macrophages by free lymphokines, however, has not been achieved. There are several reasons for this failure: (1) lymphokines injected into venous circulation have a short half-life,[192] probably because they bind with plasma proteins;[193] (2) only a small fraction of the mononuclear phagocyte system may be capable of responding to MAF; (3) macrophages can be activated by lymphokines only within a relatively short period following their emigration into tissues from the circulation;[193] (4) the tumoricidal properties of macrophages are short-lived (2 to 3 days), and macrophages are refractory to reactivation by soluble lymphokines.[193]

Studies from our laboratory[36,55,57-60,68-70,83-85] and subsequently by others[46,71-73] have shown that the phagocytic uptake by macrophages of liposomes containing macrophage-activating agents produces highly efficient activation of rodent and human macrophages in vitro. These findings raised the possibility that agents encapsulated within liposomes could be similarly efficient in activating macrophages in vivo. An attractive feature of liposomes as carriers for delivering agents to macrophages *in situ* is that most of the liposomes injected intravenously are taken up by phagocytic cells of the reticuloendothelial system. This passive targeting of liposomes offers a means of enhancing uptake of agents that stimulate mononuclear phagocyte activity.[194,195] Moreover, liposomes prepared from natural phospholipids are nonimmunogenic, and thus, they offer a way to avoid eliciting the allergic reactions commonly associated with the systemic administration of immune adjuvants.[196]

To test this possibility, mice with spontaneous pulmonary and lymph node metastases were injected intravenously with MAF encapsulated within multilamellar liposomes composed of phosphatidylcholine and phosphatidylserine. This type of liposome was chosen for several reasons. First, studies of body distribution of liposomes of different size and phospholipid composition demonstrated that these negatively charged liposomes localize and are retained in the lungs (in addition to organs rich with reticuloendothelial cell activity).[197] Second, toxicity studies in which these liposomes containing MAF were injected intravenously into mice or beagle dogs revealed no adverse reactions in recipient animals even after repeated injections.[198] Finally, another study has shown that i.v. injection of these liposomes activates murine or rat lung macrophages to become tumoricidal.[199]

In the initial studies, multiple i.v. injections of liposome-encapsulated MAF, but not soluble MAF or control liposome preparations, led to the eradication of spontaneous visceral metastases in C57BL/6 mice subsequent to surgical excision of syngeneic melanoma growing subcutaneously.[200] To initiate local tumors, each mouse was given an intrafootpad injection of viable B16-BL6 melanoma cells. When the primary tumor reached a size of 1.0 to 1.2 cm in diameter (4 weeks of growth), the tumor-bearing leg, including the draining popliteal lymph node, was amputated. Treatment of mice began 3 days after leg amputation and consisted of an i.v. injection of 2.5 μmol liposome (phosphatidylcholine and phosphatidylserine admixed at a 7:3 ratio) containing 6.25 μℓ of MAF. Mice were treated twice weekly for 4 weeks (total of 8 i.v. injections). The B16-BL6 tumor routinely metastasizes to the lungs and lymph nodes in about 90% of untreated mice, and at the start of therapy, the metastatic tumor burden in the lungs and lymph nodes may have exceeded a total body burden of 10^7 cells. Nonetheless, 70% of mice treated with liposome-encapsulated MAF survived at least 200 days. The median life span of mice implanted with 10 viable B16 cells admixed with 10^6 dead cells is 40 to 50 days.[201] For this reason, it is most likely that the tumor burden was reduced to fewer than ten viable cells in the successfully treated mice. Thus, multiple i.v. injections of liposome-encapsulated MAF brought about the complete regression of established pulmonary and lymph node metastases.

In the above studies, the use of crude lymphokine preparations with multiple immune-potentiating activities including MAF complicated delineation of the mechanism involved during the successful treatment of metastases. To investigate this issue, and to further examine the therapeutic implications of liposomes containing macrophage-activating agents in cancer metastases, we used synthetic MDP.[68] The principal target cell for immune modulation by MDP is believed to be the macrophage.[185,186] Recent studies from our laboratory have shown that MDP encapsulated within liposomes can render macrophages tumoricidal in vitro much more efficiently than free, unencapsulated MDP.[36,69] In contrast to free MDP, liposome-encapsulated MDP requires less time (2 hr) to activate macrophages, and maximum cytolytic capacity is achieved after an 8-hr incubation.[36] Furthermore, the total amount of liposome-encapsulated MDP that is delivered to macrophages is at least 4000 times lower than the total amount of free MDP necessary to render macrophages tumoricidal.[36,69] Finally, after the initial activation period, liposome-encapsulated MDP can prolong the duration of tumoricidal properties in macrophages.[69]

We have recently studied the organ distribution and retention of free and liposome-encapsulated MDP ([3H]-labeled) following i.v. administration into mice.[202] In agreement with previous studies,[187,188] we found that by 2 hr after its administration, more than 90% of free MDP was cleared from the body and excreted in the urine. However, the excretion rate of liposome-encapsulated MDP was 3 to 6%/hr and the percentage of the total dose of liposome-encapsulated MDP that localized in the liver, spleen, and lung was increased 10- to 30-fold over that of free MDP. Moreover, liposome encapsulation delayed the onset of MDP metabolite production.[202] In this regard, the injection of MDP in saline did not render alveolar macrophages of mice tumoricidal, whereas injection of MDP encapsulated in liposomes did activate the alveolar macrophages to become tumoricidal against B16-BL6 melanoma cells, and the systemic activation of macrophages by liposome-encapsulated MDP can be maintained by repeated injections.[68,69,203] Finally, in the melanoma therapy model the i.v. injection of liposome-encapsulated MDP, but not free MDP, destroyed established pulmonary and lymph node metastases.[68]

The mechanisms responsible for the regression of established metastases after the systemic administration of liposome containing MDP or MAF probably involved the activation of macrophages to become tumoricidal. Several lines of evidence tend to support this conclusion. First, lung macrophages are not activated by macrophage-activating agents encapsulated within liposomes that are not retained in the lung.[204] Second, the pretreatment of tumor-bearing animals with agents that are toxic for macrophages (silica, carrageenan, hyperchlorinated drinking water) before systemic therapy with liposome-encapsulated MDP or MAF abrogates the response to liposome therapy, and such animals rapidly die of metastatic disease.[204] Third, the possible involvement of T lymphocytes as effector cells is excluded by the finding that systemic activation of macrophages by liposome-encapsulated MDP can be accomplished in athymic nude mice and in adult thymectomized or X-irradiated mice.[205] Fourth, i.v. injection of macrophages activated in vitro by incubation with liposome-encapsulated MDP produces a reduction in metastatic burden comparable to that achieved by systemic administration of liposome-encapsulated activators.[204] Finally, direct evidence that the regression of established metastases after treatment of tumor-bearing mice with liposome-encapsulated activators was associated with tumoricidal macrophages comes from morphological and functional analysis of macrophages isolated from pulmonary metastases.[206] Immunofluorescence and electron microscopic analyses revealed that 24 hr after the tumor-bearing mice were given i.v. injections of liposomes, 15% of the alveolar macrophages and 5% of the metastasis-associated macrophages contained phagocytosed liposomes. However, only macrophages isolated from lungs or metastases of mice given injections of liposomes containing activators (treatment success), but not macrophages from mice treated with empty liposomes (treatment failure), were tumoricidal against the target cells in vitro.[206]

Since the original demonstration that the activation of tumoricidal properties in mononuclear phagocytes by liposome-encapsulated lymphokines or MDP is associated with eradication of cancer metastasis, several laboratories began to investigate novel compounds in similar and different tumor models. Such compounds include other lymphokine preparations or C-reactive protein encapsulated in liposomes for treatment of pulmonary or liver metastases arising from the T241 murine fibrosarcoma and MCA-38 colon carcinoma, respectively,[207-209] and liposome-entrapped lipophilic derivatives of MDP for macrophage activation and therapy of B16 lung metastases.[17,210,211]

Our studies have clearly shown that MDP encapsulated within liposomes renders macrophages tumoricidal much more effectively than does unencapsulated MDP.[36,68,69,203,205] Moreover, once macrophages have phagocytosed liposomes containing MDP, they remain cytotoxic for 2 to 3 days.[68,69,203] Recent studies have suggested that lipophilic derivatives of MDP, in which acyl chains are attached to the molecule, enhance the effectiveness of MDP for priming peritoneal macrophages to release superoxide anion.[212] Because low molecular solutes such as hydrophilic MDP can leak out of liposomes, we examined the possibility of whether a lipophilic derivative of MDP, N-acetylmuramyl-L-alanyl-D-isoglutamyl-L-alanyl-2(1′,2′-dipalmitoyl-sn-glycero-3′ phosphoryl)-ethylamide (MTP-PE) inserted in the phospholipid bilayers of liposomes could be retained more efficiently within macrophages, thereby promoting longer periods of tumoricidal activity.[70] The superiority of liposomes containing the lipophilic MTP-PE over liposomes containing water-soluble MDP for in vitro or in vivo activation of macrophages was demonstrated in several ways. First, the i.v. injection of liposomes containing a dose of MTP-PE equal to MDP led to higher levels of alveolar macrophage-mediated cytotoxicity. Second, alveolar macrophages harvested from mice given i.v. injections of liposomes containing MTP-PE maintained their tumoricidal activity for a longer period (5 days) than macrophages harvested from mice inoculated with liposome-encapsulated MDP (3 days). Similar results were obtained from experiments dealing with macrophage activation in vitro.

It has been suggested that once macrophages phagocytose liposomes containing MDP, the liposomes function as a slow-release depot from which encapsulated material is released over a sustained period of time.[36,69] The extent of release and the possible equilibration of MDP with the extracellular medium are determined by the integrity of liposome membranes. However, MTP-PE, which is only slightly soluble in water, would remain active for longer periods, until it is degraded. Since liposomes can be seen inside macrophages for several days after phagocytosis,[213] the degradation of MTP-PE incorporated into the liposome phospholipid bilayer is apparently relatively slow and inefficient.

The increased efficacy of lipophilic MTP-PE over MDP for the in vivo activation of macrophages was also observed for therapy of spontaneous pulmonary and lymph node metastases.[210] In these experiments, the survival of tumor-bearing mice that received liposome-entrapped MTP-PE was significantly increased and obtained with fewer treatments compared with those animals given injections of liposome-encapsulated MDP. Similar results have been reported for 2 other lipophilic derivatives of MDP, 6-O-stearoyl-N-acetylmuramyl-L-α-aminobutyryl-D-isoglutamine (6-O-S[Abu] MDP)[211] and α(N-acetylmuramyl-L-alanyl-D-isoglutaminyl), β, γ-dipalmitoyl-sn-glycerol (MDP-GDP).[71]

Liposomes could also deliver more than one agent to macrophages and previous studies from our laboratory have demonstrated that MAF and MDP entrapped within the same liposome preparation can act synergistically to render rat alveolar macrophages tumoricidal in vitro.[80] Moreover, the multiple systemic administration of liposomes containing both MAF and MDP into tumor-bearing mice produced synergistic activation of macrophages, which in turn were responsible for eradication of established lymph node and lung metastases.[81] In this study, it should be noted that we deliberately postponed the start of treatment to examine the hypothesis that MDP and MAF packaged within the same multilamellar vesicle (MLV) would synergistically activate macrophages *in situ*. Specifically, i.v. injections of MLV containing an optimal dose of MAF or MDP led to regression of metastases in at least one third of the mice treated. MLV containing diluted MAF or diluted MDP had no such effects. On the other hand, the i.v. injections of MLV containing subthreshold amounts of both MAF and MDP significantly increased the long-term survival of mice.[81]

IV. SUMMARY

The emergence of metastases resistant to conventional therapy could be a major reason for the failure to cure this disease. Tumors are heterogeneous with regard to many characteristics, including metastatic potential, and the proliferation of a minor subpopulation of cells within the primary tumor could cause treatment-resistant metastases to emerge; therefore, the successful approach to destruction of metastases will be one that circumvents tumor cell heterogeneity and does not induce resistance.

At least in vitro, appropriately activated macrophages appear able to recognize and destroy neoplastic cells regardless of other biologic phenotypes, and target cells do not appear to develop resistance to macrophage-mediated cytotoxicity. A significant effort is now under way in many laboratories to develop effective agents that will stimulate the antitumor activities of macrophages. Liposomes offer a most suitable carrier system for delivering agents to macrophages in vivo. When injected intravenously, the majority of liposomes are taken up by phagocytic reticuloendothelial cells in the liver and spleen and by circulating monocytes. This provides a highly effective mechanism for targeting of liposome-encapsulated materials to macrophages. We have exploited this mechanism to deliver lymphokines and synthetic MDP to macrophages *in situ*. Intravenous administration of lymphokines or MDP encapsulated in multilamellar liposomes activates macrophages in vivo and augments host resistance to metastases. No beneficial effects are obtained with the same materials administered in unencapsulated form. Not all mice treated with i.v. injections of liposomes containing immunomodulators survived. However, the metastases of treatment-failure animals were not populated by macrophage-resistant tumor cells, indicating that macrophage activation could overcome the fundamental problem of phenotypic heterogeneity among tumor cells.[214]

The optimal conditions for systemic therapy with liposome-encapsulated immunomodulators and the efficacy of this modality alone and in combination in treating large metastatic tumor burdens are now being defined. As with many other antitumor therapies, optimal application of macrophage treatment for metastasis will require combination with other antitumor agents. Indeed, the most likely role for tumoricidal macrophages is in the destruction of micrometastases or the few tumor cells that remain after treatment with conventional adjuvant therapies such as chemotherapy.

REFERENCES

1. **Fidler, I. J.**, The evolution of biological heterogeneity in metastatic neoplasms, in *Cancer Invasion and Metastasis: Biologic and Therapeutic Aspects*, Nicolson, G. L. and Milas, L., Eds., Raven Press, New York, 1984, 5.
2. **Fidler, I. J. and Hart, I. R.**, Biological diversity in metastatic neoplasms: origins and implications, *Science*, 217, 998, 1982.

3. **Heppner, G.,** Tumor heterogeneity, *Cancer Res.,* 214, 2259, 1984.

4. **Fidler, I. J. and Kripke, M. L.,** Metastasis results from preexisting variant cells within a malignant tumor, *Science,* 197, 893, 1977.

5. **Talmadge, J. E., Wolman, S. R., and Fidler, I. J.,** Evidence for the clonal origin of spontaneous metastases, *Science,* 217, 361, 1982.

6. **Cifone, M. A. and Fidler, I. J.,** Increasing metastatic potential is associated with increasing genetic instability of clones isolated from murine neoplasms, *Proc. Natl. Acad. Sci. U.S.A.,* 78, 6949, 1981.

7. **Hill, R. P., Chambers, A. F., Ling, V., and Harris, J. F.,** Dynamic heterogeneity: rapid generation of metastatic variants in mouse B16 melanoma cells, *Science,* 224, 998, 1984.

8. **Granger, G. A. and Weiser, R. S.,** Homograft target cells: specific destruction in vitro by contact interaction with immune macrophages, *Science,* 145, 1427, 1964.

9. **Evans, R. and Alexander, P.,** Mechanism of immunologically specific killing of tumor cells by macrophages, *Nature (London),* 236, 168, 1972.

10. **Keller, R.,** Cytostatic elimination of syngeneic rat tumor cells in vitro by nonspecifically activated macrophages, *J. Exp. Med.,* 138, 625, 1973.

11. **Hibbs, J. B., Jr., Lambert, L. H., and Remington, J. S.,** Control of carcinogenesis: a possible role for the activated macrophage, *Science,* 177, 998, 1972.

12. **Hibbs, J. B., Jr.,** Macrophage nonimmunologic recognition: target cell factors related to contact inhibition, *Science,* 180, 868, 1973.

13. **Yen, S., Thomasson, D. L., and Stewart, C. C.,** The activation of cloned macrophages by concanavalin A for tumoricidal effect: assessment of tumor cell cytotoxicity by a clonogenic assay, *J. Cell. Physiol.,* 110, 1, 1982.

14. **Meltzer, M. S., Tucker, R. W., Sanford, K. K., and Leonard, E. J.,** Interaction of BCG-activated macrophages with neoplastic and nonneoplastic cell lines in vitro: quantitation of the cytotoxic reaction by release of tritiated thymidine from prelabeled target cells, *J. Natl. Cancer Inst.,* 54, 1177, 1975.

15. **Norbury, K. and Fidler, I. J.,** In vitro tumor cell cytotoxicity by syngeneic mouse macrophages: methods for assaying cytotoxicity, *J. Immunol. Methods,* 7, 109, 1975.

16. **Wiltrout, R. H., Taramelli, D., and Holden, H. T.,** Microcytotoxicity isotope release assay using indium for assessment of macrophage-mediated cytolysis, in *Manual of Macrophage Methodology: Collection, Characterization and Function,* Herscowitz, H. B., Holden, H. T., Bellanti, J. A., and Ghaffar, A., Eds., Marcel Dekker, New York, 1981, 337.

17. **Normann, S. J. and Cornelius, J.,** Cytokinetics of macrophage-mediated cytotoxicity, *Cancer Res.,* 44, 2313, 1984.

18. **Meltzer, M. S., Tucker, R. W., and Brever, A. C.,** Interaction of BCG-activated macrophages with neoplastic and nonneoplastic cell lines in vitro: cinemicrographic analysis, *Cell. Immunol.,* 17, 30, 1975.

19. **Bucana, C. D., Hoyer, L. C., Hobbs, B., Breesman, S., McDaniel, M., and Hanna, M. G., Jr.,** Morphological evidence for the translocation of lysosomal organelles from cytotoxic macrophages into the cytoplasm of tumor target cells, *Cancer Res.,* 36, 4444, 1976.

20. **Bucana, C. D., Hoyer, L. C., Schroit, A. J., Kleinerman, E., and Fidler, I. J.,** Ultrastructural studies of the interaction between liposome-activated human blood monocytes and allogeneic tumor cells in vitro, *Am. J. Pathol.,* 112, 101, 1983.

21. **Raz, A., Fogler, W. E., and Fidler, I. J.,** The effects of experimental conditions on the expression of in vitro macrophage-mediated tumor cytotoxicity, *Cancer Immunol. Immunother.,* 7, 157, 1979.

22. **Fidler, I. J.,** The MAF dilemma, *Lymphokine Res.,* 3, 51, 1984.

23. **Wiltrout, R. H., Taramelli, D., and Holden, H. T.,** Measurement of macrophage-mediated cytotoxicity against adherent and non-adherent target cells by release of ^{111}Indium-oxine, *J. Immunol. Methods,* 43, 319, 1981.

24. **North, S. M. and Nicolson, G. L.,** Heterogeneity in the sensitivities of the 13762 NF rat mammary adenocarcinoma cell clones to cytolysis mediated by extra- and intratumoral macrophages, *Cancer Res.,* 45, 1453, 1985.

25. **Pace, J. L., Varesio, L., Russell, S. W., and Blasi, E.,** The strain of mouse and assay conditions influence whether muIFN-γ primes or activates macrophages for tumor cell killing, *J. Leukocyte Biol.,* 37, 475, 1985.

26. **Keller, R. and Jones, V. E.,** Role of activated macrophages and antibody in inhibition and enhancement of tumor growth in rats, *Lancet,* 2, 847, 1971.

27. **Hibbs, J. B., Jr., Lambert, L. H., and Remington, J. S.,** Macrophage-mediated nonspecific cytotoxicity: possible role in tumour resistance, *Nature (London) New Biol.,* 235, 48, 1972.

28. **Cleveland, R. P., Meltzer, M. S., and Zbar, B.,** Tumor cytotoxicity in vitro by macrophages from mice infected with *Mycobacterium bovis* strain BCG, *J. Natl. Cancer Inst.,* 52, 1887, 1974.

29. **Alexander, P. and Evans, R.,** Endotoxin and double stranded RNA render macrophages cytotoxic, *Nature (London),* 232, 76, 1971.

30. **Hibbs, J. B., Jr., Taintor, R. R., Chapman, H. A., Jr., and Weinberg, J. B.,** Macrophage tumor killing: influence of the local environment, *Science*, 197, 279, 1977.
31. **Doc, W. F. and Henson, P. M.,** Macrophage stimulation by bacterial lipopolysaccharides, *J. Exp. Med.*, 148, 554, 1978.
32. **Pace, J. L. and Russell, S. W.,** Activation of mouse macrophages for tumor cell killing. I. Quantitative analysis of interactions between lymphokine and lipopolysaccharide, *J. Immunol.*, 126, 1863, 1981.
33. **Peri, G., Polentarutti, N., Sessa, C., Mangioni, C., and Mantovani, A.,** Tumoricidal activity of macrophages isolated from human ascitic and solid ovarian carcinomas: augmentation by interferon, lymphokines and endotoxin, *Int. J. Cancer*, 28, 143, 1981.
34. **Juy, D. and Chedid, L.,** Comparison between macrophage activation and enhancement of nonspecific resistance to tumors by mycobacterial immunoadjuvants, *Proc. Natl. Acad. Sci. U.S.A.*, 72, 4105, 1975.
35. **Taniyama, T. and Holden, H. T.,** Direct augmentation of cytolytic activity of tumor-derived macrophages and macrophage cell lines by muramyl dipeptide, *Cell. Immunol.*, 48, 369, 1979.
36. **Sone, S. and Fidler, I. J.,** In vitro activation of tumoricidal properties in rat alveolar macrophages by synthetic muramyl dipeptide encapsulated in liposomes, *Cell. Immunol.*, 57, 42, 1981.
37. **Kripke, M. L., Budmen, M. B., and Fidler, I. J.,** Production of specific macrophage-activating factor by lymphocytes from tumor-bearing mice, *Cell. Immunol.*, 30, 341, 1976.
38. **Evans, R. and Alexander, P.,** Rendering macrophages specifically cytotoxic by a factor released from immune lymphoid cells, *Transplantation*, 12, 227, 1971.
39. **Evans, R., Grant, C. K., Cox, H., Steele, K., and Alexander, P.,** Thymus-derived lymphocytes produce an immunologically specific macrophage-arming factor, *J. Exp. Med.*, 136, 1318, 1972.
40. **Boraschi, D. and Tagliabui, A.,** Interferon-induced enhancement of macrophage-mediated tumor cytolysis and its difference from activation by lymphokines, *Eur. J. Immunol.*, 11, 110, 1981.
41. **David, J. R.,** Macrophage activation by lymphocyte mediators, *Fed. Proc. Fed. Am. Soc. Exp. Biol.*, 34, 1730, 1975.
42. **Churchill, W. H., Piessens, W. F., Sulis, C. A., and David, J. R.,** Macrophages activated as suspension cultures with lymphocyte mediators devoid of antigens become cytotoxic for tumor cells, *J. Immunol.*, 115, 781, 1975.
43. **Fidler, I. J. and Raz, A.,** The induction of tumoricidal capacities in mouse and rat macrophages by lymphokines, in *Lymphokines*, Pick, E., Ed., Academic Press, New York, 1981, 345.
44. **Schultz, R. M., Papametheakis, J. D., and Chirigos, M. A.,** Interferon: an inducer of macrophage activation by polyanions, *Science*, 197, 674, 1977.
45. **Evans, R.,** Specific and nonspecific activation of macrophages, *Activation of Macrophages*, Wagner, W. H. et al., Eds., Excerpta Medica, Amsterdam, 1974, 305.
46. **Barna, B. P., Deodhar, S. D., Gautam, S., Yen-Lieberman, B., and Roberts, D.,** Macrophage activation and generation of tumoricidal activity by liposome-associated human C-reactive protein, *Cancer Res.*, 44, 305, 1984.
47. **Munder, P. G., Weltzien, H. V., and Modelell, M.,** Lysolecithin analogs: a new class of immunopotentiators, in *Immunopathology*, Miescher, P. A., Ed., Grune & Stratton, New York, 1977, 411.
48. **Tarnowski, G. S., Mountain, I. M., Stock, C. C., Munder, P. G., Weltzien, H. L., and Westphal, O.,** Effects of lysolecithin and analogs on mouse ascites tumors, *Cancer Res.*, 38, 339, 1978.
49. **Cohn, Z. A.,** The activation of mononuclear phagocytes: fact, fancy and future, *J. Immunol.*, 121, 813, 1978.
50. **North, R. J.,** The concept of the activated macrophage, *J. Immunol.*, 121, 806, 1978.
51. **Adams, D. O. and Hamilton, T. A.,** The cell biology of macrophage activation, *Annu. Rev. Immunol.*, 2, 283, 1984.
52. **Petit, J. E. and Lemaire, G.,** Macrophage activation, *Ann. Inst. Pasteur Paris*, 137C, 191, 1986.
53. **Poste, G., Kirsh, R., and Fidler, I. J.,** Cell surface receptors for lymphokines. I. The possible role of glycolipids as receptors for macrophage migration inhibitor factor (MIF) and macrophage activating factor (MAF), *Cell. Immunol.*, 44, 71, 1979.
54. **Celada, A., Gray, P. W., Rinderknecht, E., and Schreiber, R.,** Evidence for a gamma-interferon receptor that regulates macrophage tumoricidal activity, *J. Exp. Med.*, 160, 55, 1984.
55. **Poste, G., Kirsh, R., Fogler, W. E., and Fidler, I. J.,** Activation of tumoricidal properties in mouse macrophages by lymphokines encapsulated in liposomes, *Cancer Res.*, 39, 881, 1979.
56. **Piessens, W. F., Remold, H. G., and David, J. R.,** Increased responsiveness to macrophage-activating factor (MAF) after alteration of macrophage membranes, *J. Immunol.*, 118, 2078, 1977.
57. **Sone, S., Poste, G., and Fidler, I. J.,** Rat alveolar macrophages are susceptible to free and liposome-encapsulated lymphokines, *J. Immunol.*, 124, 2197, 1980.
58. **Fidler, I. J., Raz, A., Fogler, W. E., Hoyer, L. C., and Poste, G.,** The role of plasma membrane receptors and the kinetics of macrophage activation by lymphokines encapsulated in liposomes, *Cancer Res.*, 41, 495, 1981.

59. **Fogler, W. E., Talmadge, J. E., and Fidler, I. J.,** The activation of tumoricidal properties in macrophages of endotoxin responder and nonresponder mice by liposome-encapsulated immunomodulators, *J. Reticuloendothel. Soc.,* 33, 165, 1983.

60. **Kleinerman, E. S., Schroit, A. J., Fogler, W. E., and Fidler, I. J.,** Tumoricidal activity of human monocytes activated in vitro by free and liposome-encapsulated human lymphokines, *J. Clin. Invest.,* 72, 304, 1983.

61. **Ellouz, F., Adam, A., Ciorbaru, R., and Lederer, E.,** Minimal structural requirements for adjuvant activity of bacterial peptidoglycan derivatives, *Biochem. Biophys. Res. Commun.,* 59, 1317, 1974.

62. **Kotani, S., Watanabe, Y., Shimono, T., Narita, T., Kato, K., Stewart-Tull, D. E. S., Kinoshita, F., Yokogawa, K., Kawata, S., Shiba, T., Kusumoto, S., and Tarumi, Y.,** Immunoadjuvant activities of cell walls, their water-soluble fractions and peptidoglycan subunits, prepared from various gram-positive bacteria, and of synthetic N-acetyl-muramyl peptides, *Z. Immunitaetsforsch. Exp. Ther.,* 149, 302, 1975.

63. **Tenu, J. P., Roche, A. C., Yapo, A., Kieda, C., Monsigny, M., and Petit, J. F.,** Absence of cell surface receptors for muramyl peptides in mouse peritoneal macrophages, *Biol. Cell,* 44, 157, 1982.

64. **Silverman, D. H. S., Wu, H., and Karnovsky, M. L.,** Muramyl peptides and serotonin interact at specific binding sites on macrophages and enhance superoxide release, *Biochem. Biophys. Res. Commun.,* 131, 1160, 1985.

65. **Silverman, D. H. S., Krueger, J. M., and Karnovsky, M. L.,** Specific binding sites for muramyl peptides on murine macrophages, *J. Immunol.,* 136, 2195, 1986.

66. **Fogler, W. E. and Fidler, I. J.,** The activation of tumoricidal properties in human blood monocytes by muramyl peptides requires a specific intracellular interaction, *J. Immunol.,* 136, 2311, 1986.

67. **Chapes, S. K. and Haskill, S.,** Role of *Corynebacterium parvum* in the activation of peritoneal macrophages. I. Association between intracellular *C. parvum* and cytotoxic macrophages, *Cell. Immunol.,* 70, 65, 1982.

68. **Fidler, I. J., Sone, S., Fogler, W. E., and Barnes, Z.,** Eradication of spontaneous metastases and activation of alveolar macrophages by intravenous injection of liposomes containing muramyl dipeptide, *Proc. Natl. Acad. Sci. U.S.A.,* 78, 1680, 1981.

69. **Schroit, A. J. and Fidler, I. J.,** Effects of liposome structure and lipid composition on the activation of tumoricidal properties of macrophages by liposomes containing muramyl dipeptide, *Cancer Res.,* 42, 161, 1982.

70. **Fidler, I. J., Sone, S., Fogler, W. E., Smith, D., Braun, D. G., Tarcsay, L., Gisler, R. H., and Schroit, A. J.,** Efficacy of liposomes containing a lipophilic muramyl dipeptide derivative for activating the tumoricidal properties of alveolar macrophages in vivo, *J. Biol. Resp. Modifiers,* 1, 43, 1982.

71. **Phillips, N. C., Moras, M. L., Chedid, L., Lefrancier, P., and Bernard, J. M.,** Activation of alveolar macrophage tumoricidal activity and eradication of experimental metastases by freeze-dried liposomes containing a lipophilic muramyl dipeptide derivative, *Cancer Res.,* 45, 128, 1985.

72. **Lopez-Berestein, G., Mehta, K., Mehta, R., Juliano, R. L., and Hersh, E. M.,** The activation of human monocytes by liposome-encapsulated muramyl dipeptide analogues, *J. Immunol.,* 130, 1500, 1983.

73. **Sone, S., Musuura, S., Ogawara, M., and Tsubura, E.,** Potentiating effect of muramyl dipeptide and its lipophilic analog encapsulated in liposomes on tumor cell killing by human monocytes, *J. Immunol.,* 132, 2105, 1984.

74. **Kleinerman, E. S., Erickson, K. L., Schroit, A. J., Fogler, W. E., and Fidler, I. J.,** Activation of tumoricidal properties in human blood monocytes by liposomes containing lipophilic muramyl tripeptide, *Cancer Res.,* 43, 2010, 1983.

75. **Koff, W. C., Fidler, I. J., Showalter, S. D., Chakrabarty, M. K., Hampar, B., Ceccorulli, L. M., and Kleinerman, E. S.,** Human blood monocytes activated by immunomodulators in liposomes lyse herpes virus-infected but not normal cells, *Science,* 224, 1007, 1984.

76. **Kleinschmidt, W. J. and Schultz, R. M.,** Similarities of murine gamma interferon and the lymphokine that renders macrophages cytotoxic, *J. Interferon Res.,* 2, 291, 1982.

77. **Schultz, R. M.,** Synergistic activation of macrophages by lymphokine and lipopolysaccharide: evidence for lymphokine as the primer and interferon as the trigger, *J. Interferon Res.,* 2, 459, 1982.

78. **Kleinerman, E. S., Zicht, R., Sarin, P. S., Gallo, R. C., and Fidler, I. J.,** Constitutive production and release of a lymphokine with macrophage-activating factor activity distinct from gamma-interferon by a human T-cell leukemia virus-positive cell line, *Cancer Res.,* 44, 4470, 1984.

79. **Ruco, L. P. and Meltzer, M. S.,** Macrophage activation for tumor cytotoxicity: development of macrophage cytotoxic activity requires completion of a sequence of short-lived intermediary reactions, *J. Immunol.,* 121, 2035, 1978.

80. **Sone, S. and Fidler, I. J.,** Synergistic activation by lymphokines and muramyl dipeptide of tumoricidal properties in rat alveolar macrophages, *J. Immunol.,* 125, 2454, 1980.

81. **Fidler, I. J. and Schroit, A. J.,** Synergism between lymphokines and muramyl dipeptide encapsulated in liposomes: in situ activation of macrophages and therapy of spontaneous cancer metastases, *J. Immunol.,* 133, 515, 1984.

82. **Ruco, L. P. and Meltzer, M. S.,** Macrophage activation for tumor cytotoxicity: tumoricidal activity by macrophages from C3H/HeJ mice requires at least two activation stimuli, *Cell. Immunol.,* 41, 35, 1978.

83. **Siaki, I. and Fidler, I. J.,** Synergistic activation by recombinant mouse gamma-interferon and muramyl dipeptide of tumoricidal properties in mouse macrophages, *J. Immunol.,* 135, 684, 1985.

84. **Saiki, I., Sone, S., Fogler, W. E., Kleinerman, E. S., Lopez-Berestein, G., and Fidler, I. J.,** Synergism between human recombinant gamma-interferon and muramyl dipeptide encapsulated in liposomes for activation of antitumor properties in human blood monocytes, *Cancer Res.,* 45, 6188, 1985.

85. **Fidler, I. J., Fogler, W. E., Kleinerman, E. S., and Saiki, I.,** Abrogation of species specificity for activation of tumoricidal properties in macrophages by recombinant mouse or human gamma-interferon encapsulated in liposomes, *J. Immunol.,* 135, 4289, 1985.

86. **Eppstein, D. A., Marsh, Y. V., Pas, M., Felgner, P. L., and Schreiber, A. B.,** Biological activity of liposome-encapsulated murine interferon γ is mediated by a cell membrane receptor, *Proc. Natl. Acad. Sci. U.S.A.,* 82, 3688, 1985.

87. **Hibbs, J. B., Jr.,** Discrimination between neoplastic and nonneoplastic cells in vitro by activated macrophages, *J. Natl. Cancer Inst.,* 53, 1487, 1974.

88. **Piessens, W. F., Churchill, W. H., Jr., and David, J. R.,** Macrophages activated in vitro with lymphocyte mediators kill neoplastic but not normal cells, *J. Immunol.,* 114, 293, 1975.

89. **Fidler, I. J.,** Recognition and destruction of target cells by tumoricidal macrophages, *Isr. J. Med. Sci.,* 14, 177, 1978.

90. **Fidler, I. J. and Kleinerman, E. S.,** Lymphokine-activated human blood monocytes destroy tumor cells but not normal cells under cocultivation conditions, *J. Clin. Oncol.,* 2, 937, 1984.

91. **Hamilton, T. A. and Fishman, M.,** Characterization of the recognition of target cells sensitive or resistant to cytolysis by activated macrophages, *J. Immunol.,* 127, 1702, 1981.

92. **Tucker, R. W., Meltzer, M. S., and Sanford, K. K.,** Susceptibility to killing by BCG-activated macrophages associated with "spontaneous" neoplastic transformation in culture, *Int. J. Cancer.,* 27, 555, 1981.

93. **Marino, P. A. and Adams, D. O.,** Interaction of BCG-activated macrophages and neoplastic cells in vitro. I. Conditions of binding and its selectivity, *Cell. Immunol.,* 54, 11, 1980.

94. **Marino, P. A. and Adams, D. O.,** Interaction of BCG-activated macrophages and neoplastic cells in vitro. II. The relationship of selective binding to cytolysis, *Cell. Immunol.,* 54, 26, 1980.

95. **Piessens, W. F.,** Increased binding of tumor cells by macrophages activated in vitro with lymphocyte mediators, *Cell. Immunol.,* 35, 303, 1978.

96. **Adams, D. O. and Marino, P.A.,** Evidence for a multistep mechanism of cytolysis by BCG-activated macrophages: the interrelationship between the capacity for cytolysis, target binding, and secretion of cytolytic factor, *J. Immunol.,* 126, 981, 1981.

97. **Fidler, I. J.,** Macrophages and metastasis: a biological approach to cancer therapy, *Cancer Res.,* 45, 4714, 1985.

98. **Marino, P. A., Whisnant, C. C., and Adams, D. O.,** Binding of Bacillus Calmette-Guerin-activated macrophages to tumor targets, *J. Exp. Med.,* 154, 77, 1981.

99. **Mercurio, A. M.,** Disruption of oligosaccharide processing in murine tumor cells inhibits their susceptibility to lysis by activated mouse macrophages, *Proc. Natl. Acad. Sci. U.S.A.,* 83, 2609, 1986.

100. **Brunda, M. J., Wiltrout, R. H., Holden, H. T., and Varesio, L.,** Selective inhibition by monosaccharides of tumor cell cytotoxicity mediated by mouse macrophages, macrophage-like cell lines, and natural killer cells, *Int. J. Cancer,* 31, 373, 1983.

101. **Schlepper-Schafer, J., Holl, N., Kolb-Bachofen, V., Friedrich, E., and Kolb, H.,** Role of carbohydrates in rat leukemia cell-liver macrophage cell contacts, *Biol. Cell,* 52, 253, 1984.

102. **Cameron, D. J.,** Specificity of macrophage-mediated cytotoxicity: role of target and effector cell fucose, *Immunol. Lett.,* 11, 39, 1985.

103. **Cameron, D. J. and Churchill, W. H.,** Specificity of macrophage mediated cytotoxicity: role of target cell sialic acid, *Jpn. J. Exp. Med.,* 52, 9, 1982.

104. **Fidler, I. J., Roblin, R. O., and Poste, G.,** In vitro tumoricidal activity of macrophages against virus-transformed lines with temperature-dependent transformed phenotypic characteristics, *Cell. Immunol.,* 38, 131, 1978.

105. **Bennett, D. C., Dexter, T. J., Ormerod, E. J., and Hart, I. R.,** Increased experimental metastatic capacity of a murine melanoma following induction of differentiation, *Cancer Res.,* 46, 3239, 1986.

106. **Fidler, I. J. and Cifone, M. A.,** Properties of metastatic and nonmetastatic cloned subpopulations of an ultraviolet-light-induced murine fibrosarcoma of recent origin, *Am. J. Pathol.,* 97, 633, 1979.

107. **Giavazzi, R., Bucana, C. D., and Hart, I. R.,** Correlation of tumor growth inhibitory activity of macrophages exposed to Adriamycin and the Adriamycin sensitivity of the target tumor cells, *J. Natl. Cancer Inst.,* 73, 447, 1984.

108. **Kripke, M. L., Gruys, E., and Fidler, I. J.,** Metastatic heterogeneity of cells from an ultraviolet light-induced murine fibrosarcoma of recent origin, *Cancer Res.,* 38, 2962, 1978.

109. **Reading, C. L., Kraemer, P. M., Miner, K. M., and Nicolson, G. L.,** In vivo and in vitro properties of malignant variants of RAW 117 metastatic murine lymphoma lymphosarcoma, *Clin. Exp. Metastasis,* 1, 135, 1983.

110. **Miner, K. M., Klostergaard, J., Granger, G. A., and Nicolson, G. L.,** Differences in cytotoxic effects of activated murine peritoneal macrophages and J774 monocytic cells on metastatic variants of B16 melanoma, *J. Natl. Cancer Inst.,* 70, 717, 1983.

111. **Miner, K. M. and Nicolson, G. L.,** Differences in the sensitivities of murine metastatic lymphoma/lymphosarcoma variants to macrophage mediated cytolysis and/or cytostasis, *Cancer Res.,* 43, 2063, 1983.

112. **Yamamura, Y., Fischer, B. C., Harnaha, J. B., and Proctor, J. W.,** Heterogeneity of murine mammary adenocarcinoma cell subpopulations. In vitro and in vivo resistance to macrophage cytotoxicity and its association with metastatic capacity, *Int. J. Cancer,* 33, 67, 1984.

113. **Kaplan, A. M., Brown, J., Collins, J. M., Morahan, P. S., and Snodgrass, M. J.,** Mechanisms of macrophage-mediated tumor cell cytotoxicity, *J. Immunol.,* 121, 1781, 1978.

114. **Granger, D. L., Taintor, R. R., Cook, J. L., and Hibbs, J. B., Jr.,** Injury of neoplastic cells by murine macrophages leads to inhibition of mitochondrial respiration, *J. Clin. Invest.,* 65, 357, 1980.

115. **Hibbs, J. B., Jr.,** Heterocytolysis by macrophages activated by Bacillus Calmette-Guerin: lysosome exocytosis into tumor cells, *Science,* 184, 468, 1974.

116. **Miller, M. L., Stimmett, J. D., and Clark, L. C., Jr.,** Ultrastructure of tumoricidal peritoneal exudate cells stimulated in vivo by perfluorochemical emulsions, *J. Reticuloendothel. Soc.,* 27, 105, 1980.

117. **Keller, R., Keist, R., and Groscurth, P.,** Firm persistent binding between activated macrophages and tumor cells is not a prerequisite for the mediation of cytolysis, *Int. J. Cancer,* 37, 89, 1986.

118. **Klostergaard, J.,** The role of cytotoxins in monocyte/macrophage tumor cytotoxicity in vitro, *Prog. Leukocyte Biol.,* 2, 447, 1986.

119. **Ruff, M. R. and Gifford, G. E.,** Tumor necrosis factor, in *Lymphokines,* Vol. 2, Pick, E., Ed., Academic Press, New York, 1981, 235.

120. **Ferluga, J., Schorlemmer, H. U., Baptista, C. C., and Allison, A. C.,** Production of the complement cleavage product, C3a, by activated macrophages and its tumorilytic effects, *Clin. Exp. Immunol.,* 31, 512, 1978.

121. **Nathan, C. F., Brukner, L. H., Silverstein, S. C., and Cohn, Z. A.,** Extracellular cytolysis by activated macrophages and granulocytes. I. Pharmacologic triggering of effector cells and the release of hydrogen peroxide, *J. Exp. Med.,* 149, 84, 1979.

122. **Nathan, C. F., Silverstein, S. C., Brukner, L. H., and Cohn, Z. A.,** Extracellular cytolysis by activated macrophages and granulocytes. II. Hydrogen peroxide as a mediator of cytotoxicity, *J. Exp. Med.,* 149, 100, 1979.

123. **Currie, G. A. and Basham, C.,** Differential arginine dependence and the selective cytotoxic effects of activated macrophages for malignant cells in vitro, *Br. J. Cancer,* 39, 653, 1978.

124. **Stadecker, M. J., Calderon, J., Karnovsky, M. J., and Unanue, E. R.,** Synthesis and release of thymidine by macrophages, *J. Immunol.,* 119, 1738, 1978.

125. **McIvoc, K. L. and Weiser, R. S.,** Mechanisms of target cell destruction by alloimmune peritoneal macrophages. II. Release of a specific cytotoxin from interacting cells, *Immunology,* 20, 315, 1971.

126. **Pipen, C. E. and McIvoc, K. L.,** Alloimmune peritoneal macrophages as specific effector cells: characterization of specific macrophage cytotoxin, *Cell. Immunol.,* 122, 1785, 1979.

127. **Aksamit, R. R. and Kim, K. J.,** Macrophage cell lines produce a cytotoxin, *J. Immunol.,* 122, 1785, 1979.

128. **Adams, D. O.,** Effector mechanism of cytolytically activated macrophages. I. Secretion of neutral proteases and effect of protease inhibitor, *J. Immunol.,* 124, 286, 1980.

129. **Adams, D. O., Kao, K. J., Farb, R., and Pizzo, S. V.,** Effector mechanisms of cytolytically activated macrophages. II. Secretion of a cytolytic factor by activated macrophages and its relationship to secreted neutral proteases, *J. Immunol.,* 124, 293, 1980.

130. **Sharma, S. F., Piessens, W. F., and Middlebrook, G.,** In vitro killing of tumor cells by soluble products of activated guinea pig peritoneal macrophages, *Cell. Immunol.,* 49, 379, 1980.

131. **Drysdale, B., Zacharchuk, C. M., and Shin, H. S.,** Mechanism of macrophage-mediated cytotoxicity: production of a soluble cytotoxic factor, *J. Immunol.,* 131, 2362, 1983.

132. **Klostergaard, J., Foster, W. A., Hamilton, D. A., Turpin, J., and Lopez-Berestein, G.,** Effector mechanisms of human monocyte-mediated tumor cytotoxicity in vitro: biochemical, functional, and serological characterization of cytotoxins produced by peripheral blood monocytes isolated by counterflow elutriation, *Cancer Res.,* 46, 2871, 1986.

133. **Kay, M. M. B.,** Mechanism of removal of senescent cells by human macrophages in situ, *Proc. Natl. Acad. Sci. U.S.A.,* 72, 3521, 1975.

134. **MacDonald, R. A., MacSween, R. N. M., and Pechet, G. S.,** Iron metabolism by reticuloendothelial cells in vitro: physical and chemical conditions, lipotrope deficiency, and acute inflammation, *Lab. Invest.,* 21, 236, 1969.

135. **Day, A. J.**, The macrophage system, lipid metabolism and atherosclerosis, *J. Atheroscler. Res.*, 4, 117, 1964.
136. **Cohn, Z. A.**, The structure and function of monocytes and macrophages, *Adv. Immunol.*, 9, 163, 1968.
137. **Van Furth, R.**, *Mononuclear Phagocytes in Immunity, Infection and Pathology*, Blackwell Scientific, Oxford, 1975.
138. **Nathan, C. F., Murray, H. W., and Cohn, Z. A.**, Current concepts: the macrophage as an effector cell, *N. Engl. J. Med.*, 303, 622, 1980.
139. **Nelson, D. S.**, *Immunobiology of the Macrophage*, Academic Press, New York, 1976.
140. **Fink, M. A.**, *The Macrophage in Neoplasia*, Academic Press, New York, 1976.
141. **James, K., McBride, B., and Stuart, A.**, *The Macrophage and Cancer*, University of Edinburgh Press, Edinburgh, Scotland, 1977.
142. **Adams, D. O. and Snyderman, R.**, Do macrophages destroy nascent tumors?, *J. Natl. Cancer Inst.*, 16, 1341, 1979.
143. **Lurie, H.**, *Resistance of Tuberculosis: Experimental Studies in Native and Acquired Defense Mechanisms*, Harvard University Press, Cambridge, Mass., 1964.
144. **Droller, M. J. and Remington, J. S.**, A role for the macrophage in in vivo and in vitro resistance to murine bladder tumor cell growth, *Cancer Res.*, 35, 49, 1975.
145. **Norbury, K. and Kripke, M. L.**, Ultraviolet-induced carcinogenesis in mice treated with silica, trypan blue or pyran copolymer, *J. Reticuloendothel. Soc.*, 26, 827, 1979.
146. **Jones, D. D. E. and Castro, J. E.**, Immunological mechanisms in metastatic spread and the antimetastatic effects of *C. parvum*, *Br. J. Cancer*, 35, 519, 1977.
147. **Sadler, T. E., Jones, D. D. E., and Castro, J. E.**, The effects of altered phagocytic activity on growth of primary and metastatic tumors, in *The Macrophage and Cancer*, James, K., McBride, J. F., and Stuart, A., Eds., University of Edinburgh Press, Edinburgh, Scotland, 1979, 115.
148. **Mantovani, A., Giavazzi, R., Polentanitti, N., Spreafico, F., and Gavattinni, S.**, Divergent effects of macrophage toxins of growth of primary tumors and lung metastases in mice, *Int. J. Cancer*, 25, 617, 1980.
149. **Fidler, I. J.**, Inhibition of pulmonary metastasis by intravenous injection of specifically activated macrophages, *Cancer Res.*, 34, 1074, 1974.
150. **Gorelik, E., Wiltrout, R. H., Brunda, M. J., Holden, H. T., and Herberman, R. B.**, Augmentation of metastasis formation by thioglycollate-elicited macrophages, *Int. J. Cancer*, 29, 575, 1982.
151. **Liotta, L. A., Gattozzi, C., Kleinerman, J., and Saidel, G.**, Reduction of tumor cell entry into vessels by BCG-activated macrophages, *Br. J. Cancer*, 36, 639, 1977.
152. **Fidler, I. J., Fogler, W. E., and Connor, J.**, The rationale for the treatment of established experimental micrometastases with the injection of tumoricidal macrophages, in *Immunobiology and Immunotherapy of Cancer*, Terry, W. D. and Yamamura, Y., Eds., Elsevier, Amsterdam, 1979, 361.
153. **Den Otter, W., Dullens, H. F. J., Van Lovern, H., and Pels, E.**, Antitumor effects of macrophages injected into animals: a review, in *The Macrophage and Cancer*, James, K., McBride, B., and Stuart, A., Eds., University of Edinburgh Press, Edinburgh, Scotland, 1977, 119.
154. **Blamey, R. W., Crosby, D. L., and Baker, J. M.**, Reticuloendothelial activity during the growth of rat sarcomas, *Cancer Res.*, 29, 335, 1969.
155. **Old, L. J., Clarke, D. A., Benacerraf, B., and Goldsmith, M.**, The reticuloendothelial system and the neoplastic process, *Science*, 88, 164, 1960.
156. **Rhodes, J.**, Altered expression of human monocyte Fc receptors in malignant disease, *Nature (London)*, 265, 253, 1977.
157. **Rhodes, J.**, Resistance of tumor cells to macrophages, *Cancer Immunol. Immunother.*, 7, 211, 1980.
158. **Bernstein, I. D., Zbar, B., and Rapp, H. J.**, Impaired inflammatory response in tumor-bearing guinea pigs, *J. Natl. Cancer Inst.*, 49, 1641, 1972.
159. **Eccles, S. A. and Alexander P.**, Sequestration of macrophages in growing tumors and its effect on the immunological capacity of the host, *Br. J. Cancer*, 30, 42, 1974.
160. **Meltzer, M. S. and Stevenson, M. M.**, Macrophage function in tumor-bearing mice: tumoricidal and chemotactic response of macrophages activated by infection with *Mycobacterium bovis*, strain BCG, *J. Immunol.*, 118, 2176, 1977.
161. **Meltzer, M. S. and Stevenson, M. M.**, Macrophage function in tumor-bearing mice: dissociation of phagocytic and chemotactic responsiveness, *Cell. Immunol.*, 35, 99, 1978.
162. **Normann, S. J. and Sorkin, E.**, Cell-specific defect in monocyte function during tumor growth, *J. Natl. Cancer Inst.*, 57, 135, 1976.
163. **Snyderman, R., Pike, M. C., Blaylock, B. L., and Weinstein, P.**, Effect of neoplasms on inflammation: depression of macrophage accumulation after tumor implantation, *J. Immunol.*, 116, 585, 1976.
164. **Sone, S. and Fidler, I. J.**, Activation of rat alveolar macrophages to the tumoricidal state in the presence of progressively growing pulmonary metastases, *Cancer Res.*, 41, 2401, 1981.

165. **Urban, J. L. and Schreiber, H.,** Selection of macrophage-resistant progressor tumor variants by the normal host: requirement for concomitant T cell-mediated immunity, *J. Exp. Med.,* 157, 642, 1983.

166. **Nestel, F. P., Casson, P. R., Wiltrout, R. H., and Kerbel, R. S.,** Alterations in sensitivity to nonspecific cell mediated lysis associated with tumor progression: characterization of activated macrophage- and natural killer cell-resistant tumor variants, *J. Natl. Cancer Inst.,* 73, 483, 1984.

167. **Fogler, W. E. and Fidler, I. J.,** Nonselective destruction of murine neoplastic cells by syngeneic tumoricidal macrophages, *Cancer Res.,* 45, 14, 1985.

168. **Fidler, I. J., Gersten, D. M., and Budmen, M. B.,** Characterization in vivo and in vitro of tumor cells selected for resistance to syngeneic lymphocyte-mediated cytotoxicity, *Cancer Res.,* 36, 3160, 1976.

169. **Hanna, N. and Fidler, I. J.,** Role of natural killer cells in the destruction of circulating tumor emboli, *J. Natl. Cancer Inst.,* 65, 801, 1980.

170. **Eccles, S. A. and Alexander, P.,** Macrophage content of tumors in relationship to metastatic spread, *Nature (London),* 250, 667, 1974.

171. **Eccles, S. A.,** Macrophages and cancer, in *Immunological Aspects of Cancer,* Castro, J. E., Ed., MTP Press, Lancaster, England, 1978, 123.

172. **Talmadge, J. E., Key, M., and Fidler, I. J.,** Macrophage content of metastatic and nonmetastatic rodent neoplasms, *J. Immunol.,* 126, 2245, 1981.

173. **Evans, R. and Eidler, D. M.,** Macrophage accumulation in transplanted tumors is not dependent on host immune responsiveness or presence of tumor-associated rejection antigens, *J. Reticuloendothel. Soc.,* 30, 425, 1981.

174. **Evans, R. and Lawler, E. M.,** Macrophage content and immunogenicity of C57BL/6J and BALB/cByJ methylcholanthrene-induced sarcomas, *Int. J. Cancer,* 26, 831, 1980.

175. **Key, M., Talmadge, J. E., and Fidler, I. J.,** Lack of correlation between the progressive growth of spontaneous metastases and their content of infiltrating macrophages, *J. Reticuloendothel. Soc.,* 32, 387, 1982.

176. **Dvorak, H. R., Dickersin, G. R., Dvorak, A. M., Manseau, E. J., and Pyne, K.,** Human breast carcinoma: fibrin deposits and desmoplasia. Inflammatory cell type and distribution in microvasculature and infarction, *J. Natl. Cancer Inst.,* 67, 335, 1981.

177. **Mantovani, A.,** Effects on in vitro tumor growth of murine macrophages isolated from sarcoma lines differing in immunogenicity and metastasizing capacity, *Int. J. Cancer,* 22, 741, 1978.

178. **Russell, S. W. and McIntosh, A. T.,** Macrophages isolated from regressing Moloney sarcomas are more cytotoxic than those recovered from progressing sarcomas, *Nature (London),* 268, 69, 1977.

179. **Loveless, S. E. and Heppner, G. H.,** Tumor associated macrophages of mouse mammary tumors. I. Differential cytotoxicity of macrophages from metastatic and nonmetastatic tumors, *J. Immunol.,* 131, 2074, 1983.

180. **Mahoney, K. H., Fulton, A. M., and Heppner, G. H.,** Tumor-associated macrophages of mouse mammary tumors. II. Differential distribution of macrophages from metastatic and nonmetastatic tumors, *J. Immunol.,* 131, 2079, 1983.

181. **Takeo, S., Yasumoto, K., Nagashima, A., Nakahashi, H., Sugimachi, K., and Nomoto, K.,** Role of tumor-associated macrophages in lung cancer, *Cancer Res.,* 46, 3179, 1986.

182. **Nash, J. R. G., Price, J. E., and Tarin, D.,** Macrophage content and colony-forming potential in mouse mammary carcinomas, *Br. J. Cancer,* 45, 478, 1981.

183. **Mantovani, A.,** In vitro effects on tumor cells of macrophages isolated from an early-passage chemically-induced murine sarcoma and from its spontaneous metastases, *Int. J. Cancer,* 27, 221, 1981.

184. **Allison, A. C.,** Mode of action of immunological adjuvants, *J. Reticuloendothel. Soc.,* 26, 619, 1979.

185. **Chedid, L., Audibert, F., and Johnson, A. G.,** Biological activities of muramyl dipeptide, a synthetic glycopeptide analogous to bacterial immunoregulating agents, *Prog. Allergy,* 25, 63, 1978.

186. **Fogler, W. E. and Fidler, I. J.,** Modulation of the immune response by muramyl dipeptide, in *Immune Modulation Agents and Their Mechanisms,* Chirigos, M. A. and Fenichel, R. L., Eds., Marcel Dekker, New York, 1984, 499.

187. **Parant, M., Parant, F., Chedid, L., Yapo, A., Petit, J. F., and Lederer, E.,** Fate of the synthetic immunoadjuvant, muramyl dipeptide, (^{14}C-labeled) in the mouse, *Int. J. Immunopharmacol.,* 1, 35, 1978.

188. **Ambler, L. and Hudson, A. M.,** Pharmacokinetics and metabolism of muramyl dipeptide and normuramyl dipeptide (^{3}H-labeled) in the mouse, *Int. J. Immunopharmacol.,* 6, 133, 1984.

189. **Yoshida, T. and Cohen, S.,** Lymphokine activity in vivo in relation to circulating monocyte levels and delayed skin reactivity, *J. Immunol.,* 122, 1540, 1972.

190. **Papermaster, B. W., Holterman, O. A., Rosner, D., Klein, E., Dao, T., and Djerassi, I.,** Regressions produced in breast cancer lesions by a lymphokine fraction from a human lymphoid cell line, *Res. Commun. Chem. Pathol. Pharmacol.,* 8, 413, 1974.

191. **Salvin, S. B., Younger, Y. S., Nishio, J., and Neta, R.,** Tumor suppression by a lymphokine released into the circulation of mice with delayed hypersensitivity, *J. Natl. Cancer Inst.,* 55, 1233, 1975.

192. **Donohue, J. H. and Rosenburg, S. A.,** The fate of interleukin-2 after in vivo administration, *J. Immunol.*, 130, 2203, 1983.
193. **Poste, G. and Kirsh, R.,** Rapid decay of tumoricidal activity and loss of responsiveness to lymphokines in inflammatory macrophages, *Cancer Res.*, 39, 2582, 1979.
194. **Schroit, A. J., Hart, I. R., Madsen, J., and Fidler, I. J.,** Selective delivery of drugs encapsulated in liposomes: natural targeting to macrophages involved in various disease states, *J. Biol. Resp. Modifiers*, 2, 97, 1983.
195. **Poste, G., Kirsh, R., and Bugelski, P.,** Liposomes as a drug delivery system in cancer therapy, in *New Approaches to Cancer Chemotherapy*, Academic Press, New York, 1984, 165.
196. **Allison, A. C. and Gregoriadis, G.,** Liposomes as immunological adjuvants, *Nature (London)*, 252, 252, 1979.
197. **Fidler, I. J., Raz, A., Fogler, W. E., Kirsh, R., Bugelski, P., and Poste, G.,** Design of liposomes to improve delivery of macrophage-augmenting agents to alveolar macrophages, *Cancer Res.*, 40, 4460, 1980.
198. **Hart, I. R., Fogler, W. E., Poste, G., and Fidler, I. J.,** Toxicity studies of liposome-encapsulated immunomodulators administered intravenously to dogs and mice, *Cancer Immunol. Immunother.*, 10, 157, 1981.
199. **Fogler, W. E., Raz, A., and Fidler, I. J.,** In situ activation of murine macrophages by liposomes containing lymphokines, *Cell. Immunol.*, 53, 214, 1980.
200. **Fidler, I. J.,** Therapy of spontaneous metastases by intravenous injection of liposomes containing lymphokines, *Science*, 208, 1469, 1980.
201. **Griswold, D. P., Jr.,** Consideration of the subcutaneously implanted B16 melanoma as a screening model for potential anticancer agents, *Cancer Chemother. Rep.*, 3, 315, 1972.
202. **Fogler, W. E., Wade, R., Brundish, D. E., and Fidler, I. J.,** Distribution and fate of free and liposome-encapsulated (^{3}H)nor-muramyl dipeptide and (^{3}H)muramyl tripeptide phosphatidylethanolamine in mice, *J. Immunol.*, 135, 1372, 1985.
203. **Fogler, W. E. and Fidler, I. J.,** In situ activation of tumoricidal properties in murine alveolar macrophages following the systemic administration of muramyl dipeptide encapsulated within liposomes, *Fed. Proc. Fed. Am. Soc. Exp. Biol.*, 40, 761, 1981.
204. **Fidler, I. J., Barnes, Z., Fogler, W. E., Kirsh, R., Bugelski, P., and Poste, G.,** Involvement of macrophages in the eradication of established metastases produced by intravenous injection of liposomes containing macrophage activators, *Cancer Res.*, 42, 496, 1982.
205. **Fidler, I. J.,** The in situ induction of tumoricidal activity in alveolar macrophages by liposomes containing muramyl dipeptide is a thymus-independent process, *J. Immunol.*, 127, 1719, 1981.
206. **Key, M. E., Talmadge, J. E., Fogler, W. E., Bucana, C., and Fidler, I. J.,** Isolation of tumoricidal macrophages from lung melanoma metastases of mice treated systemically with liposomes containing a lipophilic derivative of muramyl dipeptide, *J. Natl. Cancer Inst.*, 69, 1189, 1982.
207. **Deodhar, S. D., Barna, B. P., Edinger, M., and Chiang, T.,** Inhibition of lung metastases by liposomal immunotherapy in a murine fibrosarcoma model, *J. Biol. Resp. Modifiers*, 1, 27, 1982.
208. **Deodhar, S. D., James, K., Chiang, T., Edinger, M., and Barna, B.,** Inhibition of lung metastases in mice bearing a malignant fibrosarcoma by treatment with liposomes containing human c-reactive protein, *Cancer Res.*, 42, 5084, 1982.
209. **Thombre, P. and Deodhar, S. D.,** Inhibition of liver metastases in murine colon adenocarcinoma by liposomes containing human c-reactive protein or crude lymphokine, *Cancer Immunol. Immunother.*, 16, 145, 1984.
210. **Schroit, A. J. and Fidler, I. J.,** The design of liposomes for delivery of immunomodulators to host defense cells, in *Medical Applications of Liposomes*, Yagi, K., Ed., Japan Scientific Societies Press, Tokyo, Japan, 1986, 141.
211. **Lopez-Berestein, G., Milas, L., Hunter, N., Mehta, K., Hersh, E. M., Kurahara, C. G., Vanderpas, M., and Eppstein, D. A.,** Prophylaxis and treatment of experimental lung metastases in mice after treatment with liposome-encapsulated 6-O-stearoyl-N-acetylmuramyl-L-α-aminobutyryl-D-isoglutamine, *Clin. Exp. Metastasis*, 2, 127, 1984.
212. **Pabst, M. J., Cummings, N. P., Shiba, T., Kusumoto, S., and Kotani, S.,** Lipophilic derivative of muramyl dipeptide is more active than muramyl dipeptide in priming macrophages to release superoxide anion, *Infect. Immun.*, 29, 617, 1980.
213. **Raz, A., Bucana, C., Fogler, W. E., Poste, G., and Fidler, I. J.,** Biochemical, morphological, and ultrastructural studies on the uptake of liposomes by murine macrophages, *Cancer Res.*, 41, 487, 1981.
214. **Fidler, I. J. and Poste, G.,** Macrophage-mediated destruction of malignant tumor cells and new strategies for the therapy of metastatic disease, *Springer Semin. Immunopathol.*, 5, 161, 1982.

Chapter 10

STRATEGIES FOR ACTIVATION OF MACROPHAGES IN VIVO FOR THE THERAPY OF METASTATIC DISEASE

Richard Kirsh, William J. Johnson, Peter J. Bugelski, and George Poste

TABLE OF CONTENTS

I. INTRODUCTION

Since the late 1800s, when Metchnikoff[1] first described the participation of mononuclear phagocytes in the inflammatory process, a large body of evidence has been generated indicating that both fixed and free mononuclear phagocytes play pivotal roles in tissue remodeling during embryogenesis and metamorphosis; in tissue destruction and repair; in injury and inflammation, and in the clearance of dead, damaged, or senescent blood cells and foreign particulate materials from the circulation. The mechanism by which these diverse functions occur was attributed initially to the primitive phagocytic function of macrophages and the accompanying process of intracellular digestion of ingested materials. It is now recognized, however, that ingestion and digestion represent only a limited part of the repertoire of the homeostatic functions of the macrophage and its pivotal role in myriad immunological and nonimmunological processes.[2-5,164,166,170]

The role of cells of the mononuclear phagocyte system (MPS) comprising Kupffer cells in the liver; alveolar, splenic, lymph node, and bone marrow macrophages; and circulatory blood monocytes in host defense against neoplastic disease have attracted increasing attention over the past 10 years.[2,3,6-9] This reflects three categories of experimental observations. Mononuclear phagocytes, when appropriately activated,* display significant cytotoxicity towards neoplastic cells while leaving "normal" nontumorigenic cells completely unharmed.[10-12,187] Second, mononuclear phagocytes infiltrate neoplastic lesions in a number of species and, third, agents that activate the tumoricidal properties of mononuclear phagocytes, augment host defense against tumors. These observations, coupled with the disappointing results obtained to date in both clinical and experimental trials with immunologically specific therapeutic modalities mediated by T- and B-lymphocytes have led to renewed interest in the functions of macrophages in host defense against cancer, and reappraisal of the therapeutic potential of augmenting the immunologically nonspecific tumoricidal properties of mononuclear phagocytes in adjuvant therapy of cancer.

Metastasis, the process by which secondary neoplastic lesions are established in organs distant from the site of the original primary tumor is the single most devastating aspect of cancer and the principal reason for the lack of success in cancer treatment. There are several reasons for the disappointing results obtained in the treatment of metastatic tumors. First, by the time the initial diagnosis of cancer is made, many tumors have already metastasized, but the metastases are too small to be detected by routine clinical diagnostic procedures. Thus, despite significant advances in surgical techniques for the removal of primary tumors, most cancer deaths, other than those caused by infections, are caused by metastatic disease. The anatomic location and histologic organization of metastases is also a limiting factor. The presence of metastatic lesions in diverse body sites imposes taxing requirements for achieving adequate (therapeutic) drug concentrations at all sites without inducing unacceptable levels of toxicity to normal host cells. The third, and perhaps greatest obstacle to successful cancer therapy is the problem of tumor cell heterogeneity.[13-17] The phenotypic diversity of tumor cells coexisting within the same tumor at the time of diagnosis, as well as in advanced lesions, is sufficiently large that the responses of cells from a single metastatic lesion to a panel of therapeutic modalities may differ significantly from the response of cells in the primary tumor from which it originated and also from cells in other metastatic lesions.[15-17] Tumor cells in metastases proliferating in different organs, or even the same organ, may exhibit bewildering heterogeneity in the expression of numerous biological properties, including such clinically important traits as hormone receptor density, antigenicity, immunogenicity, and sensitivity to chemotherapeutic and biological response modifier

---

* In this chapter the term activated macrophage will refer to macrophages that display tumoricidal and/or microbicidal activity.

(BRM) agents.[16,18-25] The principal obstacle to effective cancer treatment thus lies not so much in the surgical removal of the primary tumor but in the elimination of widely disseminated metastases that are not amenable to surgery. Moreover, successful treatment of metastatic disease demands that the heterogeneity in tumor cell responses to various therapeutic modalities can be circumvented and against which resistance is unlikely to develop. Finally, successful treatment requires destruction of every cell in the metastasis. Survival and proliferation of even a small number of neoplastic cells means that they will eventually kill the host.

In this chapter we review the rationale for the therapeutic manipulation of macrophages as a strategy to augment host defense against neoplasia.

II. STRATEGIES FOR MACROPHAGE ACTIVATION IN CANCER THERAPY

A. The Activated Macrophage

As mentioned previously, the central role of the MPS in host defense is well documented. In addition to its classical role as a scavenging system for the clearance of foreign materials, immune complexes, dead or effete cells, and cell debris from the circulation, the functional status of the MPS is now known to be involved in determining the outcome of various forms of shock, tissue ischemia, and drug therapy.[4] Considerable attention has also been devoted to the role of activated macrophages in host defense against invading bacteria, parasites, and tumor cells.[26] The term "activated macrophage" is an operational definition and is used differently by various authors to describe acquisition of a variety of functions that are not exhibited by resident tissue macrophages. Examples of the use of the term activation can be found referring to activated macrophages as cells that show oxidative metabolism but lack microbicidal or tumoricidal activity, in other instances as macrophages that exhibit microbicidal but not tumoricidal activity, whereas other authors, including ourselves, limit the use of the term to macrophages that exhibit both microbicidal and tumoricidal properties. In this chapter the term will be used solely in the latter context to describe macrophages that have acquired both microbicidal and tumoricidal activity. Acquisition of tumoricidal properties may be accompanied by other phenotypic alterations including increased phagocytosis, secretion of neutral proteases and acid hydrolases, synthesis and release of arachadonic acid metabolites, expression of an altered ectoenzyme profile, the ability to suppress natural killer (NK)-cell activation, and an enhanced ability to kill intracellular microorganisms.[9,27,29] In this review, macrophages that display a biochemical and/or physiological profile different from resident tissue macrophages, but which do not express *tumoricidal* activity, will be referred to as stimulated macrophages.

Despite this useful general definition, the term "macrophage activation" is often the source of a great deal of confusion and misunderstanding. Of the many reasons for this confusion, the following deserve emphasis:

- Macrophages capable of killing certain microorganisms are not necessarily capable of killing tumor cells and vice versa.[162,163] Indeed, lysis of different types of tumor cells by macrophages can occur in the absence of any effect on other tumor cells, with the same being true for different microorganisms.[163-165]
- Macrophages have on their surfaces at least 30 distinct receptors and are capable of the secretion of over 75 different substances. The expression or production of most of these is alterable by stimulation or activation.[164,166,167] Preoccupation with the measurement of many of these parameters after the in vitro stimulation of macrophages with defined stimuli does not reflect what is likely to be a complex regulatory process in vivo.[9]
- No definitive evidence exists for the presence of macrophage populations with distinct

differentiation patterns.[168,169] Despite this fact, macrophage populations are quite heterogeneous in regard to expression of various phenotypic and functional markers.[169,170] This heterogeneity can make analysis of the role of regulatory signals more difficult (see Chapter 1).

- Significant differences exist in regard to phenotypic and functional parameters of macrophage activation among different species[164,171-173] and even among different strains within a species.[174] Most distressing is the observation that without standardization of animal vendors, mouse strains, tumor target types, reagent sources, and other variables, quite different results can be obtained in regard to assessments of macrophage function using mouse macrophages.[174]

- Endotoxin contamination continues to be a major difficulty in studies on the role of different cytokines in macrophage activation. This problem exists despite the increased awareness of investigators and manufacturers of media and other reagents. Investigations using human monocytes are rendered particularly difficult because of the increased sensitivity of human cells to endotoxin effects.

- In vivo studies regarding macrophage activation by cytokines have been minimal.[175,176] Because of this there is a general lack of understanding of the dose, route of administration, and kinetic requirements for macrophage activation in vivo using cytokines.

- Macrophages obtained from different anatomical sites can also vary considerably in their functional capabilities.[177-180] Thus, data obtained with one population cannot be extrapolated to another in all cases.

B. Pathways of Macrophage Activation

Macrophages can be rendered tumoricidal by a wide variety of naturally occurring and synthetic agents. Currently, there are two major classes of macrophage-activating agents that appear attractive as potential therapeutic candidates: microbial cell wall components and structural analogs related to these agents and various lymphokines. Macrophages can be activated by agents that either act directly or by agents that induce other cells to release mediators that evoke macrophage activation.

The direct activation of macrophages is induced by interaction with agents such as bacterial endotoxin (lipopolysaccharide, LPS), lentinin, glucan, picibanil, and diverse bacteria such as *Mycobacteria, Propionibacteria, Nocardia,* or subunits isolated from the cell walls of these microorganisms.[28-40]

Most of the microbial cell-wall derived materials are unsuitable for clinical use due to significant toxicities. In addition, detailed structural characterization of many of the components responsible for macrophage activation by these materials has yet to be accomplished. One notable exception is the water soluble, low molecular weight (M_r 459) synthetic dipeptide, *N*-acetyl-muramyl-L-alanyl-D-isoglutamine, referred to as muramyl dipeptide (MDP). MDP is the smallest structural unit capable of inducing all of the adjuvant activities of mycobacteria in a water in oil emulsion (complete Freund's adjuvant).[42,44] MDP has been shown to stimulate a wide variety of macrophage functions in vitro including secretion of prostaglandins and collagenase, generation of superoxide anion, release of interleukin-1 (IL-1), and to augment macrophage-mediated bacteriocidal and tumoricidal activities.[41-44] In vivo, MDP has been shown to protect experimental animals against lethal infection by a range of bacteria,[45-53] parasites,[52] fungi,[46,49] and viruses.[54,57] However, MDP, although far less toxic than intact mycobacteria, is much less effective than the intact bacteria in activating macrophages to the tumoricidal state in vivo. Its efficacy in vivo is limited by its extremely rapid clearance (90% of MDP injected intravenously can be detected in the urine within 2 hr).[43] Even when administered in high doses, it fails to stimulate significant macrophage-mediated antitumor activity.[58-60]

Indirect macrophage activation can be achieved by lymphokines released by antigen- or mitogen-stimulated lymphocytes and which interact with specific receptors on the macrophage surface.[61] This activity is referred to by the predictable designation as macrophage activating factor (MAF), but the exact identity of the mediator(s) involved and whether different subpopulations of macrophages[62-64] are activated by different mediators in lymphokine preparations is still unknown.

Current limitations in lymphokine production and purification technology dictate that the lymphokine preparations containing MAF activity are crude and vary markedly in their biological activities. In particular, the crucial question of whether there is a single, specific lymphokine that merits classification as MAF, or whether such activity can be attributed exclusively to other lymphokines such as gamma-interferon (IFN-γ), is currently an area of intense investigation. MAF activity and IFN-γ share many physicochemical and biological characteristics including co-purification by a variety of chromatographic procedures, similar chemical stabilities,[65] and abilities to induce an oxidative burst and expression of microbicidal and tumoricidal properties.[66-72] Conversely, several groups have now demonstrated MAF activity in culture supernatants from T cell lines that contain no detectable IFN-γ activity in association with materials whose physicochemical and immunological properties are distinct from IFN-γ.[73-76] The biological effects of these MAFs have some overlap with the effects of IFN-γ with respect to shared induction of macrophage-mediated cytotoxicity. However, several significant differences can be cited. First, interferon-induced macrophage-mediated cytotoxicity requires the presence of a second signal, supplied by bacterial endotoxin, for complete expression of the tumoricidal phenotype,[72] whereas MAF-induced tumoricidal activity is independent of second signals.[75] Second, MAF does not induce the expression of Fc receptors or Class I or II histocompatability antigens and does not have direct antiviral activity, whereas interferon treatment induces these effects.[161] However, formal proof of the existence of a specific non-IFN lymphokine with macrophage activation activity must await cloning of the gene and rigorous chemical analysis of the gene product.

1. Cytokine-Mediated Macrophage Activation

Because of the potential importance to immunotherapeutic applications, much recent work has focused on the ability of different cytokines to induce activation. The following list describes briefly what is known about various classes of agents in addition to interferon and their ability to directly or indirectly activate macrophages either alone or in combination with other agents.

a. Interleukins

- IL-1 has been reported to directly effect macrophage activation by promoting monocyte-mediated tumor cytotoxicity.[215] It has also been reported to induce tumor necrosis factor (TNF) in human monocytes[214] and may be an autocrine system in mouse macrophages.[216] It may also indirectly contribute to macrophage activation by inducing cytokine production in other cells.[217]
- Interleukin-2 (IL-2) has recently been described to directly activate human monocytes for tumor cytolysis.[218] It has been reported *not* to be active in inducing reactive oxygen metabolite secretion and microbicidal activity in monocytes.[219] Interestingly, IL-2 may also activate autoreactive killer cells that are cytotoxic against human monocytes.[220]
- Interleukin-4 (IL-4) B cell-stimulating factor (BSF-1) has recently been described to activate mouse macrophages for tumor cytolysis.[221]

b. Tumor Necrosis Factors (TNF)

- TNF-α induces its own production and monocyte-mediated cytotoxicity by human monocytes.[214] Again it was reported *not* to induce oxidative metabolism and microbicidal activity[219] by itself but has been reported to synergize with IFN-γ for induction of both tumoricidal and microbicidal activities in mouse macrophages.[222] TNF-α also induces cytokine production by monocytes, macrophages, and fibroblasts with the potential for inducing macrophage activation, namely IL-1[223,224] and granulocyte-macrophage colony-stimulating factor (GM-CSF).[225]

- TNF-β (lymphotoxin) synergizes with IFN-γ for induction of tumoricidal and microbicidal properties in mouse macrophages.[222]

c. Colony-Stimulating Factors (CSF)

- GM-CSF can induce tumoricidal activities in both granulocytes and macrophages[77,226,227] as well as microbicidal activity[228,229] and enhanced production of reactive oxygen[230] intermediates in murine macrophages and human monocytes.
- Colony-stimulating factor-1 (CSF-1) induces tumoricidal activity[231] and molecules with the potential for inducing activation of macrophages.[232]

d. Hormones

- 1,25-Dihydroxyvitamin D_3 has multiple immunoregulatory effects, including the ability to induce and/or augment production of IL-1 by human monocytes.[233] It is not known if a direct effect of this hormone on cytotoxic activity of the monocytes is evident.
- Neurotensin, although not capable of direct activation, markedly enhances IFN-γ-mediated cytolytic capacities of mouse macrophages.[234] Other neurohormones have the opposite effect.

Efforts to augment the tumoricidal activity of mononuclear phagocytes in vivo by the systemic administration of crude lymphokine preparations have been largely unsuccessful. Although direct intratumoral inoculation of MAF-containing preparations has been reported to induce regression in several primary skin tumors and cutaneous metastases,[77] systemic administration of MAF is probably not feasible due to its very short biological half-life caused by rapid binding to serum proteins.[10]

Therapeutic efforts to activate macrophages using agents that stimulate T-lymphocytes to produce MAF may also be unproductive. Recent data have shown that lymphocytes from animals bearing large, progressively growing tumors are deficient in their ability to release lymphokines needed for the recruitment and activation of macrophages.[10] This defect may stem, in part, from recent observations showing that the rapid emergence of suppressor T-lymphocytes during progressive tumor growth reduces T-lymphocyte-mediated antitumor mechanisms.[78-81] If such a defect is a generalized phenomenon in tumor bearing hosts, then administration of agents that seek to augment host antitumor responses via stimulation of T-lymphocytes may be of little or no value in the treatment of more advanced lesions where active immunosuppression may be prevalent. In addition, at any time a substantial fraction of the intratumoral macrophage population may be refractory to activation by lymphokines.[82]

Effective cancer therapy with macrophage-activating agents will thus, require compounds that are not only nontoxic and nonimmunogenic, but are capable of activating those macrophages that are refractory to lymphokine-mediated activation either as a result of an active suppression phenomenon imposed by other immune cell subsets or the passive decline in the responsiveness of macrophages to activation by lymphokines that accompany their migration from the blood stream into the tissue.[83,121]

C. Markers of the Stages of Macrophage Activation

Most models of the stages of activation of macrophages emphasize the progressive acquisition of the ability to perform complex functions.[164,170,172] These models also tend to emphasize the difference between resident tissue macrophages and inflammatory macrophages either stimulated with various potential activators or not. How the peripheral blood monocyte fits into this scheme has not been addressed to a large extent. Recent work suggests that murine monocytes closely resemble macrophages taken from sites of inflammation, and are distinct from resident peritoneal macrophages.[164,181-183] Many studies in the murine system have emphasized the importance of the inflammatory macrophage in regard to responsiveness to signals for induction of tumoricidal activity.[172-184] Others demonstrate clearly that resident macrophages are capable of being activated to both the microbicidal[185] as well as tumoricidal states.[186] The type of assay used, as well as the strain of mouse and animal vendor, are potential variables in these analyses.[165,174]

Macrophages taken from sites of inflammation (stimulated macrophages) are readily distinguished from resident macrophages based on several functional characteristics including increased phagocytosis and pinocytosis, increased secretion of lysosomal enzymes, increased expression of several receptors, decreased expression of certain ectoenzymes, and many others.[164,166,170] These types of changes in functional and biochemical markers are also associated with primed and activated macrophage populations.[172] Primed macrophages can be defined as macrophages that are prepared to complete a complex function such as microbicidal or tumoricidal functions, but require an additional signal. Activated macrophages are capable of mediating such functions.[164] Since many of the functional and biochemical changes seen in inflammatory macrophages are also seen in primed and activated cells (see Table 2 from Reference 164), many of these parameters are not useful markers for the tumoricidal or microbicidal phenotype. Attention, therefore, is focused on properties related to the completion of the complex function such as the selective recognition and binding of tumor cells or the secretion of cytolytic effector molecules.[187]

At present no marker exists for the activated phenotype which is absolutely predictive of microbicidal or tumoricidal activity. The following, however, represent recent descriptions of markers that are associated with the activated phenotype:

- The selective augmentation of S-adenosylmethionine in murine macrophages after activation by IFN-γ,[188] as well as a decreased level of RNA synthesis[189] and alteration in ribosomal RNA accumulation.[190]
- The activation and translocation of protein kinase C during activation.[191,192]
- The elevated selective recognition and capture of tumor target cells by activated macrophages[193] and the potential involvement of lymphocyte function associated 1 (LFA-1) antigen in this process.[201]
- The induction of specific receptors for IL-2 on both human peripheral blood monocytes[194-196] and alveolar macrophages.[196]
- The release of neopterin from macrophages activated by IFN-γ.[197] Although this is used as an indicator of T cell function in vivo[198] it should be emphasized that patients with certain psychiatric disorders,[199] as well as normal pregnant women,[200] show elevated levels of secreted neopterin.
- Protein changes associated with the stages of activation have been identified by two different groups. Specific changes in two proteins are associated with the acquisition of tumoricidal activity (p47b and p71/73).[202] Similarly, a 120 kDa protein has been identified to be expressed upon activation.[203] The synthesis of other proteins,[204] as well as altered phosphorylation of several proteins,[205] has also been associated with activation. The identity and function of these proteins are not yet known.
- Similarly, alterations in oncogene expression during macrophage activation have received recent attention.[206-208]

III. AUGMENTATION OF MACROPHAGE-MEDIATED ANTITUMOR ACTIVITY IN VIVO

A. Animal Models of Metastatic Disease

As emphasized, the single most important factor contributing to the lack of current success in cancer treatment is the propensity of malignant tumors to metastasize. Drug delivery to metastases, located in different organs including the brain, represents a considerably greater technical challenge than the therapy of more localized primary tumors. Animal tumor models adopted for evaluating new therapeutic protocols must address the problem of metastasis. In evaluating any potential regimen for therapeutic efficacy against metastatic disease, it is imperative that activity be measured against established metastatic lesions.[82,84-87] Test systems in which potential antineoplastic agents are administered concurrently with tumor cells, or within a few hours of tumor implantation, have little relevance to the clinical setting, where the oncologist must deal with established metastases. Unfortunately, too large a fraction of the reported studies in experimental therapeutics ignores this issue and reports on the therapy of intraperitoneal (i.p.) ascites tumors using agents administered coincident with, or within 24 to 48 hr of inoculating tumor cells into the peritoneal cavity are still abundant in journals purported to be concerned with cancer therapy. Similarly, experimental protocols in which the test agent is administered in the direct vicinity of the tumor cells would seem to have little relevance to the demands of clinical oncology. Unfortunately, all animal tumors are flawed in some regard as models for human neoplasms.[82-87] However, this does not mean that an effort should not be made to evaluate new treatment modalities in models that share as many features as possible with human malignancies, not the least of which is the challenging task of achieving a pharmacodisposition consistent with achieving therapeutic concentrations of the candidate treatment agent at the diverse sites required for successful therapy of disseminated disease.

Intraperitoneal therapy of a minimal ascites tumor burden localized in the peritoneal cavity does not meet this requirement since the drug or the drug carrier can gain immediate access to tumor cells without interference from anatomical barriers. Similarly, well-vascularized, transplanted tumors growing subcutaneously or intramuscularly, though more difficult to eradicate than i.p. tumors, also fail to provide a sufficiently demanding model for evaluating the effectiveness of agents in treating metastases. Implantation of tumor cells into host tissues by injection disrupts the local tissue microvasculature and enhances vascular permeability at the injection site. Not surprisingly, the effects which persist until vascular repair is achieved within 2 to 3 days influence the efficiency with which materials injected intravenously localize in the tumor. Administration of drug within 24 to 48 hr of tumor implantation can, therefore, result in unusually high concentrations of drug within the tumor. Furthermore, the blood supply of transplanted tumors is established by emigration of new capillary sprouts into the tumor from surrounding host vessels.[90] During this initial angiogenic response, the newly forming capillary sprouts are highly permeable because of gaps between adjacent endothelial cells and open terminal ends.[89] The sprouts allow virtually unlimited passage of materials, including erythrocytes, into the surrounding extravascular tissue.[88] Penetration of transplanted tumors not only by drugs but also by macromolecules such as antibodies and even relatively large particulate materials such as liposomes or circulating blood cells may thus, be artificially high. Little or no insight is provided into the behavior of these materials in the vascular bed of human tumors or spontaneous animal tumors in which the vascular supply has evolved in an entirely different fashion during progressive enlargement of the tumor cell population.[88]

In the formation of hematogenous metastases, circulating tumor cells arrest in capillaries, extravasate, and grow initially as pericapillary colonies in the extravascular parenchyma (micrometastases) before the angiogenic response needed to support the additional cell growth and formation of clinically significant metastases occurs.[86,87,90,91] There is no evidence that capillary permeability is drastically altered by tumor cell extravasation in micrometastasis formation. Thus, if drugs, drug carriers, or cells are to gain access to micrometastases, they must cross structurally intact microvessels.[89]

We consider that at a minimum these events dictate that experimental chemotherapy regimens be evaluated for their activity against established metastases in adjuvant therapy protocols comparable to those undertaken routinely in the clinic following removal or reduction of the primary tumor.

Our rationale in proposing that experimental therapies be tested for activity against established metastases is not based on the premise that the therapeutic responses of cells in metastases may differ from tumor cells in the primary lesion. The fact that tumors are heterogeneous and contain subpopulations of cells with differing metastatic abilities and responses to therapeutic agents is well documented.[13-25,85] However, it is not established that metastatic tumor cell subpopulations exhibit unique responses to therapeutic agents that are not seen in nonmetastatic cells. Both nonmetastatic and metastatic cells appear to display an extraordinary level of diversity in their responses to various anticancer modalities, but no correlation with metastatic ability is evident. Consequently, there is no reason to assume that the sensitivity of metastatic tumor cell subpopulations to any given modality could not be determined by merely assaying the response of a heterogeneous tumor cell population containing both metastatic and nonmetastatic cell subpopulations implanted subcutaneously or intramuscularly.

The more compelling rationale for using metastatic tumor models is to establish that the disposition and pharmacokinetics of a drug or a delivery system used to "target" materials to tumors are consistent with achieving therapeutic concentrations in the organs typically affected by metastases in the neoplasm of interest. Since metastases in the same host vary significantly in their size, growth rates, cell growth fraction, and vascular supply, the use of metastatic models also yields useful secondary information about the efficacy of therapeutic modalities in circumventing these factors.

Numerous metastatic animal tumors are available that could be used for this purpose.[83,86,91] In addition, methods have been described recently that permit reproducible metastasis of human tumor xenografts in nude mice,[151] and this approach will probably find increasing use in the testing of new antineoplastic agents.

B. Augmentation of Macrophage-Mediated Tumoricidal Activity In Vivo

The clinical appeal and the therapeutic advantages of targeting drugs to different cell types in the body do not need to be stated. Cancer probably represents the most obvious, and is certainly the most quoted, example of a disease in which targeted drug delivery and selective destruction of tumor cells would produce truly dramatic therapeutic gains. Thus, it comes as no surprise that targeting is the stated goal of most current experimental approaches to drug delivery in vivo, whether via liposomes and other particulate carriers or via antibody-drug conjugates or immunotoxins.

A wide variety of cellular, macromolecular, and particulate carriers have been investigated as potential drug delivery systems with the stated objective of improving cancer chemotherapy. These include erythrocytes, leukocytes, antibodies, nucleic acids, heat- or chemically denatured plasma proteins, and a diverse array of particulate carriers of differing sizes and biodegradability prepared from various polymeric materials including dextran, gelatin, agarose, cellulose, albumin, or phospholipids.[93,94,152-155] Many have failed to fulfill their initial promise, but interest in drug delivery systems remains high in both academic and commercial laboratories. Among these systems, liposomes have attracted considerable interest, at least as judged by the number of published papers and patents issued concerning their potential value as a drug carrier.[89,93,108]

The successful targeting of liposomes (or any carrier) to a specific cell type in vivo requires successful completion of several independent steps: (1) access to the appropriate target cell, (2) recognition and selective interaction with the target cell, and (3) selective uptake by the target cell with little or no uptake by nontarget cells.[92,97] In addition, the liposome-drug combination must not produce unacceptable levels of toxicity, and the drug must remain associated with the liposome for a sufficient time to enable therapeutically effective drug concentrations to be delivered to the target cells.

1. Passive-Targeting of Liposomes to Mononuclear Phagocytes In Vivo

Liposomes and other particulates offer a very efficient system for the delivery of materials to mononuclear phagocytes in vivo. Studies on the disposition of intravenously injected liposomes have demonstrated that in common with other particulate materials, liposomes localize selectively in organs with high levels of mononuclear phagocyte activity[92,95-97] such as the liver, spleen, and bone marrow, as well as circulating to blood monocytes.[92,95-98] This passive localization of liposomes within macrophages and monocytes thus, facilitates selective delivery of liposome-associated materials to these cells in vivo. The term passive targeting is used[89] since liposome-mediated drug delivery to mononuclear phagocytes merely exploits the natural disposition of these particles to this cell type. In contrast, active targeting refers to systems in which the drug carrier is associated with some form of cell-recognition ligand, typically a cell-specific antibody, in an effort to alter the pharmacodisposition of the drug to the target cell in question. In addition to delivery of materials to mononuclear phagocytes, entrapment of materials in liposomes serves several other useful functions. Encapsulation of biologically labile materials within liposomes will protect them from premature inactivation or degradation within the circulation. Furthermore, compounds such as MDP that show rapid clearance kinetics when administered as a "free" compound may show extended retention in vivo when administered within liposomes.

Macrophage-activating agents such as MDP, MAF, C-reactive protein, or poly-inosinic-cytodylic acid (I.C.), encapsulated within liposomes are highly efficient in rendering macrophages tumoricidal in vitro.[10,96,98-101,103] Murine peritoneal, alveolar, and subcutaneous (s.c.) tissue macrophages as well as human monocytes incubated with liposomes containing either MAF or MDP become cytotoxic toward syngeneic, allogeneic or xenogeneic tumor cells while leaving nonneoplastic cells unharmed.[96,100,104-106] Although accurate dose-response comparisons between "free" unencapsulated MAF and liposome-encapsulated MAF are hampered by the lack of a direct biochemical assay for MAF, the efficacy of "free" (unencapsulated) MAF vs. encapsulated MAF may be determined by comparing the volume of MAF-containing preparation required to elicit a defined response. Such dose-response determinations indicate that liposome-encapsulated MAF can activate macrophages at significantly lower doses than the amount of free MAF required to elicit an equivalent level of tumoricidal activity.[100] Similar reductions in dose-response relationships have been observed with IFN and polyinosinic-polycytodylic acid[101] or MAF and MDP encapsulated in liposomes.[107]

2. Macrophage-Mediated Destruction of Established Micrometastases

As the lung is a major site for metastatic disease in man, we have been interested in: (1) identifying factors that influence the retention of liposomes within the pulmonary microvasculature and (2) achieving efficient uptake of liposome-encapsulated BRM agents by alveolar macrophages *in situ*. Analyses of the effect of liposome size, surface charge, and lipid composition have demonstrated that large (0.5 to 3.0 μm diameter) multilamellar vesicle (MLV) and reverse phase evaporation vesicle (REV) liposomes are arrested in the lung more efficiently than small unilamellar vesicles (SUVs) of identical lipid composition. In addition, liposomes containing negatively charged lipids arrest more efficiently in the lung than neutral liposomes or liposomes containing positively charged phospholipids.[96,98] Comparison of a variety of negatively charged lipids has demonstrated that liposomes prepared from phosphatidylserine and phosphatidylcholine (3:7 molar ratio) show the most efficient arrest within the lung.[98,102] Alveolar macrophages recovered by pulmonary lavage after i.v. injection of liposome-encapsulated MAF resulted in significant tumoricidal activity associated with the isolated macrophage population.[98,102] In contrast, macrophages recovered from control animals receiving either unencapsulated MAF, "empty" liposomes, or neutral (PC) liposomes containing MAF which are not efficiently retained within the lung, were ineffective in activating macrophages *in situ*.[92,102]

Since our ultimate goal is the *in situ* activation of tumoricidal macrophages for the therapy of metastatic disease, the liposome preparations in the following discussion will be limited to multilamellar liposomes composed of phosphatidylcholine and phosphatidylserine in a 7:3 ratio unless stated otherwise.

Liposomes containing MAF, MDP, or human C-reactive protein (CRP) cause significant destruction of established metastases caused by a range of murine tumors.[102-104,107,131] In these systems spontaneous pulmonary and lymph node metastases arising from tumors implanted in the footpad were well established at the start of liposome therapy. Multiple metastatic lesions containing several thousand tumor cells were present at the onset of therapy, which in the absence of therapy, progressed rapidly to form large colonies exceeding 2 to 3 mm in diameter at the time of death. However, when a 3-week protocol of therapy was initiated with liposome-encapsulated macrophage-activity agents (within 3 to 4 days) after removal of the "primary" lesion in the footpad, the majority (about 70%) of treated animals were free of macroscopic or microscopic tumors. Furthermore, in treated animals that still exhibited residual metastatic disease, the median number of metastatic colonies was still significantly reduced compared with both the untreated control group and animals treated with unencapsulated "free" activating agents.[3,102,103]

The therapeutic efficacy of liposome-encapsulated BRM in rendering pulmonary macrophages tumoricidal is very encouraging since the lung is a major site of metastatic disease. Studies on the residual metastatic lesions from experimental animals treated with liposomes containing BRM indicate that the residual tumor cells are not resistant to killing by activated macrophages.[3,107,131] This is consistent with the lack of success in selecting tumor cell clones with increased resistance to macrophage-mediated killing[3] and hence, reinforces the suggestion that the most important potential factor limiting the clinical use of this approach will not be due to the emergence of resistant subpopulations but due to the extent of tumor burden at the outset of therapy.

The optimal conditions for therapy with liposome-encapsulated macrophage-activating agents and the efficacy of this modality for treatment of metastatic burdens of increasing severity have still to be defined. In addition to the use of clinically relevant tumor models with predictive value, evaluation and development of immunotherapeutic BRM agents will require reappraisal and modification of existing antineoplastic test protocols. In contrast to conventional cytotoxic chemotherapeutic agents, which are routinely evaluated at the maximum tolerated dose (MTD), BRM agents may exhibit complex response curves, often with biphasic or multiphasic responses. Agents with this profile may often be more effective at lower doses than high dose levels.[109,110] In most instances to date, however, optimum dose-response relationships for clinical studies have not been quantified in detail and clinical trials with BRM agents are all too frequently conducted using a dose seemingly selected in arbitrary fashion, other than with the obvious prerequisite of accordance of extreme toxicity. The superior efficacy of low doses of BRM agents (compared to those BRM agents administered at their MTD) has recently been demonstrated in three experimental rodent tumor models using recombinant IL-2, the interferon inducer poly-I.C., and a low molecular weight semisynthetic microbial cell wall fragment FK565.[109,110] Similarly, dosing frequency and the duration of treatment can also have profound influences on the therapeutic efficacy of BRM agents.[110] Critical evaluation of BRM agents and optimization of immunotherapeutic protocols, will, therefore, require a thorough evaluation of the complex pharmacodynamic properties of the BRM agents with respect to the combination of dose, dosage frequency, and duration of treatment on acquisition and maintenance of the activated phenotype in vivo.

In addition to the prerequisite of successfully augmenting macrophage-mediated tumoricidal activity in vivo, a further critical issue in the design of BRM agent-mediated therapies concerns the number and physiological status of tumor-infiltrating macrophages. At this point, it seems highly unlikely that liposome-encapsulated activating agents could serve as a single modality in treating advanced metastatic disease. For example, in mice, even allowing for maximal macrophage recruitment into the lung, there are insufficient numbers of pulmonary macrophages to eradicate more than 10^8 tumor cells per lung.[3] As tumor burdens of this size are easily attained, the potential application of macrophage activation is almost certainly not in the elimination of large tumor masses, but in the eradication of the residual tumor following cytoreductive therapy (also see next section). Thus, in common with many other antineoplastic regimens, optimal application will involve use in conjunction with other antitumor modalities.

IV. FACTORS INFLUENCING THE EFFICACY OF MACROPHAGE-MEDIATED ANTINEOPLASTIC THERAPY

Several factors have been identified that limit the therapeutic potential of macrophage-activation protocols *in situ*. These include the effect of the rate and extent of monocyte production by the bone marrow on the total number of macrophages; the kinetics of macrophage recruitment into metastases; and the presence of chemical signals in the tumor microenvironment that can suppress monocyte recruitment, impair macrophage responsiveness to activation stimuli or impede expression of macrophage-mediated tumoricidal activity.

A. Macrophage Content of Metastases

The content of mononuclear phagocytes in both primary tumors and their metastases is highly variable and does not correlate with the antigenicity, immunogenicity, or the metastatic capabilities of the tumor cells.[111-113] In some tumor systems, the extent of macrophage infiltration is related inversely to the rate of tumor growth and metastasis.[113-116] However, in other tumor systems, including human tumors, the absence of an extensive mononuclear infiltrate in the primary tumor is not necessarily suggestive of a high propensity for metastasis.[111,117,119,120] For example, Talmadge[111] has demonstrated convincingly the absence of significant macrophage infiltration in s.c. tumors established from poorly metastatic clones of the B16 melanoma. In this system the absence of a macrophage infiltrate does not compensate for the inability of tumor cells with intrinsically low metastatic capability to invade stromal tissue, enter the blood stream, survive transit within the circulation, and extravasate and grow into metastatic lesions. The maturational and functional status of tumor infiltrating macrophages is of equal importance to the number of tumor-infiltrating macrophages.[118,122] As discussed below (see next section), mononuclear phagocytes are responsive to activation signals for only a short time after their emigration from the circulation into the tissues.[83,121] Thus, if the majority of tumor-associated macrophages represent older, more "mature" cells, they may lack the ability to undergo activation to the tumoricidal state.

The factors influencing the recruitment of macrophages into tumors are poorly understood. It is clear, however, that in addition to recruitment signals for macrophages produced by immunologically specific T cell-mediated responses against tumor-associated antigens that generate the production of chemotactic lymphokines, nonimmune responses also influence macrophage accumulation in neoplastic lesions.[112] For example, under conditions of cytoreductive chemotherapy and subsequent necrosis of tumor tissue, the onset of nonspecific inflammatory reactions can serve as a stimulus for macrophage recruitment and/or activation.[112]

B. Macrophage Recruitment into Metastatic Tumors

As emphasized above, the mere presence of macrophages within a tumor does not mean that they are tumoricidal. Work from our laboratory has shown that mononuclear phagocytes are susceptible to activation signals for only a short time (3 to 5 days) after their emigration from the circulation.[83,122] Furthermore, the tumoricidal properties of activated macrophages decay rapidly, after which the cells become refractory to additional cycles of activation.[83] Measurement of the absolute number of tumor-associated macrophages provides little or no useful information regarding the fraction of tumoricidal macrophages. Since newly emigrated macrophages represent an important category of cells in antitumor defense mechanisms, the ability to monitor accurately the kinetics of macrophage recruitment into tumors is an essential requirement for evaluating macrophage-mediated host defense against tumors and in evaluating potential therapeutic modalities designed to augment macrophage-mediated destruction of tumor cells *in situ*.

Traditionally, macrophage recruitment into tumors has been estimated by examining single-cell suspensions prepared from enzymatic or mechanical disaggregation of tumor nodules of varying size.[112] Although widely employed, this method is hampered by the need to use large macroscopic tumors, the variable loss of cells during processing, the inability to distinguish pre-existing and newly recruited macrophages, and the inability to determine the topographic location of macrophages in the tumor.

Existing methods for the identification, localization, and characterization of tissue macrophages in both frozen and paraffin tissue sections based on histochemical identification of macrophage-associated markers such as enzymes, cell-surface receptors, or antigens are hampered by the lack of absolute specificity for macrophages together with technical difficulties in preserving these markers during tissue processing.[122-124] In addition, techniques involving pulse labeling in vivo with [³H] thymidine followed by autoradiographic analysis of histological sections, although appropriate for estimating macrophage recruitment and turnover in tissues with steady-state cell kinetics,[125,126] are clearly not relevant when dealing with tumors in which a high proportion of the tumor cells may be cycling.

Recently, we have described a new double-label histochemical technique that allows the macrophage content of tumors to be quantified in histologic sections and also permits simultaneous measurement of macrophage recruitment into metastatic tumor colonies.[127-129] This procedure exploits two well-known macrophage functions: phagocytic uptake of particulate materials and the storage of nonheme iron. The method involves the sequential systemic administration of two markers, colloidal iron and lanthanum, to tumor-bearing animals at different times during tumor development. These colloidal metal probes are cleared from blood passing through the tumor vascular bed by tumor-associated macrophages. Thus, if colloidal iron is administered to a tumor-bearing animal on day 1 and colloidal lanthanum is administered on day 5, macrophage recruitment during the 4-day period can be estimated based on differential counts of iron- (macrophages pre-existing in the lesion) and lanthanum-stained cells (newly recruited macrophages) within an individual tumor nodule.

Morphometric analysis of serial sections of several hundred lung metastases produced by the murine B16 melanoma has revealed marked heterogeneity in the macrophage content of individual metastases present in the same animal (Figure 1).[128] Furthermore, this study also revealed that the macrophage density in individual metastases drops rapidly as the lesions increase in size, reaching a uniformly low level in lesions with median cross-sectional areas of 0.01 mm² or greater.[128] Lesions of this size typically contain between 400 and 1000 melanoma cells. Assuming that cells within metastases exhibit exponential cell growth

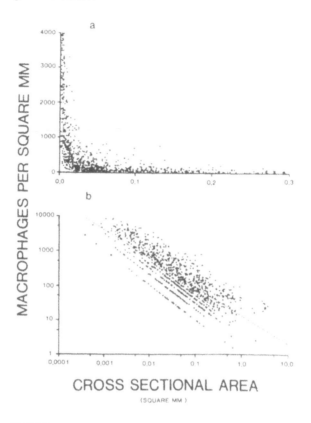

FIGURE 1. (a) Scatter diagram showing macrophage density vs. cross-sectional area. Each point represents a section from an individual metastasis. Data were collected from 9 sets of lungs, from which 954 metastases sections were evaluated. A strong negative correlation between area of metastasis and macrophage density is evident. (b) Data shown in a log-log plot. The dotted line shows the results of linear regression analysis of these data. Coefficient of correlation, −0.82. (From Bugelski, P., Kirsh, R., and Poste, G., *Am. J. Pathol.*, 118, 419, 1985. With permission.)

kinetics, it would take only 8 to 10 days to generate a metastasis of this size from a single cell for tumor cells with doubling times of 24 hr.

These findings provide a possible explanation for the failure of nonspecific immunotherapy in the treatment of large tumor burdens.[130,131] Of particular interest is the recent investigation on the optimization of therapy with liposomes containing muramyl-tripeptide phosphatidy-lethanolamine (MTP-PE).[130] In this study, primary tumors were established by s.c. inoculation of suspensions of B16 melanoma cells. Therapy with MTP-PE was started at various times after removal of the primary tumor. The success of this modality in eradicating pulmonary metastases was reduced significantly when therapy was initiated 10 days after therapy compared to day 3 or 7 after excision of the primary tumor. This observation, in concert with our results on the macrophage content of established metastatic lesions of different sizes,[128,129] suggests that successful macrophage-mediated therapy of established metastatic disease will not be useful for treatment of large tumor burdens and will more likely be of utility in eradicating residual tumor cells following conventional cytoreductive therapy.

C. Tumor Cell Escape from Macrophage-Mediated Cytotoxic Activity

Expression of the tumoricidal activity of activated macrophages in vitro or in vivo depends not only on variation in the responsiveness of the macrophages to "activation" signals depending upon their maturational status but is also regulated by a complex interplay of stimulating and suppressive signals in the microenvironment.[132] For example, E-series prostaglandins (PGE) have been shown to be potent inhibitors of several macrophage activities including release of plasminogen activator, secretion of lysosomal hydrolases, collagenase production, chemokinesis, and tumoricidal activity.[132-138] Since macrophages produce PGE and production is enhanced after activation, PGE may act as a negative-feedback signal to regulate the expression of the activated phenotype. A large number of experimental animal tumors, and also human cancers, have been shown to synthesize and contain significant amounts of PGE.[139-141] This raises the possibility that tumor-associated PGE may contribute to the lack of success obtained with immunotherapeutic treatment protocols.

Tumors may also escape detection and/or destruction by subversion of normal immunological control mechanisms mediated by suppressor T cells. Currently, little is known about suppressor T cell-mediated down regulation of macrophages. However, immune complexes of antibody and tumor-associated antigens have been demonstrated to induce a set of suppressor inducer T-lymphocytes, which following interaction with normal T-lymphocytes, induces a set of suppressor cells that can inhibit Fc receptor expression on macrophages.[142,143] Whether this set of suppressor cells can also inhibit the tumoricidal activity of macrophages is unknown. This suggests, however, that suppressor cells present in the tumor microenvironment may inhibit macrophage-mediated tumoricidal activity, and hence, play an important role in the therapy of established tumors.

Glucocorticoids have also been shown to suppress macrophage functions, including inhibition of tumoricidal activity.[138,144,145] The exact mechanism by which glucocorticoids inhibit macrophage-mediated cytotoxicity is not known. Both tissue macrophages and circulating blood monocytes have saturable corticosteroid-binding proteins with specificity for cortisol and related synthetic derivatives. Although the relationship between glucocorticoids and macrophage activation is unclear, Schultz et al.[146] demonstrated that acute stress decreased the ability of macrophages to become tumoricidal in vitro and in vivo.

In addition to physiological inhibitors of macrophage-tumoricidal activity, several groups have demonstrated that macrophage functions can be altered by peptides released by tumor cells. Snyderman and his co-workers[147,148] and Poste et al.[88,89] have demonstrated that subcutaneously growing tumors can inhibit macrophage recruitment into inflammatory lesions in vivo and reduce responsiveness to chemotactic stimuli in vitro. These effects are apparently mediated by a low molecular weight peptide released by growing tumors. Chemotactic hyporesponsiveness has often been observed in human peripheral blood monocytes from patients with cancer of the breast, lung, and prostate,[158-160] but the relationship of this effect to factors released by tumor cells has yet to be demonstrated.

V. COMMERCIAL DEVELOPMENT OF LIPOSOME-ASSOCIATED MACROPHAGE ACTIVATORS

A. Safety

The safety of a drug carrier system must be evaluated from two standpoints: the toxicity of the carrier itself and the risk of novel, drug-induced toxicities arising from differences in the disposition, pharmacokinetics, and metabolism of carrier-associated drug compared with conventional drug formulations. These criteria must be evaluated under test conditions that mimic, as closely as possible, the dose, frequency, and route of administration envisaged for clinical use.

Single doses of biodegradable particles such as liposomes and albumin microspheres are tolerated well by many animal species.[92,151-154] However, repeated dosing with particulate carriers can impair RES clearance functions. The onset, extent, and duration of RES failure is affected by particle size, dose, number, and frequency of doses. For liposomes, phospholipid composition is also relevant. Impairment of reticuloendothelial system (RES) function results from sequential saturation and exhaustion of particle clearance capacities in the liver, spleen, and bone marrow.[95] Histologic evidence of bone marrow hypoplasia and alterations in hematopoiesis have been observed in extended i.v. dosing with liposomes.[89] It is, therefore, necessary to assess the toxic liabilities associated with each proposed dosing schedule and also to evaluate the possibility of novel toxicities associated with each individual phospholipid mixture and activation mediator.

The disposition, pharmacokinetics, and metabolic fate of drugs administered in association with a carrier may differ substantially from conventional formulations of the same agents, and the risk of novel toxicities must, therefore, be considered. Perhaps the most obvious example concerns the use of liposomes and other particulate carriers to deliver anticancer drugs. By delivering high concentrations of cytotoxic drugs to mononuclear phagocytes in the blood and the RES, this approach may induce toxic ablation of a vital element of host defense. Inhibitors of DNA synthesis might be expected to have little toxic effect on nondividing macrophage populations, but drugs that impair RNA and protein synthesis may be toxic to such cells. Recent studies have shown that this fear is justified.[92,95] Systemic administration of several antitumor drugs encapsulated within liposomes enhanced the metastatic spread of mouse tumors.[95] This effect was not induced by liposomes injected subcutaneously or intramuscularly and it was reversed by injecting syngeneic macrophages 12 hr after each treatment cycle, indicating that the iatrogenic enhancement of metastases was probably caused by toxic destruction of mononuclear phagocytes.[92] The case for using liposomes or other particulate carriers for drug delivery in cancer treatment may be seriously flawed if the drug in question destroys host macrophages.

The ability of certain cytotoxic antitumor drugs to destroy the RES when administered in association with liposomes was perhaps predictable in light of existing data that identified the RES as the major site of liposome localization in vivo. This phenomenon is not unique to liposomes. Impairment of RES function has been reported in mice injected intravenously with erythrocyte ghosts containing encapsulated bleomycin.[156]

In our opinion, the potential risk posed by drug carriers that show appreciable localization in the RES is of sufficient magnitude to preclude their clinical use as carriers for cytotoxic antineoplastic drugs until extensive toxicology studies show that ablation of the RES is not induced by the specific drug(s) to be used in clinical studies. Multiple dosing with particulate carriers for long periods also presents the additional risk of RES toxicity induced by the carrier itself.

B. Commercialization of Liposome-Based Drug Carriers

Widespread application of liposomes or any other particulate drug carriers in clinical therapeutics will obviously require successful commercialization. As with all potential pharmaceutical products, the decision to embark on the high risk, lengthy, and expensive development process necessitates not only a clear definition of the scientific and technical merits of the proposed drug design, but a careful examination of both the medical need, alternative approaches, and the economic demands of product development.

The potential therapeutic advantages of a liposome-based drug delivery system for activating macrophages in vivo have been the subject of numerous scientific reports and need not be discussed further. However, the technological and economic feasibility of commercial development of liposomes for use as drug carriers is far from certain. In order to be successful within the foreseeable future, liposome production must be adapted to convenient, cost-effective, large-scale preparative methods that will not require extensive process development or a substantial capital investment in ultraspecialized instrumentation. Furthermore, the manufacturing process must be carried out under conditions acceptable to the regulatory agencies. The final product must be homogeneous, amenable to large scale production, have at least a 12 to 18 month shelf-life, and offer maximum convenience to the medical community.

Additional uncertainties arise when one considers that the response of the regulatory agencies that govern the manufacturing and marketing of pharmaceutical products to liposomes or other particulate carrier vehicles has largely gone untested. Although there are no clear precedents, the response of the Food and Drug Administration (FDA) in the U.S. to both pro-drugs and implantable controlled-release polymeric matrices suggests that liposome-associated drugs will be treated as new chemical entities (NCE) and be required to undergo the full range of toxicologic, metabolic, and pharmaceutic evaluations required for approval of any new drug administered to patients.

Although the demands of solving the scientific, technical, and economic problems associated with liposome production seem formidable, there has been extensive U.S. and international patent activity concerning the utilization and production of liposome-mediated drug delivery systems. However, with few exceptions, these patents do not address the methodological problems associated with the large-scale preparation of pharmaceutically acceptable liposomes. Furthermore, the technical and economic demands of preparing large batches of ultrapure synthetic phospholipids for use in liposome preparation do not appear to be fully appreciated. For example, assuming that experimental studies indicate that an effective liposome dose is 10 mg phospholipid per kg, then the total amount of phospholipid required for a complete pathology/toxicology evaluation of the liabilities of a liposome-based dosage form, including acute and subacute pathology at 3 dose levels in rats and dogs, as well as reproductive toxicology in rats, will be approximately 100 kg. In addition to pathology/toxicology, preclinical development will also require a complete metabolic and pharmacokinetic profile of the liposome-based drug formulation and a thorough physico-chemical characterization of the final formulation to be administered to patients. This coupled with the amount of phospholipid required for production of clinical supplies for phase I, II, and III clinical trials prior to launch into the market, dictates that several hundred kilograms of purified phospholipid must be available for each drug tested.

Economic considerations such as this clearly suggest that other particulate microcarrier systems such as multiphase emulsions and biodegradable polymeric nanoparticles, which share many of the advantageous properties of liposomes, deserve careful evaluation. Prevailing commercial factors currently favor these alternative drug carriers because they can be produced as pharmaceutically acceptable formulations at far less cost than liposomes using existing equipment and manufacturing processes universally available within the pharmaceutical industry. In this regard, one emulsion-based drug delivery system containing diazapam is currently available commercially for parenteral use.

VI. SUMMARY

The mechanisms by which mononuclear phagocytes discriminate between self and nonself, recognize foreign materials, senescent, damaged, old or effete cells, and tumor cells are unknown. However, irrespective of the mechanism(s) involved, once activated by the appropriate signals, macrophages demonstrate the capability to selectively recognize and destroy neoplastic cells in vitro and in vivo.

Liposomes injected intravenously, in common with other particulate or polymeric matrices localize preferentially in organs with high mononuclear phagocyte activity and also circulating blood monocytes. As such, microparticulates offer convenient systems for the selective delivery of encapsulated drugs to cells of the mononuclear phagocyte series in vivo. Liposomes are a particularly attractive experimental system because of their capacity to incorporate a wide variety of water-soluble and lipid-soluble drugs, however, at this time there is no reason to assume that a liposome-based drug delivery system will offer any significant therapeutic advantage compared to other microparticulate drug delivery systems.

Liposomes containing macrophage-activating agents are highly effective at augmenting macrophage-mediated tumoricidal activity in vitro and eradicating tumor metastasis in vivo. The effectiveness of this modality is highly encouraging when one considers that metastatic disease is the major cause of treatment failure in cancer therapeutics.

Analysis of metastatic lesions from animals that have residual metastatic disease (albeit reduced compared with untreated control mice) following treatment with liposome-encapsulated macrophage activating agents has revealed that the tumor cells present in these lesions are still fully susceptible to destruction by activated macrophages. This is consistent with the evidence discussed earlier which suggests that tumor cell resistance to killing by activated macrophages is not likely to be a rate-limiting factor in the effectiveness of liposome-encapsulated macrophage activators. The more challenging problem will be the extent of the tumor burden at the time that therapy is initiated and the possibility that signals that suppress the activated phenotype are present in sufficient concentrations to suppress any therapeutic effect.

In order to successfully utilize liposome-encapsulated immunomodulators it will most likely be necessary to evaluate this modality in combination with conventional antineoplastic chemo- and radiotherapeutic protocols. In addition to the obvious advantages of reducing tumor burden, cytoreductive therapy can offer several other benefits. First, tumor necrosis and release of nonspecific chemoattractants could augment the recruitment of macrophages into the lesion, thereby improving the efficacy of this modality by increasing the intralesional macrophage-to-tumor cell ratio. Second, the reduced antigen load could serve to decrease immune complex-mediated generation of suppressor inducer cells, and third, as T-suppressor cells present in tumors are known to be radiosensitive, γ irradiation could serve to abolish the detrimental effects of T-suppressor cells on macrophage-mediated host defenses. Studies to evaluate the efficacy of liposome-encapsulated host defenses in combination with chemo- and radiotherapeutic regimens in treating metastatic disease are currently in progress.

Although the demands of solving the scientific and technical problems associated with liposome development are substantial, the extraordinary rate of scientific achievement in both biology and pharmaceutics greatly enhances the prospect of success with at least several aspects of liposome-mediated drug delivery. The next few years will be crucial in determining whether the commercial development of liposomes is feasible or whether they will join the ranks of other drug carrier designs that have failed to fulfill their initial promise.

REFERENCES

1. **Metchnikoff, E.,** *Immunity in Infectious Disease,* Cambridge University Press, London, 1905.
2. **Eccles, S. A.,** Macrophages and cancer, in *Immunological Aspects of Cancer,* Castro, J. E., Ed., University Park Press, Baltimore, 1978, 123.
3. **Fidler, I. J. and Poste, G.,** Macrophage-mediated destruction of malignant tumor cells and new strategies for the therapy of metastastic disease, *Springer Semin. Immunopathol.,* 5, 161, 1982.
4. **Altura, B. M.,** Reticuloendothelial cells and host defense, *Adv. Microcirc.,* 9, 252, 1980.
5. **Chirigos, M. A., Mitchell, M., Mastrangelo, M. J., and Krim, M., Eds.,** *Modulation of Cellular Immunity in Cancer by Immune Modifiers,* Raven Press, New York, 1981.
6. **Witz, I. P. and Hanna, M. G., Jr., Eds.,** In situ expression of tumor immunity, *Contemp. Top. Immunobiol.,* 10, 1, 1980.
7. **Norbury, K. and Kripke, M. L.,** Ultraviolet-induced carcinogenesis in mice treated with silica, trypan blue or pyran copolymer, *J. Reticuloendothel. Soc.,* 26, 827, 1979.

8. **Mantovani, A., Giavazzi, R., Polentanitti, N., Spreafico, F., and Garattini, S.,** Divergent effects of macrophage toxins on growth of primary tumors and lung metastases in mice, *Int. J. Cancer,* 25, 617, 1980.
9. **North, R. J.,** The concept of activated macrophages, *J. Immunol.,* 121, 806, 1978.
10. **Fidler, I. J. and Raz, A.,** The induction of tumoricidal capacities in mouse and rat macrophages by lymphokines, in *Lymphokines,* Pick E., Ed., Academic Press, New York, 1981, 345.
11. **Poste, G., Kirsh, R., Fogler, W. E., and Fidler, I. J.,** Activation of tumoricidal properties in mouse macrophages by lymphokines encapsulated in liposomes, *Cancer Res.,* 39, 881, 1979.
12. **Kleinerman, E. S. and Fidler, I. J.,** Macrophage activation by lymphokines: usefulness as antineoplastic agents, in *Novel Approaches to Cancer Chemotherapy,* Sunkara, P. S., Ed., Academic Press, Orlando, Fla., 1984, 232.
13. **Fidler, I. J. and Cifone, M. A.,** Properties of metastatic and nonmetastatic cloned subpopulations of an ultraviolet light-induced murine fibrosarcoma of recent origin, *Am. J. Pathol.,* 97, 633, 1979.
14. **Fidler, I. J. and Kripke, M. L.,** Biological variability within murine neoplasms, *Antibiot. Chemother.,* 28, 123, 1980.
15. **Poste, G. and Greig, R.,** On the genesis and regulation of cellular heterogeneity in malignant tumors, *Invasion and Metastasis,* 2, 137, 1982.
16. **Kerbel, R. S.,** Implications of immunological heterogeneity of tumors, *Nature (London),* 280, 358, 1979.
17. **Owens, A. H., Coffey, D. S., and Baylin, S. B., Eds.,** in *Tumor Cell Heterogeneity: Origins and Implications,* Academic Press, New York, 1982.
18. **Sluyser, M. and Van Nie, R.,** Estrogen receptor content and hormone responsive growth of mouse mammary tumors, *Cancer Res.,* 34, 3252, 1974.
19. **Sluyser, M., Evers, S. G., and DeGoey, C. C.,** Sex hormone receptors in mammary tumours of GR mice, *Nature (London),* 263, 386, 1976.
20. **Prehn, R. T.,** Analysis of antigenic heterogeneity within individual 3-methylcholanthrene-induced mouse sarcomas, *J. Natl. Cancer Inst.,* 45, 1039, 1970.
21. **Sugarbaker, E. V. and Cohen, A. M.,** Altered antigenicity in spontaneous pulmonary metastases from an antigenic murine sarcoma, *Surgery,* 72, 155, 1972.
22. **Miller, F. R. and Heppner, G. H.,** Immunologic heterogeneity of tumor cell subpopulations from a single mouse mammary tumor, *J. Natl. Cancer Inst.,* 63, 1457, 1979.
23. **Heppner, G. H., Dexter, D. L., DeNucci, T., Miller, F. R., and Calabresi, P.,** Heterogeneity in drug sensitivity among tumor cell subpopulations of a single mammary tumor, *Cancer Res.,* 38, 3758, 1978.
24. **Trope, C.,** Different sensitivity to cytostatic drugs of primary tumor and metastasis of the Lewis carcinoma, *Neoplasma,* 22, 171, 1975.
25. **Trope, C.,** Different susceptibilities of tumor cell subpopulations to cytotoxic agents, in *Design of Models for Testing Cancer Therapeutic Agents,* Fidler, I. S. and White, R. J., Eds., Van Nostrand Reinhold, New York, 1981, 64.
26. **Rose, N. and Siegel, B. V., Eds.,** The reticuloendothelial system: a comprehensive treatise, in *Immunopathology,* Vol. 4, Plenum Press, New York, 1983.
27. **Hanna, N.,** Role of natural killer cells in control of cancer metastasis, *Cancer Metastasis Rev.,* 1, 45, 1982.
28. **Cohn, Z. A.,** The activation of mononuclear phagocytes: fact, fancy and future, *J. Immunol.,* 121, 813, 1978.
29. **Alexander, P. and Evans, R.,** Endotoxin and double stranded RNA render macrophages cytotoxic, *Nature (London),* 232, 76, 1971.
30. **Cleveland, R. P., Meltzer, M. S., and Zbar, B.,** Tumor cytotoxicity in vitro by macrophages from mice infected with *Mycobacterium bovis* strain BCG, *J. Natl. Cancer Inst.,* 52, 1887, 1974.
31. **Droller, M. J. and Remington, J. S.,** A role for the macrophage in the in vivo and in vitro resistance to murine bladder tumor cell growth, *Cancer Res.,* 35, 49, 1975.
32. **Kaplan, A. M., Morahan, P. S., and Regilson, W.,** Induction of macrophage mediated tumor cell cytotoxicity by pyran copolymer, *J. Natl. Cancer Inst.,* 52, 1919, 1974.
33. **Scott, M. T.,** In vivo cortisone sensitivity of nonspecific antitumor activity of *Corynebacterium parvum* activated mouse peritoneal macrophages, *J. Natl. Cancer Inst.,* 54, 789, 1975.
34. **Sone, S. and Fidler, I. J.,** In situ activation of tumoricidal properties in rat alveolar macrophages and rejection of experimental lung metastases by intravenous injections of *Nocardia rubra* cell wall skeleton, *Cancer Immunol. Immunother.,* 12, 203, 1982.
35. **Chihara, G., Maeda, Y. Y., Hamuro, J., Sasaki, T., and Fukuoka, F.,** Inhibition of mouse sarcoma 180 by the polysaccharide from *Lentinus erodes, Nature (London),* 222, 687, 1969.
36. **Chirigos, M. A., Ed.,** Immune modulation and control of neoplasia by adjuvant therapy, *Progress in Cancer Research and Therapy,* Vol. 7, Raven Press, New York, 1978.
37. **Fenichel, R. and Chirigos, M. A., Eds.,** *Immune Modulating Agents and Their Mechanisms,* Vol. 25, Marcel Dekker, New York, 1985.

38. **Halper, B.**, *Corynebacterium parvum: Applications in Experimental and Clinical Oncology*, Plenum Press, New York, 1975.

39. **Hersh, E., Chirigos, M. A., and Mastrangelo, A.**, Eds., Augmenting agents in cancer therapy, *Progress in Cancer Research and Therapy*, Vol. 16, Raven Press, New York, 1981.

40. **Mihich, E.**, Ed., *Immunological Approaches to Cancer Therapeutics*, John Wiley & Sons, New York, 1982.

41. **Okamoto, H., Shoin, S., and Kashimura, S.**, Streptomycin S-forming and anti-tumor activities of group A streptococci, in *Bacterial Toxins and Cell Membranes*, Jeljaszewica, J. and Waldstrom, T., Eds., Academic Press, New York, 1978, 259.

42. **Lederer, E.**, Synthetic immunostimulants derived from the bacterial cell wall, *J. Med. Chem.*, 23, 819, 1980.

43. **Parant, M., Parant, F., Chedid, L., Yapo, A., Petit, J. F., and Lederer, L.**, Fate of the synthetic immunoadjuvant, muramyl dipeptide (^{14}C-labelled) in the mouse, *Int. J. Immunopharmacol.*, 1, 35, 1979.

44. **Chedid, L. and Audibert, F.**, New approaches for control of infections using synthetic or semi-synthetic constructs containing MDP, *Springer Semin. Immunopathol.*, 8, 401, 1985.

45. **Chedid, L., Parant, M., Parant, F., Lefrancier, P., Choay, J., and Lederer, E.**, Enhancement of nonspecific immunity to *Klebsiella pneumoniae* infection by a synthetic immunoadjuvant (N-acetyl-mura-myl-L-alanyl-D-isoglutamine) and several analogs, *Proc. Natl. Acad. Sci. U.S.A.*, 74, 2089, 1977.

46. **Dietrich, F. M., Sackmann, W., Zak, O., and Dukor, P.**, Synthetic muramyl dipeptide immunosti-mulants: protective effects and increased efficacy antibiotics in experimental bacterial and fungal infections in mice, in *Current Chemotherapy and Infectious Disease*, Vol. 2, Nelson, J. D. and Grassi, C., Eds., Am. Soc. Microbiol., Washington, D. C., 1980, 1730.

47. **Fraser-Smith, E. B. and Matthews, T. R.**, Protective effects of muramyl dipeptide analogs against infections of *Pseudomonas aeruginosa* or *Candida albicans* in mice, *Infect. Immunol.*, 34, 676, 1981.

48. **Humphries, R. C., Heniki, P. R., Ferraresi, R. W., and Krahenbuhl, J. L.**, Effects of treatment with muramyl dipeptide and certain of its analogs on resistance to *Listeria monocytogenes* in mice, *Infect. Immunol.*, 30, 462, 1980.

49. **Matthews, T. R. and Fraser-Smith, E. B.**, Protective effect of muramyl dipeptide and analogs against *Pseudomonas aeruginosa* and *Candida albicans* infections in mice, *Current Chemotherapy of Infectious Disease*, Vol. 2, Am. Soc. Microbiol., Washington D.C., 1980, 1734.

50. **Onozuka, K., Saito-Taki, T., and Nakano, M.**, Effect of muramyl dipeptide analog on *Salmonella enteritidis* infection in beige mice with Chediak-Higashi syndrome, *Microbiol. Immunol.*, 28, 1211, 1984.

51. **Parant, M., Parant, F., and Chedid, L.**, Enhancement of the neonate's nonspecific immunity to Klebsiella infection by muramyl dipeptide, a synthetic immunoadjuvant, *Proc. Natl. Acad. Sci. U.S.A.*, 75, 3395, 1978.

52. **Kierszenbaum, F. and Ferraresi, R. W.**, Enhancement of host resistance against *Trypanosoma cruzi* infection by the immunoregulatory agent muramyl dipeptide, *Infect. Immunol.*, 25, 273, 1979.

53. **Krahenbuhl, J. L. and Humphries, R. C.**, Effects of treatment with muramyl dipeptide on resistance to *Mycobacterium leprae* and *Mycobacterium marinum* infection in mice, *Immunopharmacology*, 5, 329, 1983.

54. **Dietrich, F. M., Lukas, B., and Schmidt-Rupin, K. H.**, MTP-PE (synthetic muramyl peptide): prophy-lactic and therapeutic effects in experimental viral infections, Commun. 13th Int. Cong. Chemother., Vienna, August 28, 1983.

55. **Lukas, B., Schmidt-Rupin, K. H., and Dietrich, F. M.**, Prophylactic and therapeutic effects of MTP-PE, a synthetic muramyl peptide, in experimental virus infections, Proc. Int. Symp. on Immunomodulation by Chemically-Defined Adjuvants, Sapporo, Japan, 1983, 42.

56. **Koff, W. C., Showalter, S. D., Seniff, D. A., and Hampar, B.**, Lysis of herpesvirus-infected cells by macrophages activated with free or liposome-encapsulated lymphokine produced by murine T cell hybridoma, *Infect. Immun.*, 42, 1067, 1983.

57. **Koff, W. C., Fidler, I. J., Showalter, S. D., Chakrabarty, M. K., Hampar, B., Ceccorulli, L. M., and Kleinerman, E. S.**, Human monocytes activated by immunomodulators in liposomes lyse herpesvirus-infected but not normal cells, *Science*, 224, 1007, 1984.

58. **Fidler, I. J.**, In situ induction of tumoricidal activity in alveolar macrophages by liposomes containing muramyl dipeptide is a thymus-independent progress, *J. Immunol.*, 127, 1719, 1981.

59. **Fidler, I. J. and Poste, G.**, Macrophage destruction of micrometastases, in *Manual of Macrophage Methodology*, Herscowitz, H. B., Holden, H. T., Bellanti, J. A., and Ghaffar, A., Eds., Marcel Dekker, New York, 1981, 509.

60. **Fidler, I. J. and Poste, G.**, Treatment of spontaneous murine metastases by the systemic administration of liposomes containing macrophage-activating agents, in *Cancer: Achievements, Challenges and Prospects for the 1980's*, Vol. 2, Burchenal, J. H. and Oettgen, H. F., Eds., Grune & Stratton, New York, 1981, 77.

61. **Poste, G., Kirsh, R., and Fidler, I. J.**, Cell surface receptors for lymphokines, *Cell. Immunol.*, 44, 71, 1979.
62. **Andreesen, R., Bross, K. J., Osterholz, J., and Emmrich, F.**, Human macrophage maturation and heterogeneity: analysis with a newly generated set of monoclonal antibodies to differentiation antigens, *Blood*, 67(5), 1257, 1986.
63. **Shen, H. H., Talle, M. A., Goldstein, G., and Chess, L.**, Functional subsets of human monocytes defined by monoclonal antibodies. A distinct subset of monocytes contains the cells capable of inducing the autologous mixed lymphocytes culture, *J. Immunol.*, 130, 698, 1983.
64. **Zembala, M., Uracz, W., Ruggiero, I., Mytar, B., and Pryjma, J.**, Isolation and functional characterization of FcR$^+$ and FcR$^-$ human monocyte subsets, *J. Immunol.*, 133, 1293, 1984.
65. **Schreiber, R. D., Pace, J. L., Russell, S. W., Altman, A., and Katz, D. H.**, Macrophage-activating factor produced by a T cell hybridoma: physiochemical and biosynthetic resemblance of γ-interferon, *J. Immunol.*, 131, 826, 1983.
66. **Le, J., Prensky, W., Yip, Y. K., Chang, Z., Hoffman, T., Stevenson, H. C., Balazs, I., Sadlik, J. R., and Vilcek, J.**, Activation of human monocyte cytotoxicity by natural and recombinant immune interferon, *J. Immunol.*, 131, 2821, 1984.
67. **Schultz, R. M.**, Macrophage activating by interferons, in *Lymphokine Reports*, Vol. 1, Pick, E., Ed., Academic Press, New York, 1980, 63.
68. **Pace, J. L., Russell, S. W., Schreiber, R. D., Altman, A., and Katz, D. H.**, Macrophage activation: priming activity from a T-cell hybridoma is attributable to interferon-γ, *Proc. Natl. Acad. Sci. U.S.A.*, 80, 3782, 1983.
69. **Schreiber, R. D., Pace, J. L., Russell, S. W., Altman, A., and Katz, D. H.**, Macrophage activating factor produced by a T cell hybridoma: physiochemical and biosynthetic resemblance to γ-interferon, *J. Immunol.*, 131, 826, 1983.
70. **Roberts, W. K. and Vasil, A.**, Evidence for the identity of murine gamma interferon and macrophage activating factor, *J. Interferon Res.*, 2, 519, 1982.
71. **Kleinschmidt, W. J. and Schultz, R. M.**, Similarities of murine gamma interferon and the lymphokine that renders macrophages cytotoxic, *J. Interferon Res.*, 2, 291, 1982.
72. **Kleinerman, E. S., Zicht, R., Sarin, P. S., Gallo, R. C., and Fidler, J.**, Constitutive production and release of a lymphokine with macrophage activating factor activity distinct from γ-interferon by a human T cell leukemia virus-positive cell line, *Cancer Res.*, 44, 4470, 1984.
73. **Meltzer, M. S., Gilbreath, M., Nacy, C. A., and Schreiber, R. D.**, Macrophage activation factor from EL-4 cells distinct from murine gamma interferon (IFN), *Fed. Proc. Fed. Am. Soc. Exp. Biol.*, 44, (Abstr.), 1697, 1985.
74. **Crawford, R., Hoover, D., Finbloom, D., Gilbreath, M., Nacy, C., and Meltzer, M.**, Physicochemical properties of a human lymphokine (LK) distinct from gamma interferon (IFN) that activates monocytes to kill *Leishmania donovani*, *Fed. Proc. Fed. Am. Soc. Exp. Biol.*, 44 (Abstr.), 1697, 1985.
75. **Lee, J. C., Rebar, L., Young, P., Ruscetti, R. W., Hanna, N., and Poste, G.**, Identification and characterization of a human T cell line-derived lymphokine with MAF-like activity distinct from interferon-γ, *J. Immunol.*, 136, 1322, 1986.
76. **Pace, J. L., Russell, S. W., Torres, B. A., Johnson, H. M., and Gray, P. W.**, Recombinant mouse interferon induces the priming step in macrophage activation for tumor cell killing, *J. Immunol.*, 130, 2011, 1983.
77. **Grabstein, K. H., Urdal, D. L., Tushinski, R. J., Mochizuki, D. Y., Price, V. L., Cantrell, M. A., Gillis, S., and Conlon, P. J.**, Induction of macrophage tumoricidal activity by granulocyte-macrophage colony-stimulating factor, *Science*, 232, 506, 1986.
78. **Papermaster, B. W., Holterman, O. A., and Klein, E.**, Preliminary observations on tumor regressions induced by local administration of a lymphoid cell culture supernatant fraction in patients with cutaneous metastatic lesions, *Clin. Immunol. Immunopathol.*, 5, 31, 1976.
79. **North, R. J. and Bursuker, I.**, The generation and decay of the immune response to a progressive fibrosarcoma. I. Lyl$^+$2$^-$ suppressor T cells down regulate and generation of Lyl$^-$2$^+$ effector T cells, *J. Exp. Med.*, 159, 1295, 1984.
80. **Dye, E. S. and North, R. J.**, Specificity of T cells that mediate and suppress adoptive immunotherapy of an established tumor, *J. Leukocyte Biol.*, 36, 27, 1984.
81. **North, R. J. and Dye, E. S.**, Ly-1$^+$2$^-$ suppressor T cells down-regulate the generation of Ly-1$^-$2$^+$ effector T cells during progressive growth of the P815 mastocytoma, *Immunology*, 54, 47, 1985.
82. **Bursuker, I. and North, R. J.**, Suppression of generation of concomitant immunity by passively transferred suppressor T cells from tumor-bearing donors, *Cancer Immunol. Immunother.*, 19, 215, 1985.
83. **Poste, G. and Kirsh, R.**, Rapid decay of tumoricidal activity and loss of responsiveness to lymphokines in inflammatory macrophages, *Cancer Res.*, 39, 2582, 1979.
84. **Poste, G.**, Experimental systems for analysis of the malignant phenotype, *Cancer Metastasis Rev.*, 1, 141, 1982.

85. **Fidler, I. J. and White, R. W., Eds.,** *Design of Models for Testing Cancer Chemotherapeutic Agents,* Van Nostrand Reinhold, New York, 1982.

86. **Poste, G.,** Tumor cell heterogeneity and the pathogenesis of cancer metastasis, in *Basic Mechanisms and Clinical Treatment of Tumor Metastasis,* Torisu, M. and Yoshida, T., Eds., Academic Press, New York, 1985, 79.

87. **Poste, G. and Greig, R.,** Experimental models for studying the pathogenesis and therapy of metastatic disease, in *Mechanisms of Cancer Metastasis: Potential Therapeutic Implications,* Honn, K. V., Ed., Martinus Nijhoff, Boston, 1986, 41.

88. **Poste, G.,** Pathogenesis of metastatic disease: implications for current therapy and for the development of new therapeutic strategies, *Cancer Treatment Rep.,* 70, 183, 1986.

89. **Poste, G., Kirsh, R., and Bugelski, P.,** Liposomes as a drug delivery system in cancer therapy, in *Novel Approaches to Cancer Chemotherapy,* Sunkara, P., Ed., Academic Press, Orlando, Fla., 1984, 166.

90. **Folkman, J. and Haudenschild, C.,** Induction of capillary growth in vitro, in *Cellular Interactions,* Dingle, J. T. and Gordon, J. L., Eds., Elsevier, Amsterdam, 1981, 119.

91. **Poste, G. and Fidler, I. J.,** The pathogenesis of cancer metastasis, *Nature (London),* 283, 139, 1980.

92. **Poste, G., Kirsh, R., and Koestler, T.,** The challenge of liposome targeting in vivo, in *Lipsome Technology,* Gregoriadis, G., Ed., CRC Press, Boca Raton, Fla., 1983, 1.

93. **Gregoriadis, G., Senior, J., and Trouet, A., Eds.,** *Targeting of Drugs,* NATO Advanced Studies Institute Series, Vol. A47, Plenum Press, New York, 1982.

94. **Gregoriadis, G., Senior, J., Poste, G., and Trouet, A., Eds.,** *Receptor-Mediated Targeting of Drugs,* Plenum Press, New York, in press, 1985.

95. **Poste, G.,** Liposome targeting in vivo: problems and opportunities, *Biol. Cell,* 47, 19, 1983.

96. **Poste, G., Kirsh, R., Fogler, W. E., and Fidler, I. J.,** Analysis of the fate of systemically administered liposomes and implications for their use in drug delivery, *Cancer Res.,* 42, 1412, 1982.

97. **Poste, G. and Kirsh, R.,** Site-specific (targeted) drug delivery in cancer therapy, *Biotechnology,* 1, 869, 1983.

98. **Fidler, I. J., Raz, A., Fogler, W. E., Bugelski, P., Kirsh, R., and Poste, G.,** Design of liposomes to improve delivery of macrophage-augmenting agents to alveolar macrophages, *Cancer Res.,* 40, 4460, 1980.

99. **Fidler, I. J., Raz, A., Fogler, W. E., Hoyer, L. C., and Poste, G.,** The role of plasma membrane receptors and the kinetics of macrophage activation by lymphokines encapsulated in liposomes, *Cancer Res.,* 41, 495, 1981.

100. **Poste, G., Kirsh, R., Raz, S., Bucana, C., Fogler, W. E., and Fidler, I. J.,** Activation of tumoricidal properties in macrophages by liposome-encapsulated lymphokines: in vitro studies, in *Liposomes and Immunology,* Tom, B. H. and Six, H. R., Eds., Elsevier, Amsterdam, 1980, 93.

101. **Pidgeon, C., Schreiber, R. D., and Schultz, R. M.,** Macrophage activation: synergism between hybridoma MAF and poly (I)-poly (C) delivered by liposomes, *J. Immunol.,* 131, 311, 1983.

102. **Fidler, I. J., Hart, I. R., Raz, A., Fogler, W. E., Kirsh, R., and Poste, G.,** Activation of tumoricidal properties in macrophages by liposome-encapsulated lymphokines: in vivo studies, in *Liposomes and Immunobiology,* Tom, B. H. and Six, H. R., Eds., Elsevier, Amsterdam, 1980, 109.

103. **Deodhar, S. D., Barna, B. P., Edinger, M., and Chiang, T.,** Inhibition of lung metastases by liposomal immunotherapy in a murine fibrosarcoma model, *J. Biol. Response Modif.,* 1, 27, 1982.

104. **Kleinerman, E. S. and Fidler, I. J.,** Macrophage activation by lymphokines: usefulness as antimetastatic agents, in *Novel Approaches to Cancer Chemotherapy,* Sunkara, P., Ed., Academic Press, New York, 1984, 234.

105. **Kleinerman, E. S. and Fidler, I. J.,** Production and utilization of human lymphokines containing macrophage-activating factor (MAF) activity, *Lymphokine Res.,* 2, 7, 1983.

106. **Kleinerman, E. S., Schroit, A. J., Fogler, W. E., and Fidler, I. J.,** Tumoricidal activity of human monocytes activated in vitro by free and liposome-encapsulated human lymphokines, *J. Clin. Invest.,* 72, 1, 1983.

107. **Schroit, A. J. and Fidler, I. J.,** The design of liposomes for delivery of immunomodulators to host defense cells, in *Medical Applications of Liposomes,* Yagi, K., Ed., Japan Scientific Societies Press, Tokyo, 1986, 141.

108. **Yagi, K.,** *Medical Application of Liposomes,* Japan Scientific Societies Press, Tokyo, 1986.

109. **Talmadge, J. E., Adams, J., Phillips, H., Collins, M., Lenz, B., Schnedier, M., and Chirigos, M.,** Immunotherapeutic potential of poly ICLC in murine tumor models, *Cancer Res.,* 45, 1066, 1985.

110. **Talmadge, J. E. and Chirigos, M. A.,** Comparison of immunomodulatory and immunotherapeutic properties of biologic response modifiers, *Springer Semin. Immunopathol.,* 8, 429, 1985.

111. **Talmadge, J. E., Key, M., and Fidler, I. J.,** Macrophage content of metastatic and nonmetastatic rodent neoplasms, *J. Immunol.,* 126, 2245, 1981.

112. **Key, M. E.,** Macrophages of cancer metastases and their relevance to metastatic growth, *Cancer Metastasis Rev.,* 2, 75, 1983.

113. **Eccles, S. A. and Alexander, P.**, Macrophage content of tumours in relation to metastatic spread and host immune reaction, *Nature (London)*, 250, 667, 1974.
114. **Eccles, S. A. and Alexander, P.**, Sequestration of macrophages in growing tumors and its effect on the immunological capacity of the host, *Br. J. Cancer*, 30, 42, 1974.
115. **Birbeck, M. S. and Carter, R. L.**, Observations of the ultrastructure of two hamster lymphomas with particular reference to infiltrating macrophages, *Int. J. Cancer*, 9, 249, 1972.
116. **Wood, G. W. and Gillespie, G. Y.**, Studies on the role of macrophages in regulation of growth and metastasis of murine chemically induced fibrosarcoma, *Int. J. Cancer*, 16, 1022, 1975.
117. **Evans, R. and Lawler, E. M.**, Macrophage content and immunogenicity of C57BL/6J and BALB/cBYJ methylcholanthrene induced sarcomas, *Int. J. Cancer*, 26, 831, 1980.
118. **Mahoney, K. H., Fulton, A. M., and Heppner, G. H.**, Tumor associated macrophages of mouse mammary tumors. II. Differential distribution of macrophages form metastatic and non-metastatic tumors, *J. Immunol.*, 131, 2079, 1983.
119. **Vose, B. M.**, Cytotoxicity of adherent cells associated with some human tumors and lung tissues, *Cancer Immunol. Immunother.*, 5, 173, 1978.
120. **Gauci, C. L. and Alexander, P.**, The macrophage content of some human tumors, *Cancer Lett.*, 1, 29, 1975.
121. **Poste, G.**, The tumoricidal properties of inflammatory tissue macrophages and multinucleate giant cells, *Am. J. Pathol.*, 96, 95, 1979.
122. **Ault, K. A. and Springer, T. A.**, Cross reaction of a rat antimouse phagocyte-specific monoclonal antibody (Anti Mac-I) with human monocytes and natural killer cells, *J. Immunol.*, 126, 359, 1981.
123. **Brown, R. and Wolman, M.**, Differentiation of macrophages from Lewis lung carcinoma tumor cells in tissue sections by their α-naphthyl butyrate esterase activity, *Histochem. J.*, 13, 975, 1981.
124. **Wood, G. W. and Gollahon, K. A.**, Detection and quantitation of macrophage infiltration into primary human tumors with the use of cell surface markers, *J. Natl. Cancer Inst.*, 59, 1081, 1977.
125. **van Furth, R. and Blusse van Oud Alblas, A.**, The current view on the origin of pulmonary macrophages, *Pathol. Res. Pract.*, 174, 38, 1982.
126. **Blusse van Oud Alblas, A. and van Furth, R.**, The origin, kinetics and characteristics of pulmonary macrophages in the normal steady state, *J. Exp. Med.*, 149, 1504, 1979.
127. **Bugelski, P., Kirsh, R., and Poste, G.**, A new histochemical method for measuring intratumoral macrophages and macrophage recruitment into experimental metastases, *Cancer Res.*, 43, 5493, 1983.
128. **Bugelski, P., Kirsh, R., and Poste, G.**, Changes in the macrophage content of lung metastases at different stages in tumor growth, *Am. J. Pathol.*, 118, 419, 1985.
129. **Bugelski, P. J., Kirsh, R., Buscarino, C., Corwin, S. P., and Poste, G.**, Recruitment of exogenous macrophages into metastases at different stages of tumor growth, *Cancer Immunol. Immunother.*, 24, 93, 1987.
130. **Hollinshead, A.**, Immunotherapy trials: current status and future directions with special emphasis on biologic drugs, *Springer Semin. Immunopathol.*, 9, 85, 1986.
131. **Fidler, I. J.**, Optimization and limitations of systemic treatment of murine melanoma metastases with liposomes containing muramyl tripeptide phosphatidylethanolamine, *Cancer Immunol. Immunother.*, 21, 169, 1986.
132. **Hibbs, J. B., Taintor, R. R., Chapman, H. A., and Weinberg, J. B.**, Macrophage tumor killing: influence of the local environment, *Science*, 197, 279, 1977.
133. **Bonney, R. J., Wightman, P. D., Davies, P., Sadoneski, S. J., Keuh, F. A., and Humes, S. L.**, Regulation of prostaglandin synthesis and of elective release of lysosomal hydrolases by mouse peritoneal macrophages, *Biochem. J.*, 176, 433, 1978.
134. **Gallin, J. I., Sandler, J. A., Clyman, R. I., Manganiello, V. C., and Vaughn, M.**, Agents that increase cyclic-AMP inhibit accumulation of CGMP and depress human monocyte locomotion, *J. Immunol.*, 114, 1472, 1978.
135. **Schultz, R. M., Stoychkov, J. N., Pavlidis, N., Chirgos, M., and Olkowski, Z. L.**, Role of E-type prostaglandins in the regulation of interferon-treated macrophage cytolytic activity, *J. Reticuloendothel. Soc.*, 26, 93, 1979.
136. **Snyder, D. S., Beller, D. I., and Unanue, E. R.**, Prostaglandins modulate macrophage Ia expression, *Nature (London)*, 299, 163, 1982.
137. **Weissman, G., Zurier, R. B., Spieler, P. J., and Goldstein, I. M.**, Mechanisms of lysosomal enzyme release from leukocytes exposed to immune complexes and other particles, *J. Exp. Med.*, 134, 149, 1981.
138. **Vasalli, J., Hamilton, J., and Reich, E.**, Macrophage plasminogen activator: modulation of enzyme production by antiinflammatory steroids, mitotic inhibitors and cyclic nucleotides, *Cell*, 8, 271, 1976.
139. **Stamford, I. F., MacIntyre, J., and Bennett, A.**, Human breast carcinomas release prostaglandin-like material into the blood, in *Advances in Prostaglandin and Thromboxane Research*, Vol. 6, Samuelson, B., Ramwell, P. W., and Paoletti, R., Eds., Raven Press, New York, 1980, 571.

140. **Fiedler, L., Zahrandnik, H. P., and Schlegel, G.,** Perioperative behavior of prostaglandin E$_2$ and 13, 14-dihydro-15-keto-PGF$_2$ in serum of bronchial carcinoma patients, in *Advances in Prostaglandin and Thromboxane Research,* Samuelson, B., Ramwell, P. W., and Paoletti, R., Eds., Raven Press, New York, 1980, 585.

141. **Bennett, A., Berstock, D. A., Harris, M., Raja, B., Rowe, D. J. F., Stamford, I. F., and Wright, J. E.,** Prostaglandins and their relationships to malignant and benign human breast tumors, in *Advances in Prostaglandin and Thromboxane Research,* Vol. 6, Samuelson, B., Ramwell, P. W., and Paoletti, R., Eds., Raven Press, New York, 1980, 595.

142. **Rao, V. S., Bennett, J. A., Grodzicki, R. L., and Mitchell, M. S.,** Suppressor T cells induced by immune complexes can adoptively transfer inhibition of cytophilic antibody receptors on macrophages, *Cell. Immunol.,* 46, 227, 1979.

143. **Rao, V. S., Mokyr, M. B., Gershon, R. K., and Mitchell, M. S.,** Specific T cell dependent, antigen-antibody induced suppression of macrophages: abrogation by non-specifically stimulated T cells, *J. Immunol.,* 118, 2117, 1977.

144. **Bray, M. A. and Gordon, D.,** Prostaglandin production by macrophages and the effect of antiinflammatory drugs, *Br. J. Pharmacol.,* 63, 635, 1978.

145. **Reinhart, S., Sagone, A. L., Balcerzak, S. P., Ackerman, G. A., and LoBuglio, P.,** Effects of corticosteroid therapy on human monocyte function, *N. Engl. J. Med.,* 292, 236, 1975.

146. **Schultz, R. M., Chirgos, M. A., Stoychkov, J. N., and Pavlidis, N. A.,** Factors affecting macrophage cytolytic activity with particular emphasis on corticosteroids and acute stress, *J. Reticuloendothel. Soc.,* 26, 83, 1979.

147. **Snyderman, P., Meadows, L., Holder, W., and Wells, S.,** Abnormal monocyte chemotaxis on breast cancer: evidence for a tumor mediated effect, *J. Natl. Cancer Inst.,* 60, 737, 1978.

148. **Snyderman, R. and Pike, M. C.,** An inhibitor of macrophage chemotaxis produced by neoplasms, *Science,* 192, 370, 1976.

149. **Stevenson, M. M. and Meltzer, M. S.,** Depressed chemotactic responses in vitro of peritoneal macrophages from tumor bearing mice, *J. Natl. Cancer Inst.,* 57, 847, 1976.

150. **Normann, S. J.,** Tumor cell threshold required for suppressor of macrophage inflammation, *J. Natl. Cancer Inst.,* 60, 1091, 1978.

151. **Hanna, N.,** Role of natural killer cells in control of cancer metastasis, *Cancer Metastasis Rev.,* 1, 45, 1982.

152. **Bruck, S. D., Ed.,** *Controlled Drug Delivery,* CRC Press, Boca Raton, Fla., 1982.

153. **Chien, Y. W., Ed.,** *Novel Drug Delivery Systems,* Marcel Dekker, New York, 1982.

154. **Counsell, R. E. and Ponland, R. C.,** Lipoproteins as potential site-specific delivery systems for diagnostic and therapeutic agents, *J. Med. Chem.,* 25, 1115, 1982.

155. **Levy, R. and Miller, R. A.,** Tumor therapy with monoclonal antibodies, *Fed. Proc. Fed. Am. Soc. Exp. Biol.,* 42, 2650, 1983.

156. **Lynch, W. E., Sartiano, G. P., and Ghaffar, A.,** Erythrocytes as carriers of chemotherapeutic agents for targeting to the reticuloendothelial system, *Am. J. Hematol.,* 9, 249, 1980.

157. **Poste, G. and Nicolson, G. L.,** Experimental systems for analysis of the surface properties of metastatic tumor cells, in *Biomembranes,* Vol. 2, Nowotny, A., Ed., Plenum Press, New York, 1983, 341.

158. **Snyderman, R., Meadows, L., Holder, W., and Wells, S.,** Abnormal monocyte chemotaxis in patients with breast cancer: evidence for a tumor-mediated effect, *J. Natl. Cancer Inst.,* 60, 737, 1978.

159. **Hausman, M. S., Brosman, S., and Snyderman, R.,** Defective monocyte function in patients with genitourinary carcinoma, *J. Natl. Cancer Inst.,* 55, 1047, 1975.

160. **Boetcher, D. A. and Leonard, E. J.,** Abnormal monocyte chemotactic response in cancer patients, *J. Natl. Cancer Inst.,* 52, 1091, 1974.

161. **Lee, J. C., Badger, A. M., Johnson, W. J., Sung, C. P., and Horan, P.,** Human non-gamma interferon macrophage activating actor (MT-2/MAF) elicits multiple and cross-species effects on macrophage activations, *Abstr. Sixth Int. Congr. Immunol.,* 1986.

162. **Axline, S. G.,** Functional biochemistry of the macrophages, *Semin. Hematol.,* 7, 142, 1970.

163. **Nacy, C. A., James, S. L., Osler, C. N., and Meltzer, M. S.,** Activation of macrophages to kill Rickettsiae and Leishmania: dissociation of intracellular microbicidal activities and extracellular destruction of neoplastic cells and helminths, *Contemp. Top. Immunobiol.,* 14, 147, 1984.

164. **Adams, D. O. and Hamilton, T. A.,** The cell biology of macrophage activation, *Annu. Rev. Immunol.,* 2, 283, 1984.

165. **Koestler, T. P., Johnson, W. J., Rieman, D., Dalton, B. J., Greig, R. G., and Poste, G.,** Differential expression of murine macrophage-mediated tumor cytotoxicity induced by interferons, *Cancer Res.,* 47, 2804, 1987.

166. **Nathan, C. F. and Cohn, Z. A.,** Cellular components of inflammation: monocytes and macrophages, in *Textbook of Rheumatology,* Kelley, W., Harris, E., Ruddy, S., and Sledge, C., Eds., W. B. Saunders, Philadelphia, 1985, 144.

167. **Takemura, R. and Werb, Z.**, Secretory products of macrophages and their physiological functions, *Am. J. Physiol.*, 246, C1, 1984.
168. **Gordon, S. and Hirsch, S.**, Differentiation antigens and macrophage heterogeneity, in *Macrophages and Natural Killer Cells*, Norman, S. and Sorkin, E., Eds., Plenum Press, New York, 1982, 391.
169. **Walker, W. S.**, Functional heterogeneity of macrophages, in *Immunobiology of the Macrophage*, Nelson, D., Ed., Academic Press, Orlando, Fla., 1986, 91.
170. **Adams, D. O. and Marino, P. A.**, Activation of mononuclear phagocytes for destruction of tumor cells as a model for study of macrophage development, in *Contemporary Topics in Hematology-Oncology*, Gordon, A., Silber, R., and LoBue, J., Eds., Plenum Press, New York, 1984, 69.
171. **Fischer, D. G., Hubbard, W. J., and Koren, H. S.**, Tumor cell killing by freshly isolated peripheral blood monocytes, *Cell. Immunol.*, 58, 426, 1981.
172. **Johnson, W. J., Marino, P. A., Schrieber, R. D., and Adams, D. O.**, Sequential activation of murine mononuclear phagocytes for tumor cytolysis: differential expression of markers by macrophages in the several stages of development, *J. Immunol.*, 131, 1038, 1983.
173. **Johnson, W. J., DiMartino, M. J., and Hanna, J.**, Macrophage activation in rat models of inflammation and arthritis: determination of markers of stages of activation, *Cell. Immunol.*, 103, 54, 1986.
174. **Pace, J. L., Varesio, J., Russell, S. W., and Blasi, E.**, The strain of mouse and assay conditions influence whether muIFN-γ primes or activates macrophages for tumor killing, *J. Leukocyte Biol.*, 37, 475, 1985.
175. **Murray, H. W., Spitalny, G. L., and Nathan, C. F.**, Activation of mouse peritoneal macrophages *in vitro* and *in vivo* by interferon-γ, *J. Immunol.*, 134, 1619, 1985.
176. **Black, C. M., Catterall, J. R., and Remington, J. S.**, *In vivo* and *in vitro* activation of alveolar macrophages by recombinant interferon-γ, *J. Immunol.*, 138, 491, 1987.
177. **Lehrer, R. I., Ferrari, L. G., Patterson-Delafield, J., and Sorrell, T.**, Fungicidal activity of rabbit alveolar and peritoneal macrophages against *Candida albicans*, *Infect. Immun.*, 28, 1001, 1980.
178. **Collins, F. M., Niederbuhl, C. J., and Campbell, S. G.**, Bactericidal activity of alveolar and peritoneal macrophages exposed *in vitro* to three strains of *Pasteurella multocida*, *Infect. Immun.*, 39, 779, 1983.
179. **Schaffner, A., Douglas, H., Braude, A. I., and Davis, C. E.**, Killing of Aspergillus spores depends on the anatomical source of the macrophage, *Infect. Immun.*, 42, 1109, 1983.
180. **Black, C. M., Beaman, B. L., Donovan, R. M., and Goldstein, E.**, Intracellular acid phosphatase content and ability of different macrophage populations to kill *Nocardia asteroides*, *Infect. Immun.*, 47, 375, 1985.
181. **Beller, D. I. and Ho, K.**, Regulation of macrophage populations. V. Evaluation of the control of macrophage Ia expression *in vitro*, *J. Immunol.*, 129, 971, 1982.
182. **Pawlowski, N. A., Kaplan, G., Hamill, G. A., Cohn, Z. A., and Scott, W. A.**, Arachidonic acid metabolism by human monocytes. Studies with platelet-depleted cultures, *J. Exp. Med.*, 158, 393, 1983.
183. **Weiel, J. E., Adams, D. O., and Hamilton, T. A.**, Murine monocytes express transferrin receptors: evidence for similarity to inflammatory macrophages, *Cell. Immunol.*, 88, 343, 1984.
184. **Ruco, L. P. and Meltzer, M. A.**, Macrophage activation for tumor cytotoxicity: increased lymphokine responsiveness of peritoneal macrophages during acute inflammation, *J. Immunol.*, 120, 1054, 1978.
185. **Nacy, C. A., James, S. L., Osler, C. N., and Meltzer, M. S.**, Activation of macrophages to kill Rickettsiae and Leishmania: disassociation of intracellular microbicidal activities and extracellular destruction of neoplastic cells and helminths, *Contemp. Top. Immunobiol.*, 14, 147, 1984.
186. **Pace, J. L. and Russell, S. W.**, Activation of mouse macrophages for tumor cell killing. I. Quantitative analysis of interactions between lymphokine and LPS, *J. Immunol.*, 126, 1863, 1981.
187. **Adams, D. O. and Nathan, C. F.**, Molecular mechanisms operative in cytolysis of tumor cells by activated macrophages, *Immunol. Today*, 4, 166, 1983.
188. **Bonvini, E., Hoffman, T., Herberman, R. B., and Varesio, L.**, Selective augmentation by recombinant interferon-γ of the intracellular content of S-adenosylmethionine in murine macrophages, *J. Immunol.*, 136, 2596, 1986.
189. **Varesio, L.**, Down regulation of RNA labeling as a selective marker for cytotoxic but not suppressor macrophages, *J. Immunol.*, 132, 2683, 1984.
190. **Varesio, L.**, Imbalanced accumulation of ribosomal RNA in macrophages activated *in vivo* or *in vitro* to a cytolytic stage, *J. Immunol.*, 134, 1262, 1985.
191. **Hamilton, T. A., Becton, D. B., Somers, S. D., Gray, P. W., and Adams, D. O.**, Interferon gamma modulates protein kinase C activity in murine peritoneal macrophages, *J. Biol. Chem.*, 260, 1378, 1985.
192. **Celada, A. and Schrieber, R. D.**, Role of protein kinase C and intracellular calcium mobilization in the induction of macrophage tumoricidal activity by interferon-γ, *J. Immunol.*, 137, 2373, 1986.
193. **Somers, S. D. and Adams, D. O.**, Enhancement of selective tumor cell binding by activated murine macrophages in response to phorbol myristate acetate, *J. Immunol.*, 136, 2323, 1986.
194. **Herrmann, F., Cannistra, S. A., Levine, H., and Griffin, J. D.**, Expression of IL-2 receptors and binding of IL-2 by gamma interferon-induced human leukemic and normal monocytic cells, *J. Exp. Med.*, 162, 1111, 1985.

195. **Holter, W., Grunow, R., Stockinger, H., and Knapp, W.,** Recombinant interferon-γ induces IL-2 receptors on human peripheral blood monocytes, *J. Immunol.,* 136, 2171, 1986.

196. **Hancock, W. W., Muller, W. A., and Cotran, R. S.,** IL-2 receptors are expressed by alveolar macrophages during pulmonary sarcoidosis and are inducible by lymphokine treatment of normal human lung macrophages, blood monocytes and monocyte cell lines, *J. Immunol.,* 138, 185, 1987.

197. **Huber, C., Batchelor, J. R., Fuchs, D., Hausen, A., Lang, A., Neiderweiser, D., Reinbnegger, G., Swetly, P., Tropmair, J., and Wachter, H.,** Immune response-associated production of neopterin. Release from macrophages primarily under control of interferon-gamma, *J. Exp. Med.,* 160, 310, 1984.

198. **Woloszcuk, W., Troppmair, T., and Leiter, E.,** Relationship of interferon gamma and neopterin levels during stimulation with alloantigens *in vivo* and *in vitro, Transplantation,* 41, 716, 1986.

199. **Garbutt, J. C., Duch, D. S., Nichol, C. A., and Woolf, J. H.,** Urinary biopterin and neopterin excretion and pituitary-adrenal activity in psychiatric patients, *Psychiatr. Res. Rep.,* 16, 181, 1985.

200. **Bichler, A., Fuchs, A., and Hausen, A.,** Measurement of urinary neopterin in normal pregnant and non-pregnant women and in women with benign and malignant genital tract neoplasms, *Arch. Gynaekol.,* 233, 121, 1983.

201. **Strassmann, G., Springer, T. A., Somers, S. D., and Adams, D. O.,** Mechanisms of tumor cell capture by activated macrophages: evidence for involvement of lymphocyte function-associated (LFA)-1 antigen, *J. Immunol.,* 136, 4328, 1986.

202. **MacKay, R. J. and Russell, S. W.,** Protein changes associated with stages of activation of mouse macrophages for tumor cell killing, *J. Immunol.,* 137, 1392, 1986.

203. **Johnston, P. A., Somers, S. D., and Hamilton, T. A.,** Expression of a 120 Kd protein during tumoricidal activation in murine peritoneal macrophages, *J. Immunol.,* 138, 2739, 1987.

204. **Hamilton, T. A., Jansen, M. M., Somers, S. D., and Adams, D. O.,** Effects of bacterial lipopolysaccharide on protein synthesis in murine peritoneal macrophages: relationship to activation for macrophage tumoricidal function, *J. Cell. Physiol.,* 128, 9, 1986.

205. **Weiel, J. E., Hamilton, T. A., and Adams, D. O.,** LPS induces altered phosphate labeling of proteins in murine peritoneal macrophages, *J. Immunol.,* 136, 3012, 1986.

206. **Muller, R., Curran, T., Muller, D., and Guilbert, L.,** Induction of c-fos during myelomonocytic differentiation and macrophage proliferation, *Nature (London),* 314, 546, 1985.

207. **Martinet, Y., Bitterman, P. B., and Mornex, J.-F.,** Activated human monocytes express the c-sis proto-oncogene and release a mediator showing PDGF-like activity, *Nature (London),* 319, 158, 1986.

208. **Introna, M., Hamilton, T. A., Kaufman, R. E., Adams, D. O., and Bast, R. C.,** Treatment of murine peritoneal macrophages with bacterial LPS alters expression of c-fos and c-myc oncogenes, *J. Immunol.,* 137, 2711, 1986.

209. **Nathan, C. F., Murray, H. W., Wiebe, M. E., and Rubin, B. Y.,** Identification of interferon-γ as the lymphokine that activates human macrophage oxidative metabolism and antimicrobial activity, *J. Exp. Med.,* 159, 670, 1983.

210. **Le, J., Prensky, W., Yipp, Y. K., Chang, Z., Hoffman, T., Stevenson, H. C., Balazs, I., Sadlik, S. R., and Vilce, K. J.,** Activation of human monocyte cytotoxicity by natural and recombinant immune interferon, *J. Immunol.,* 131, 2821, 1983.

211. **Kleinerman, E. S., Ceccorulli, L. M., Bonvini, E., Zicht, R., and Gallin, J. I.,** Lysis of tumor cells by human blood monocytes by a mechanism independent of activation of the oxidative burst, *Cancer Res.,* 45, 2058, 1985.

212. **Utsugi, T. and Sone, S.,** Comparative analysis of the priming effect of human interferon γ, α, β on synergism with a MDP analog for anti-tumor expression of human blood monocytes, *J. Immunol.,* 136, 1117, 1986.

213. **Chen, A. R., Whitaker, F. S., McKinnon, K. P., and Koren, H. S.,** LPS exposure during purification of human monocytes by adherence increases their recovery and cytolytic activity, *Cell. Immunol.,* 103, 120, 1986.

214. **Philip, R. and Epstein, L. B.,** TNF as immunomodulator and mediator of monocyte cytotoxicity induced by itself, IFN-γ and IL-1, *Nature (London),* 323, 86, 1986.

215. **Onozaki, K., Matsushima, K., Kleinerman, E. S., Saito, T., and Oppenheim, J. J.,** Role of IL-1 in promoting human monocyte-mediated tumor cytotoxicity, *J. Immunol.,* 135, 314, 1985.

216. **Masuda, T. and Watanabe, T.,** Autocrine mechanism of IL-1 production in murine macrophage cell lines, M₁, *Lymphokine Res.,* 6(Abstr.), 1214, 1987.

217. **Billian, A., Damme, J. V., Opdenakker, G., Fibbe, W. E., Falkenburg, J. H. F., and Content, J.,** IL-1 as a cytokine inducer, *Immunobiology,* 172, 323, 1986.

218. **Malkovsky, M., Loveland, B., North, M., Asherton, G. L., Gao, L., Ward, P., and Fiers, W.,** Recombinant IL-2 directly augments the cytotoxicity of human monocytes, *Nature (London),* 325, 262, 1987.

219. **Nathan, C. F., Prendergast, T. J., Wiebe, M. E., Stanley, E. R., Platzer, E., Remold, H. B., Welte, K., Rubin, B. Y., and Murray, H. W.,** Activation of human macrophages. Comparison of their cytokines with interferon-γ, *J. Exp. Med.*, 160, 600, 1984.

220. **Djeu, J. Y. and Blanchared, D. K.,** Generation of autoreactive killer cells against human monocytes/macrophages by IL-2, *Lymphokine Res.*, 6(Abstr.), 1705, 1987.

221. **Meltzer, M. S., Crawford, R. M., Finbloom, D. S., Ohara, J., and Paul, W. E.,** BSF-1: a macrophage activation factor, *Lymphokine Res.*, 6(Abstr.), 1719, 1987.

222. **Esparza, I., Mannel, D., Ruppel, A., Falk, W., and Krammer, P. H.,** IFN-γ and lymphotoxin or TNF synergize to activate macrophages for tumoricidal and schistosomulicidal functions, *Lymphokine Res.*, 6(Abstr.), 1715, 1987.

223. **Hoffman, M. K.,** The effects of TNF on the production of IL-1 by macrophages, *Lymphokine Res.*, 5, 255, 1986.

224. **Bachwich, P. R., Chensue, S. W., Larrick, J. W., and Kunkel, S. L.,** TNF stimulates IL-1 and PGE_2 production in resting macrophages, *Biochem. Biophys. Res. Commun.*, 136, 94, 1986.

225. **Munker, R., Gasson, J., Ogawa, M., and Koeffer, H. P.,** Recombinant human TNF induces production of GM-CSF, *Nature (London)*, 323, 79, 1986.

226. **Wing, E. J., Waheed, A., Shadduck, R. K., Magle, L. S., and Stephenson, K.,** Effect of CSF on murine macrophages, *J. Clin. Invest.*, 69, 270, 1982.

227. **Metcalf, D.,** The granulocyte-macrophage colony stimulating factors, *Science*, 229, 16, 1985.

228. **Grabstein, K., Reed, S., Shanebeck, K., and Morrisey, P.,** Induction of macrophage microbicidal activity by GM-CSF, *Lymphokine Res.*, 6(Abstr.), 1707, 1987.

229. **Weiser, W. Y., Van Niel, A., Clark, S. C., David, J. R., and Remold, H. G.,** Recombinant human GM-CSF activates intracellular killing of *Leishmania donovani* by human monocytes, *Lymphokine Res.*, 6(Abstr.), 1706, 1987.

230. **Wing, E. J., Ampel, N. M., Waheed, A., and Shadduck, R. K.,** Macrophage CSF enhances the capacity of murine macrophages to secrete oxygen reduction products, *J. Immunol.*, 135, 2052, 1985.

231. **Ralph, P., Warren, M. K., Nakoinz, I., Lee, M. T., Brindley, L., Sampson-Johannes, A., Kawaski, E. S., Ladner, M. B., Stickler, J. E., Boosman, A., Csejtey, J., and White, T. J.,** Biological properties and molecular biology of the human macrophage growth factor, CSF-1, *Immunobiology*, 172, 194, 1986.

232. **Warren, M. K. and Ralph, P.,** CSF-1 stimulates human monocyte production of interferon, TNF and colony stimulating activity, *J. Immunol.*, 137, 2281, 1986.

233. **Bhalla, A. K., Amento, E. P., and Krane, S. M.,** Differential effects of 1,25-dihydroxyvitamin D_3 on human lymphocytes and monocyte/macrophages: inhibition of IL-2 and augmentation of IL-1 production, *Cell. Immunol.*, 98, 311, 1986.

234. **Koff, W. C. and Dunegan, M. A.,** Modulation of macrophage-mediated tumoricidal activity by neuropeptides and neurohormones, *J. Immunol.*, 135, 350, 1985.

Chapter 11

MACROPHAGES AND DEVELOPMENT OF CANCER

Gloria Heppner and Leslie Dorcey

TABLE OF CONTENTS

I. INTRODUCTION: INFLAMMATION AND CANCER

The idea that there is a relationship between inflammatory and associated processes and the development of cancer is as old as it is elusive. Similar to those postulated links between "nutrition and cancer" and "stress and cancer", the evidence that inflammation somehow influences carcinogenesis and cancer growth is often anecdotal, impossible to quantitate, and, especially, difficult to place in a mechanistic framework. Yet there remains the strong suspicion that "something is going on" and, indeed, in recent years the recognition of the great complexity of neoplastic development has suggested points of attack towards understanding the ultimate mechanism.

The purpose of this chapter is to discuss the possible roles of macrophages in the development of cancer. Other chapters in this book stress the protective or therapeutic activity of macrophages; this review will focus on their inducing or stimulatory activities. Since much of the work in this area involves processes shared by phagocytic cells in general, results obtained with polymorphonuclear leukocyte (PMNs) will be included.

One difficulty in assessing the role of inflammatory cells per se in cancer development is the confounding factor of the many other events that accompany inflammation and that may also be instrumental in neoplasia. The cellular proliferation and regenerative hyperplasia that accompany wound healing may contribute to neoplastic growth by, for example, altering target cell susceptibility to carcinogen or by providing paracrine growth factors, independently of any contributions from inflammatory cells.

Furthermore, cancer development is multifactorial. Despite the enthusiasm of many present-day "oncogenologists", no one event is responsible for overt neoplasia. It is the result of a matrix of interconnecting processes. At any given point some participants in the matrix play a dominant role. At another time, or in another cancer, different participants assume importance. At this stage of our understanding, there are always multiple explanations for any set of experimental observations. Despite these reservations, there are numerous intriguing reports that call attention to the importance of host responses in tumorigenesis. Many of these focus on the phase of development known as promotion (see below). Boone and associates showed that the nontumorigenic, but apparently "preneoplastic", permanent cell lines, Balb/c/3T3 and $C_3H/10T 1/2$, would produce tumors in syngeneic mice if the cells were attached to glass or plastic beads prior to implantation.[1,2] Beads alone did not produce tumors, at least under the conditions of the experiment. These observations relate to an older literature on the ability of "foreign bodies" of different chemical composition to induce sarcomas in rodents. Foreign body carcinogenesis remains unexplained, but there is the possibility that an inflammatory component is involved.

Argyris and Slaga[3] have reported that repeated abrasion of the skin of strain Sencar mice, which had previously been exposed to low, initiating doses of 7,12-dimethylbenz(a)anthracene (DMBA), led to the appearance of papillomas, and eventually, epidermal carcinomas. Neither DMBA alone nor abrasion alone produced tumors.

Wainberg and co-workers[4] found that injection of Bacillus Calmette-Guerin (BCG) into the wing webs of chickens 1 week before injection of avian sarcoma virus (ASV) into the same site potentiated the development of tumors at that site alone. Pretreatment with BCG at other sites had no effect on tumor development. Wainberg et al.[4] suggested that by inducing a local granuloma, BCG produced an influx of potential target cells, i.e., macrophages, susceptible to ASV transformation. Other explanations are also possible.

In a more recent study Dolberg and co-workers[5] reported that in chickens Rous Sarcoma Virus (RSV)-induced tumors form at the site of a noninjected wound, as well as at the site of virus inoculation, but not at other sites even though the birds are viremic and exhibit nonmalignant hemorrhagic lesions throughout their tissues.

In all these experiments it is difficult to separate effects on tumor growth from those on tumor development. Clinically, localized recurrent growth of cancers can occur in the wound scar following surgical removal of the primary neoplasm. Vasiliev and Moizhess[6] reported that implantation of a foreign body in the form of a polyvinyl chloride film prior to, or simultaneously with, local implantation of syngeneic tumor cells increased the incidence of successful tumor takes and decreased their latency. Removal of the film after 24 hr did not abolish its effect which, indeed, remained for many months in its absence. Although the stimulating ability of the film continued long after morphological evidence of reactive inflammation had receded, the investigators could not rule out a more subtle, continuing inflammatory process.

These reports, which are only a sampling of the literature on the subject, are presented here as a starting rationale for looking further into the possible, albeit nonexclusive, involvement of inflammatory cells in cancer development. It is now necessary to provide a more substantial mechanistic rationale.

II. CANCER DEVELOPMENT

Cancer development is usually described as a series of stages, defined operationally by the spectrum of chemical and other effectors that can influence tumorigenesis when introduced at varying times in the sequence. Initiation is the first stage. It is signaled by the induction of essentially irreversible genetic changes. There is a close correlation between ability to initiate and ability to cause mutation. The second phase in the process is promotion. Promotion involves the clonal expansion of initiated cells up to the appearance of benign tumors.[7] Promotion itself has been defined as consisting of two stages. During promotion the combined effects of alterations in the gene expression of initiated cells, via direct or epigenetic mechanisms, and of host selective forces are active. Classically, promotion has been thought not to involve alterations in DNA. This view is now changing as a result of the demonstration that tumor promoters can alter DNA through the generation of active oxygen metabolites.[8-10] Progression is the third and final major phase in the scheme. As commonly employed, progression refers to the acquisition of malignant characteristics, such as invasiveness and ability to metastasize, increased genetic lability, and loss of control, either by endogenous regulators, such as hormones, or by therapeutic intervention, as seen by the emergence of drug resistance. As in promotion, both genetic and epigenetic events are thought to be involved.

Several caveats need to accompany this scheme.

1. The initiation-promotion concept has most clearly been demonstrated for cancers of the skin. Although other types of cancers can fit into the scheme,[11] it may not be universal.

2. As stated above, the various stages are defined operationally. As the concepts are adapted to more cancer systems and to different classes of chemical effectors, new stages emerge and distinctions between old ones fade. Furthermore, as more is learned about the mechanisms of mutation and gene regulation, meaningful distinctions between genetic and epigenetic events become less clear. It is probable that neoplastic change is a continuum and that the interplay between genetic and external factors is a shifting, but constant, influence.

3. Descriptions of the initiation-promotion-progression concept tend to focus attention on the ''target'' cells of a particular reaction. In fact, it is a multicellular process involving the evolution of populations of cells that may differ in many characteristics but which coexist as a tissue. This cellular heterogeneity, which involves both normal and neoplastic cells, appears to increase as a function of progression. In assessing the role of any one component in the process, it is necessary to know not only its own

activity, but to see how it can influence and be influenced by other components as well. Practically, this means that experiments aimed at dissecting out the role of one factor in such a complex network will seldom be definitive.

Despite these caveats, the initiation-promotion-progression scheme is useful in that it provides a framework to seek a place for the action of inflammatory phagocytes in cancer development.

III. MACROPHAGES AND PROOXIDANT STATES IN CANCER DEVELOPMENT

What then are the mechanisms by which macrophages and PMNs may affect neoplastic development? The most commonly proposed mechanisms involve the series of active oxygen metabolites that are released during the respiratory burst that accompanies activation, namely, superoxide, singlet oxygen, hydroxyl radical, and hydrogen peroxide. A second radical-generating mechanism is the cyclooxygenase pathway of arachidonate metabolism. Either way, this places the inflammatory phagocytes into a large class of oxygen radical producing factors that can contribute to "prooxidant" states in which the intracellular concentration of active oxygen radicals is increased in target cells, leading to a variety of untoward biological consequences, including mutation, sister chromatid exchanges, chromosomal aberrations, cellular degeneration, and, if severe enough, cell death.[12-14] As detailed in an excellent review by Cerutti,[15] other agents that induce prooxidant states include hyperbaric oxygen, radiation, various known complete carcinogens, anticancer drugs such as daunorubicin, adriamycin, mitomycin C, and bleomycin, and a host of membrane-active agents such as the well known tumor promoters TPA (12-*O*-tetradecanoylphorbol-13-acetate) and mezerein, asbestos and silica, and prostaglandins. Agents which contribute to the intracellular defense system, the enzymes superoxide dismutase (SOD), catalase, glutathione peroxidase, and the low molecular weight nonprotein sulfhydryls (glutathione, cysteine, and cysteinyl-glycine), can likewise, induce prooxidant states. Interestingly, TPA and other promoters also fall into this class.[15] (Under normal conditions cells have strong intracellular defense mechanisms against oxygen radicals; however, very little such activity seems to exist in extracellular fluids[16] where challenge from macrophage and PMN-released radicals would be expected to occur. Furthermore, some studies report that tumor cells have unusually low levels of antioxidant enzymes.[17])

Although active oxygen radicals are capable of inducing genetic change, most investigators do not ascribe much significant activity to their role during initiation.[18] However, there is extensive evidence linking prooxidant states to promotion. Readers are referred to the reviews of Ames,[19] Troll and Wiesner,[11] Marx,[10] and Cerutti[15] for detailed discussion. Less evidence exists for a role of free radicals in tumor progression. Indeed, little work seems to have been directed specifically towards establishing such a role. Recently, however, O'Connell et al.[7] have reported that the free-radical generator, benzoyl peroxide, which is known to be a promoter of skin carcinogenesis in the Sencar mouse, can also enhance the progression of skin papillomas to epidermal carcinomas. As will be described below, we have biological evidence linking oxygen radical production by macrophages to progression in a mouse mammary tumor system.

Delineation of the molecular mechanisms, whereby active oxygen radicals confer genetic changes in sensitive target cells, is confused by the great wealth of possibilities. In the case of phagocytic cells it is necessary to see how free radicals external to the target cell can induce the prooxidant state. Since the active moieties are shortlived, it is reasonable to postulate the need for close contact between the inflammatory and the target cell. Lipid peroxidation of the polyunsaturated fatty acid side chains of membrane lipids, a process driven by enzyme-catalyzed reactions of arachidonate metabolism, is one possibility. Not only would lipid peroxidation in itself be expected to produce a variety of phenotypic alterations, lipid hydroperoxides and their metabolic products such as malondialdehyde, as well as active oxygen species generated by arachidonate metabolism, can damage DNA, leading to mutation, single- and double-strand breaks, apurinic and apyrimidinic sites, and base damage products such as 5,6-dihydroxy dihydrothymine.[15,20] Other types of membrane effects, however, can also lead to DNA alteration and chromosomal damage. TPA, which acts through its receptor protein kinase C, but also alters membrane conformation, causes a variety of chromosomal lesions, including polyadenosine diphosphate ribosylation of chromosomal proteins, gene amplification, and DNA strand breaks.[8,9,15] The inhibition of metabolic cooperation (intercellular communication), as by the radical generating promoter benzoyl peroxide, may also be a consequence of lipid peroxidation.[21]

An added complication is the role of oxygen radicals as intermediates in the formation of so-called "clastogenic factors" (CFs), i.e., diffusible cellular products that bring about chromosomal damage.[10,11,15,22] CFs can be inhibited by antioxidant inhibitors and by arachidonic acid metabolism inhibitors such as indomethacin.[22] They are induced by promoters such as TPA. Their composition apparently varies with the cell type from which they originate.

The overall picture that emerges from this murky story (again consult the above reviews for details) is that inflammatory cells can generate active oxygen species through two broad categories of reaction. One involves respiratory metabolism, the other arachidonate metabolism. Once generated the free-radicals must somehow react with the target cell; a likely mechanism is by lipid peroxidation of cell membranes, resulting in the formation of a number of reactive degradation products. Since lipid peroxidation interfaces with arachidonate metabolism, free radicals may be also generated secondarily within the target cells and CFs may also be produced. How any of these pathways leads ultimately to genetic damage is unknown. In addition to the obvious outcomes of the physical disruption of DNA, activation of cellular oncogenes by rearrangement or by amplification may be important.[9] Because of the complexity of the intermediary metabolism involved and the unique physiologies of the cell types affected by any particular circumstance, the relevant oxygen species and pathway will likely vary with different experimental models. Suffice it to say that activated phagocytic cells are known to be sources of several species and compounds of known activity in cancer development, including superoxide radicals, hydrogen peroxide (H_2O_2), arachidonic acid metabolites, and CFs.[16,23-26]

In addition to acting as direct agents in tumor promotion and progression, it is possible that macrophages interact with other promoting agents. TPA has been shown to have a number of effects on macrophages, including enhancement of phagocytosis and cytotoxicity.[25-28] TPA is a chemoattractant for mouse macrophages[29] and also induces release of prostaglandins[30], H_2O_2, and superoxide.[25,26,31] Macrophages have receptors for TPA[32] and structure-activity studies with a variety of related phorbol-ester analogs show that the ability to induce these effects in macrophages correlates with tumor-promoting activity.[28] Lewis and Adams[33] have shown that TPA-stimulated macrophages can induce the formation of 5,6 ring-saturated thymine bases in the DNA of 3T3 cells. As mentioned above, these base damage changes can be terminal products of lipid peroxidation. This effect was inhibited by catalase. Dutton and Bowden[24] reported that TPA can stimulate the release of CFs by leukocytes and that this activity was also inhibited by catalase. One can speculate, then, that in vivo one of the many effects of TPA is to recruit and stimulate macrophages to participate in promotion.

An additional effect of TPA on macrophages is stimulation of plasminogen-activator release.[11,34] Plasminogen-activators are serine proteases which have been implicated in promotion in mouse skin.[11] A number of protease inhibitors that are able to antagonize tumor promotion are also inhibitory to superoxide production by PMNs and macrophages.[35,36]

TPA not only can influence macrophage activity directly, it may also affect target cells in such a way as to alter macrophage-target cell interactions. Fishman and Gunther[37] have reported that preincubation of tumor cells with tumor-promoting phorbol esters resulted in their loss of sensitivity to macrophage-mediated cytolysis. Thus, TPA simultaneously may stimulate macrophage-promoter activity and interfere with macrophage-surveillance function.

IV. DIRECT EVIDENCE FOR MACROPHAGE INVOLVEMENT IN MUTAGENESIS AND CANCER DEVELOPMENT

The above section describes, indirectly, how macrophages could be involved in tumor induction and progression. Direct evidence for this involvement, although incomplete, has recently come from several sources.

Using the Ames assay, Weitzman and Stossel[38,39] demonstrated that human peripheral blood leukocytes can be mutagenic. Suspensions of mixed leukocytes or mixed mononuclear cells increased the revertant frequency of histidine-requiring *Salmonella typhimurium* strain TA100 to exogenous histidine independence, whereas lymphocyte suspensions or heat-killed cells did not. Leukocytes from patients with chronic granulomatous disease, which is characterized by a defect in the nicotinamide adenine dinucleotide phosphate (NADPH)-oxidase (reactive oxygen generating) system, were unable to increase the revertant frequency, suggesting a role for reactive oxygen intermediates in phagocyte-induced mutagenesis. This suggestion was strengthened by the demonstration that free radical scavengers, principally those of hydroxyl radicals, could inhibit mutagenesis.[39]

Barak et al.,[40] using a different bacterial mutation system, also demonstrated that human leukocytes can be mutagenic. Looking at reversion to luminescence of a dark mutant of *Photobacterium fisheri*, these investigators showed that neutrophils or leukocytes increased the reversion rate 1000-fold, whereas lymphocytes, or heat-killed or detergent disrupted phagocytes did not. Supernatants from the test system, taken after 60 min of phagocytosis under aerobic conditions, showed mutagenic activity. This could be increased by detergent disruption after phagocytosis. Although phagocytosis could occur under anerobic conditions, test supernatants did not have mutagenic activity.

Our own interest in the ability of phagocytes to cause genetic change came about as a result of some surprising observations on the nature of macrophage infiltrates in tumors produced by a series of cell lines that had been derived originally from a single, spontaneously arising strain BALB/cfC₃H mouse mammary tumor. As described in detail elsewhere in this volume (see Chapter 6), tumors produced by metastatic lines in this system contain a greater proportion of larger, more mature, more activated tumoricidal macrophages than do tumors from less malignant, nonmetastatic lines.[41-43] Since this preferential association of activated macrophages and metastatic tumors is a stable tumor characteristic, since activated macrophages are known sources of agents that cause DNA and chromosomal damage (see above), and since there is some evidence to suggest that metastatic tumors are either more genetically unstable[44] or more sensitive to genetic assault[45] than are nonmetastatic tumors, we postulated that tumor-infiltrating macrophages could be the source of endogenous mutagens which contribute to the induction of cellular heterogeneity within developing neoplasms and, consequently, to the evolution of new tumor characteristics over time, i.e., progression. In experiments modeled after those of Weitzman and associates,[38] Fulton et al.[46] demonstrated that phagocytes isolated from solid mammary tumor infiltrates could be mutagenic in the Ames assay. Whole suspensions of certain tumors increased the revertant frequency of *S. typhimurium* strain TA98 (a frame-shift detector) and/or TA100 (base-pair substitutions); the major mutagenic activity was associated with adherent, macrophage-enriched populations (>90% nonspecific esterase positive). Not all tumor-associated macrophages were equally effective in the assay, nor equally active against the two tester strains. Although macrophages from two highly metastatic tumor lines were active, whereas those of a poorly metastatic line were not, activity was found in macrophages from another nonmetastatic line. Thus, there is not a perfect correlation with metastasis, but clearly, given the multifactoral nature of metastasis, there can be numerous reasons for this.

Demonstrating that macrophages can cause genetic changes in bacteria is only the starting point for showing that they may be involved in neoplastic development. The next step is to show that they can also alter mammalian cells. Weitzman and Stossel examined the ability of human neutrophils to induce resistance to the drug 6-thioguanine (6-TG) in Chinese hamster ovary (CHO) cells.[47] At an effector to target cell ratio of 100:1, neutrophils increased the frequency of 6-TG-resistant colonies threefold. Addition of TPA or opsonized zymosan, which increases the secretion of reactive oxygen intermediates by phagocytes,[48] further increased the frequency.

In our laboratory, Yamashina et al.[49] examined the ability of peritoneal exudate macrophages to induce resistance to 6-TG in a mouse mammary tumor line, designated as line 66. The ability of macrophages to induce resistance was a function of both the effector-to-target cell ratio and the degree of effector cell activation. Effector-to-target cell ratios of at least 50:1 were required to induce resistance, but no straightforward dose response curve was seen above that ratio. (This lack of a dose-response relationship has been commented on by a number of investigators in this field[39,40,46] and may indicate the presence of suppressor mechanisms in the phagocyte populations.) Macrophage-induction of 6-TG resistance was inhibitable by oxygen radical scavengers. Methyl-vinyl-ether-2 (MVE-2, a fraction of pyran)-elicited macrophages induced a higher frequency of 6-TG resistant cells than did thioglycollate-elicited peritoneal cells. Resident peritoneal macrophages did not induce resistance.

In addition to activated peritoneal macrophages, Yamashina et al.[49] also showed that infiltrating macrophages, isolated directly from solid mammary tumor implants, could induce production of 6-TG resistant variants in line 66 cells. The mean activity of macrophages isolated from metastatic line 66 tumors was comparable to that of MVE-2-activated peritoneal macrophages. More experiments are necessary to see whether this characteristic can be generalized to other metastatic tumors in this, or any other, system.

The nature of the macrophage-mediated alteration that leads to 6-TG resistance in line 66 cells has been compared to that produced by the more "classic" mutagen, ethyl methanesulfonate (EMS).[49] In both cases resistance is accompanied by a significant decrease in the enzyme hypoxanthine-guanine phosphoribosyl transferase, (HGPRT) suggesting that a mutation has occurred at the HGPRT locus. Further evidence that the alteration has, in fact, a genetic basis is the stability of the change: the spontaneous reversion frequency of an EMS-induced 6-TG resistant clone of line 66 is 2×10^{-7}, as compared to the frequencies for 5 macrophage-induced clones, which ranged from 1.3×10^{-6} to 3×10^{-7}. Thus, by analogy, the ability of activated macrophages to induce 6-TG resistance in line 66 cells appears to be due to production of base-pair mutations.

Although, in general, oxidant mutagens can induce base-pair mutations, these are not their most frequent kinds of genetic alterations, nor, indeed, the easiest type of change to detect following their exposure.[15] Rather DNA strand breaks and chromosomal alterations are more common. Weitberg et al.[50] showed that stimulated phagocytes can cause significantly increased numbers of sister chromatid exchanges in CHO cells. This was seen after 30 min co-incubation with human peripheral blood leukocytes that had been stimulated with various concentrations of TPA or of opsonized zymosan. TPA, alone, had no effect, nor did stimulated leukocytes from a patient with chronic granulomatous disease, again implicating reactive oxygen intermediates in the induction of genetic lesions. Additional support for this mechanism comes from the observation that the enzyme-mediated production of superoxide by hypoxanthine and xanthine oxidase also induced significant sister chromatid exchange in CHO cells. Additionally, Weitberg and Calabresi,[51] looking at the effect of exogeneous arachidonic acid in the CHO system, found an increase in sister chromatid exchange, and further TPA augmentation of this effect, by TPA stimulated white blood cells.

As mentioned above lipid peroxidation by oxygen metabolites can lead to the appearance of base damage products. Accordingly, Lewis and Adams[33] demonstrated that inflammatory macrophages can induce 5,6-saturated thymidine bases in NIH-3T3 cells. Casein-elicited peritoneal exudate macrophages alone induced very low concentrations of saturated thymidine bases, but the addition of TPA resulted in a much larger and significant increase. It was shown that the concentration of H_2O_2 secreted into the medium rose proportionately with the extent of formation of the saturated bases. Addition of H_2O_2 alone also was effective. Much of the DNA damage (70%) was repaired in 2 hr. Lewis et al.[52] went on to investigate the ability of phagocytes elicited by different agents to induce saturated thymidine bases. They found that BCG-activated macrophages produced the highest amounts of H_2O_2, had the lowest capacity to produce arachidonic acid metabolites, and induced the lowest levels of saturated bases. Resident macrophages produced the lowest amounts of H_2O_2, had the highest capacity to produce arachidonic acid metabolites, and produced higher levels of saturated thymidine bases than did BCG-activated macrophages. Casein-elicited macrophages produced intermediate levels of H_2O_2 and arachidonic acid metabolites and produced the highest levels of saturated thymidine bases. The lipoxygenase inhibitor, nordihydroguaiaretic acid, completely inhibited, and the cyclooxygenase inhibitor, indomethacin, markedly enhanced, the induction of saturated thymidine bases by zymosan stimulated peritoneal exudate macrophages. Thus, although effector cell secretion of reactive oxygen intermediates does not correlate with induction of this type of genetic damage, other factors, such as metabolism of arachidonic acid, may be influential.

As with the bacterial systems, showing that macrophages can cause genetic changes in mammalian cells is only one step to eventually establishing a mechanistic link between macrophages and neoplasia. At least two other steps must be made. One is showing, directly, that macrophage activity can result in cancer development and/or malignant change and the other is demonstrating that any of these changes can occur in vivo. Recently, Weitzman and colleagues[54] have made progress on both steps.

Mouse fibroblastic 10T 1/2 cells were exposed, in vitro, to human leukocytes with or without stimulation by TPA.[53] The appearance of significant numbers of transformed colonies, reminiscent of those seen after exposure to conventional carcinogens, was evident after some 6 to 8 weeks in culture. Similar, although less impressive, effects were seen in cultures treated with a cell-free, superoxide-generating system of hypoxanthine plus xanthine oxidase. Interestingly, TPA stimulation was not necessary since 10T 1/2 cells could directly stimulate release of superoxide by neutrophils from at least a proportion of the donors.

If the 10T 1/2 cells were not cultured after exposure to leukocytes, but instead injected into nude mice, tumors grew up in about 25% of the animals after 13 to 22 weeks. Both benign and histologically malignant tumors developed. Thus, in these experiments, phagocytes have been linked to carcinogenesis and the tumor development, and, perhaps, malignant progression phases have been observed in vivo.

Even more recently, Weitzman et al.[54] developed a system to attempt to study the role of phagocytes in cancer induction entirely in vivo. Ulcerative colitis, an inflammatory condition known to be a risk factor for colon cancer, was induced by repeated enemas of the PMN chemoattracting peptide, formyl-norleucyl-leucyl-phenylalanine (FNLP), in mice given the carcinogen 1,2-dimethylhydrazine (DMH). Thirty-two percent of the mice given DMH and control enemas developed adenocarcinomas of the colon, as compared to 76% of the DMH plus FNLP group. Dietary vitamin E reduced the test incidence to 57%, but this was not a significant effect, perhaps because of the low number of animals used. Although there are many experiments that need to be done to show, definitively, that phagocytic cells were involved in the increased cancer incidence, and, if so, to learn the relevant mechanism of action, this work is a significant step in the elucidation of the role of phagocytes in cancer development.

V. MECHANISMS OF MACROPHAGE MUTAGENICITY

Altogether, there is a growing body of direct evidence that phagocytes are capable of inducing heritable changes in both prokaryotic and eukaryotic cells. As with other prooxidants, the mechanisms by which these changes occur appear to be variable, but involve free radicals and H_2O_2. Lewis et al.[52] demonstrated that the phagocyte-mediated induction of saturated thymidine bases in NIH 3T3 cells could be inhibited by catalase, but was increased by the addition of SOD. This supports their earlier data that suggested that H_2O_2 is the initiator of this type of genetic lesion. Weitzman and Stossel found that phagocyte-induced mutation in bacteria was inhibited by either SOD, catalase, or the hydroxyl radical scavengers, mannitol and benzoate.[39] Barak et al.[40] reported that phagocyte-induced mutation in bacteria was inhibited by the addition of SOD, benzoate, mannitol, or the oxygen radical scavenger β-carotene. Catalase induced a lag in the time required for mutation,[40] which may have been due to the inactivation of the enzyme by superoxide anion. In the studies of Weitberg et al., in which phagocytes induced sister chromatid exchanges in CHO cells, the observed genetic changes were inhibited by SOD, catalase, or mannitol.[55] Similarly, we have shown that SOD, catalase, or mannitol inhibits the induction by activated macrophages of 6-TG resistant variants in line 66 mammary tumor cells.[49]

Although 5,6-saturated thymidine bases appear to be induced by H_2O_2, it is not known if this type of genetic lesion ultimately results in mutant phenotypes since it is subject to rapid repair. In systems which directly measure either induction of sister chromatid exchange or increased frequency of mutant phenotype, inhibitors of superoxide anion or hydrogen peroxide, both of which are required for the production of hydroxyl radical via the Haber-Weiss reaction, or hydroxyl radical scavengers per se inhibit phagocyte-induced changes. Taken together it appears that hydroxyl radical is most likely the mediator of phagocyte induced mutation, however, the exact mechanism by which it induces change is not clear. Proposed mechanisms by which reactive oxygen intermediates can mediate cell damage are discussed earlier in this review.

VI. ADDITIONAL MACROPHAGE ROLES IN CANCER DEVELOPMENT

The focus of this chapter is on the direct involvement of macrophages in the genetic events of carcinogenesis and progression, but it is well to remember the numerous other potential roles for macrophages in cancer development. Macrophages may play a role in the metabolic activation of chemical carcinogens.[56] Surveillance against neoplasia has been often discussed[57] and the possibility that macrophage selection can result in more malignant variants has been proposed by De Baetselier and associates.[58] Macrophages may also be the source of a variety of tumor growth factors;[57,59,60] indeed, a previously undescribed macrophage-derived growth factor may be the explanation for the necessary involvement of inflammatory cells in the induction of mouse plasmacytomas by mineral oils or by pristane.[61,62] The influence of macrophages on normal cell proliferation and function may also be important to tumor development. Macrophage production of vasoactive amines, endothelial cell growth factors, platelet activating factors, fibronectin, collagenase, and other proteases, etc., may come into play during the establishment and spread of neoplastic growths.[57] Neovascularization, an essential step in tumor formation,[63] can be induced by activated macrophages.[64,65] Thus, there exists a wealth of possible mechanisms, whereby macrophages can influence cancer development in addition to the generation of active oxygen radicals. In this, macrophages are no different than the more classical tumor promoters which are all highly pleiotrophic in their effects.[10]

VII. CONCLUSION

In the introduction to this chapter, mention was made of the anecdotal evidence that links inflammation and cancer. The purpose of this chapter was to provide a mechanistic basis for this link. It is apparent that, although a firm basis has not yet been established, macrophages could be a driving factor at all stages of cancer development — initiation, promotion, and progression. Macrophages can also interact with other carcinogens and promoters and, furthermore, interface with many aspects of the tissue biology of cancer development. Clearly, macrophage function is not exclusively that of host defense. Hopefully, a full understanding of the role in macrophages in cancer will lead to ways to channel their diverse activities for benefit, rather than harm.

ACKNOWLEDGMENTS

Supported by grants CA27437, CA22453, and CA09421 from the National Cancer Institute, by a grant from Concern Foundation, by the E. Walter Albachten Bequest and by the United Foundation of Greater Detroit.

REFERENCES

1. **Boone, C. W.,** Malignant hemangioendotheliomas produced by subcutaneous inoculation of Balb/3T3 cells attached to glass beads, *Science,* 188, 68, 1975.
2. **Boone, C. W. and Jacobs, J. F.,** Sarcomas routinely produced from putatively nontumorigenic BALB/3T3 and C₃H/10T 1/2 cells by subcutaneous inoculation attached to plastic platelets, *J. Supramol. Struct.,* 5, 131, 1976.
3. **Argyris, T. S. and Slaga, T. J.,** Promotion of carcinomas by repeated abrasion in initiated skin of mice, *Cancer Res.,* 41, 5193, 1981.
4. **Wainberg, M. A., Beiss, B., Fong, H., Beaupre, S., and Menezes, J.,** Involvement of macrophage-like cells in growth of tumors induced by avian sarcoma virus, *Cancer Res.,* 43, 1550, 1983.
5. **Dolberg, D. S., Hollingsworth, R., Hertle, M., and Bissell, M. J.,** Wounding and its role in RSV-mediated tumor formation, *Science,* 230, 676, 1985.
6. **Vasiliev, J. M. and Moizhess, T. G.,** Tumorigenicity of sarcoma cells is enhanced by the local environment of implanted foreign body, *Int. J. Cancer,* 30, 525, 1982.
7. **O'Connell, J. F., Klein-Szanto, A. J. P., DiGiovanni, D. M., Fries, J. W., and Slaga, T. J.,** Enhanced malignant progression of mouse skin tumors by the free-radical generator benzoyl peroxide, *Cancer Res.,* 46, 2863, 1986.
8. **Birnboim, H. C.,** DNA strand breakage in human leukocytes exposed to a tumor promoter, phorbol myristate acetate, *Science,* 215, 1247, 1982.
9. **Varshavsky, A.,** Phorbol ester dramatically increases incidence of methotrexate-resistant mouse cells: possible mechanisms and relevance to tumor promotion, *Cell,* 25, 561, 1981.
10. **Marx, J. L.,** Do tumor promoters affect DNA after all?, *Science,* 219, 158, 1983.
11. **Troll, W. and Wiesner, R.,** The role of oxygen radicals as a possible mechanism of tumor promotion, *Annu. Rev. Pharmacol. Toxicol.,* 25, 509, 1985.
12. **Emerit, I., Levy, A., and Cerutti, P.,** Suppression of tumor promoter phorbol myristate acetate-induced chromosome breakage by antioxidants and inhibitors of arachidonic acid metabolism, *Mutat. Res.,* 110, 327, 1983.
13. **Phillips, B. J., James, T. E. B., and Anderson, D.,** Genetic damage in CHO cells exposed to enzymically generated active oxygen species, *Mutat. Res.,* 126, 265, 1984.
14. **Simon, R. H., Scoggin, C. H., and Patterson, D.,** Hydrogen peroxide causes the fatal injury to human fibroblasts exposed to oxygen radicals, *J. Biol. Chem.,* 256, 7181, 1981.

15. **Cerutti, P. A.**, Prooxidant states and tumor promotion, *Science*, 227, 375, 1985.
16. **McCord, J. M.**, Free radicals and inflammation: protection of synovial fluid by superoxide dismutase, *Science*, 185, 529, 1974.
17. **Oberly, L. W. and Buettner, G. R.**, Superoxide dismutase in cancer: a review, *Cancer Res.*, 39, 1141, 1979.
18. **Rao, M. S., Lalwani, N. D., Watanabe, T. K., and Reddy, J. K.**, Inhibitory effect of antioxidants ethoxyquin and 2(3)-*tert*-butyl-4-hydroxyanisole on hepatic tumorigenesis in rats fed ciprofibrate, a peroxisome proliferator, *Cancer Res.*, 44, 1072, 1984.
19. **Ames, B. N.**, Dietary carcinogens and anticarcinogens, *Science*, 221, 1256, 1983.
20. **Mukai, F. H. and Goldstein, B. D.**, Mutagenicity of malonaldehyde, a decomposition product of peroxidized polyunsaturated fatty acids, *Science*, 191, 868, 1976.
21. **Slaga, T. J., Klein-Szanto, A. J. P., Triplett, L. L., Yotti, L. P., and Trosko, J. E.**, Skin tumor-promoting activity of benzoyl peroxide, a widely used free radical-generating compound, *Science*, 213, 1023, 1981.
22. **Emerit, I. and Cerutti, P. A.**, Tumor promoter phorbol 12-myristate 13-acetate induces a clastogenic factor in human lymphocytes, *Proc. Natl. Acad. Sci. U.S.A.*, 79, 7509, 1982.
23. **Metzger, Z., Hoffeld, J. T., and Oppenheim, J. J.**, Suppression of fibroblast proliferation by activated macrophages: involvement of H_2O_2 and a non-prostaglandin E product of the cyclooxygenase pathway, *Cell. Immunol.*, 100, 501, 1986.
24. **Dutton, D. R. and Bowden, G. T.**, Indirect induction of a clastogenic effect in epidermal cells by a tumor promoter, *Carcinogenesis*, 6, 1279, 1985.
25. **Nathan, C. F., Brukner, L. H., Silverstein, S. C., and Cohn, Z. A.**, Extracellular cytolysis by activated macrophages and granulocytes. I. Pharmacologic triggering of effector cells and the release of hydrogen peroxide, *J. Exp. Med.*, 149, 84, 1979.
26. **Nathan, C. F., Silverstein, S. C., Brukner, L. H., and Cohn, Z. A.**, Extracellular cytolysis by activated macrophages and granulocytes. II. Hydrogen peroxide as a mediator of cytotoxicity, *J. Exp. Med.*, 149, 100, 1979.
27. **Laskin, D. L., Laskin, J. D., Weinstein, I. B., and Carchman, R. A.**, Modulation of phagocytosis by tumor promoters and epidermal growth factor in normal and transformed macrophages, *Cancer Res.*, 40, 1028, 1980.
28. **Laskin, D. L., Laskin, J. D., Kessler, F. K., Weinstein, I. B., and Carchman, R. A.**, Enhancement of macrophage-induced cytotoxicity by phorbol ester tumor promoters, *Cancer Res.*, 41, 4523, 1981.
29. **Laskin, D. L., Laskin, J. D., Weinstein, I. B., and Carchman, R. A.**, Induction of chemotaxis in mouse peritoneal macrophages by phorbol ester tumor promoters, *Cancer Res.*, 41, 1923, 1981.
30. **Brune, K. and Kalin, H.**, Inflammatory, tumor initiating and promoting activities of polycyclic aromatic hydrocarbons and diterpene esters in mouse skin as compared with their prostaglandin releasing potency in vitro, *Cancer Lett.*, 4, 333, 1978.
31. **Pick, E. and Keisari, Y.**, Superoxide anion and hydrogen peroxide production by chemically elicited peritoneal macrophages — induction by multiple nonphagocytic stimuli, *Cell. Immunol.*, 59, 301, 1981.
32. **Sturm, R. J., Smith, B. M., Lane, R. W., Laskin, D. L., Harris, L. S., and Carchman, R. A.**, Antagonist of phorbol ester receptor-mediated chemotaxis in mouse peritoneal macrophages, *Cancer Res.*, 43, 4552, 1983.
33. **Lewis, J. G. and Adams, D. O.**, Induction of 5,6-ring-saturated thymine bases in NIH-3T3 cells by phorbol ester-stimulated macrophages: role of reactive oxygen intermediates, *Cancer Res.*, 45, 1270, 1985.
34. **Vassalli, J.-D., Hamilton, J., and Reich, E.**, Macrophage plasminogen activator: induction by concanavalin A and phorbol myristate acetate, *Cell*, 11, 695, 1977.
35. **Goldstein, B. D., Witz, G., Amoruso, M., and Troll, W.**, Protease inhibitors antagonize the activation of polymorphonuclear leukocyte oxygen consumption, *Biochem. Biophys. Res. Commun.*, 88, 854, 1979.
36. **Hoffman, M. and Autor, A. P.**, Effect of cyclooxygenase inhibitors and protease inhibitors on phorbol-induced stimulation of oxygen consumption and superoxide production by rat pulmonary macrophages, *Biochem. Pharmacol.*, 31, 775, 1982.
37. **Fishman, M. and Gunther, G.**, Induction of tumor cell resistance to macrophage-mediated lysis by phorbol esters: a postbinding event, *Cell. Immunol.*, 100, 374, 1986.
38. **Weitzman, S. A. and Stossel, T. P.**, Mutation caused by human phagocytes, *Science*, 212, 546, 1981.
39. **Weitzman, S. A. and Stossel, T. P.**, Effects of oxygen radical scavengers and antioxidants on phagocyte induced mutagenesis, *J. Immunol.*, 128, 2770, 1982.
40. **Barak, M., Ulitzur, S., and Merzbach, D.**, Phagocytosis-induced mutagenesis in bacteria, *Mutat. Res.*, 121, 7, 1983.
41. **Loveless, S. E. and Heppner, G. H.**, Tumor-associated macrophages of mouse mammary tumors. I. Differential cytotoxicity of macrophages from metastatic and nonmetastatic tumors, *J. Immunol.*, 131, 2074, 1983.

42. **Mahoney, K. H., Fulton, A. M., and Heppner, G. H.,** Tumor-associated macrophages of mouse mammary tumors. II. Differential distribution of macrophages from metastatic and nonmetastatic tumors, *J. Immunol.*, 131, 2079, 1983.

43. **Mahoney, K. H., Miller, B. E., and Heppner, G. H.,** FACS quantitation of leucine aminopeptidase and acid phosphatase on tumor-associated macrophages from metastatic and nonmetastatic mouse mammary tumors, *J. Leukocyte Biol.*, 38, 573, 1985.

44. **Cifone, M. A. and Fidler, I. J.,** Increasing metastatic potential is associated with increasing genetic instability of clones isolated from murine neoplasms, *Proc. Natl. Acad. Sci. U.S.A.*, 78, 6949, 1981.

45. **Yamashina, K. and Heppner, G. H.,** Correlation of induced mutation and metastatic potential in tumor cell lines from a single mouse mammary tumor, *Cancer Res.*, 45, 4015, 1985.

46. **Fulton, A. M., Loveless, S. E., and Heppner, G. H.,** Mutagenic activity of tumor-associated macrophages in *Salmonella typhimurium* strains TA98 and TA100, *Cancer Res.*, 44, 4308, 1984.

47. **Weitzman, S. A. and Stossel, T. P.,** Phagocyte-induced mutation in Chinese hamster ovary cells, *Cancer Lett.*, 22, 337, 1984.

48. **Drath, D. B.,** Enhanced superoxide release and tumoricidal activity by a postlavage, in situ pulmonary macrophage population in response to activation by *Mycobacterium bovis* BCG exposure, *Infect. Immun.*, 49, 72, 1985.

49. **Yamashina, K., Miller, B. E., and Heppner, G. H.,** Macrophage-mediated induction of drug-resistance variants in a mouse mammary tumor cell line, *Cancer Res.*, 46, 2396, 1986.

50. **Weitberg, A. B., Weitzman, S. A., Destrempes, S. A., Latt, S. A., and Stossel, T. P.,** Stimulated human phagocytes produce cytogenetic changes in cultured mammalian cells, *N. Engl. J. Med.*, 308, 26, 1983.

51. **Weitberg, A. B. and Calabresi, P.,** The effect of arachidonic acid on oxygen radical-induced sister chromatid exchanges, *Proc. Am. Assoc. Cancer Res.*, 27, 372, 1986.

52. **Lewis, J. G., Hamilton, T., and Adams, D. O.,** The effect of macrophage development on the release of reactive oxygen intermediates and lipid oxidation products, and their ability to induce oxidative DNA damage in mammalian cells, *Carcinogenesis*, 7, 813, 1986.

53. **Weitzman, S. A., Weitberg, A. B., Clark, E. P., and Stossel, T. P.,** Phagocytes as carcinogens: malignant transformation produced by human neutrophils, *Science*, 227, 1231, 1985.

54. **Chester, J. F., Gaissert, H. A., Ross, J. S., Malt, R. A., and Weitzman, S. A.,** Augmentation of 1,2-dimethylhydrazine-induced colon cancer by experimental colitis in mice: role of dietary vitamin E, *J. Natl. Cancer Inst.*, 76, 939, 1986.

55. **Weitberg, A. B., Weitzman, S. A., Clark, E. P., and Stossel, T. P.,** Effects of antioxidants on oxidant-induced sister chromatid exchange formation, *J. Clin. Invest.*, 75, 1835, 1985.

56. **Harris, C. C., Hus, I. C., Stoner, G. D., Trump, B. F., and Selkirk, J. K.,** Human pulmonary alveolar macrophages metabolize benzo(a)pyrene to proximate and ultimate mutagens, *Nature (London)*, 272, 633, 1978.

57. **Evans, R.,** Macrophages and neoplasms: new insights and their implication in tumor immunobiology, *Cancer Metastasis Rev.*, 1, 227, 1982.

58. **De Baetselier, P., Kapon, A., Katzav, S., Tzehoval, E., Dekegel, D., Segal, S., and Feldman, M.,** Selecting, accelerating and suppressing interactions between macrophages and tumor cells, *Invasion Metastasis*, 5, 106, 1985.

59. **Salmon, S. and Hamburger, A. W.,** Immunoproliferation and cancer: a common macrophage-derived promoter substance, *Lancet*, 1, 1289, 1978.

60. **Nagashima, A., Yasumoto, K., Nakahashi, H., Furukawa, T., Inokuchi, K., and Nomoto, K.,** Establishment and characterization of high- and low-metastatic clones derived from a methylcholanthrene-induced rat fibrosarcoma, *Cancer Res.*, 46, 4420, 1986.

61. **Potter, M., Wax, J. S., Anderson, A. O., and Nordan, R. P.,** Inhibition of plasmacytoma development in BALB/c mice by indomethacin, *J. Exp. Med.*, 161, 996, 1985.

62. **Nordan, R. P. and Potter, M.,** A macrophage-derived factor required by plasmacytomas for survival and proliferation in vitro, *Science*, 233, 566, 1986.

63. **Folkman, J.,** How is blood vessel growth regulated in normal and neoplastic tissue?, *Cancer Res.*, 46, 467, 1986.

64. **Martin, B. M., Gimbrone, M.A., Jr., Unanue, E. R., and Cotran, R. S.,** Stimulation of nonlymphoid mesenchymal cell proliferation by a macrophage-derived growth factor, *J. Immunol.*, 126, 1510, 1981.

65. **Koch, A. E., Polverini, P. J., and Leibovich, S. J.,** Induction of neovascularization by activated human monocytes, *J. Leukocyte Biol.*, 39, 233, 1986.

INDEX

Milton Keynes UK
Ingram Content Group UK Ltd.
UKHW051951071024
449327UK00026B/2271